Dosage Calculations

made Incredibly Easy!®

Sixth Edition

Dosage Calculations made Incredibly Easy!®

Sixth Edition

Clinical Editor
Kimberly Giddings, MSN, RN, PCCN

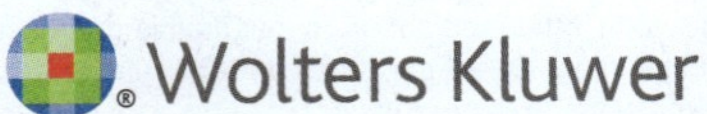

Philadelphia • Baltimore • New York • London
Buenos Aires • Hong Kong • Sydney • Tokyo

Vice President and Publisher: Julie K. Stegman
Senior Acquisitions Editor: Joyce Berendes
Director of Nursing Education and Practice Content: Jamie Blum
Senior Development Editor: Jacquelyn Saunders
Editorial Coordinator: Arvind Siddharth J
Editorial Assistant: Sara Thul
Marketing Manager: Amy Whitaker
Production Project Manager: Frances Gunning
Manager, Graphic Arts & Design: Stephen Druding
Art Director, Illustration: Jennifer Clements
Manufacturing Coordinator: Bernard Tomboc
Prepress Vendor: Aptara, Inc.

9 8 7 6 5 4 3 2 1

Printed in Mexico

Library of Congress Cataloging-in-Publication Data

Names: Giddings, Kimberly, editor.
Title: Dosage calculations made incredibly easy! / clinical editor, Kimberly Giddings.
Description: Sixth edition. | Philadelphia, PA : Wolters Kluwer, [2025] | Includes bibliographical references and index. | Summary: "Calculate correct dosages with safety and confidence, with the easy-to-follow nursing expertise of Dosage Calculations Made Incredibly Easy! 6th edition. This fully illustrated guide offers the complete how-to on calculating dosages for all drug forms and administration routes, with numerous practice exercises and seasoned guidance on interpreting drug orders accurately. Understand class materials more fully, get ready for the NCLEX or certification exam, or refresh your calculation skills with this enjoyable, colorful text"– Provided by publisher.
Identifiers: LCCN 2024024073 (print) | LCCN 2024024074 (ebook) | ISBN 9781975236601 (paperback) | ISBN 9781975236625 (epub)
Subjects: MESH: Drug Dosage Calculations | Pharmaceutical Preparations–administration & dosage | Nurses Instruction | BISAC: MEDICAL / Nursing / Reference
Classification: LCC RS57 (print) | LCC RS57 (ebook) | NLM QV 748 | DDC 615/.1401513–dc23/eng/20240702
LC record available at https://lccn.loc.gov/2024024073
LC ebook record available at https://lccn.loc.gov/2024024074

shop.lww.com

QUADM0924

Dedication

This book is dedicated to all the math phobics in the world whose dream it is to become a nurse. It is for those who may struggle with math problems and are looking for an incredibly easy solution to help them! No more guessing, no more doubts, just more confidence! This book was written for you.

Contributors

Lisa Benson, MSN, RN-BC
Adjunct Faculty
Leighton School of Nursing/
Marian University
Fountaintown, Indiana

Cheryl L. DeGraw, EdS, MSN, RN, CRNP
Nursing Instructor
Central Carolina Technical College
Florence, South Carolina

MaryAnn Edelman, MS, RN
Adjunct Professor
Kingsborough Community College
Department of Nursing
Brooklyn, New York

Kimberly Giddings, MSN, RN, PCCN
Nurse Educator
Holy Family Hospital
Methuen, Massachusetts

Sharon Nelson, MSN, RN
Lead Nurse Educator
Holy Family Hospital
Methuen, Massachusetts

Sarah Wallace, PhD, RN, CPN, CNE
Clinical Assistant Professor
Purdue University
Covington, Indiana

Megan Wince, MSN, MBA, BSN, RN
Program Faculty Manager
Western Governors University
Salt Lake City, Utah

Foreword

Struggle with med math?

Do you fear math or dread having to perform math calculations? Do you feel like you struggle to figure out math problems while others don't? Looking for simple and easy explanations to help with math concepts including med math and administration? If so, then you made the right choice in choosing this book! This book was designed to help health care professionals who are looking for a simple, step-by-step approach to math calculations. Don't understand dimension analysis? No worries! This book explains how to work with different formulas such as ratios, proportions, ratio proportions, and the most popular, desired over have formula. Whether you have a little experience or have a lot of experience with working with formulas, conversions, or rounding numbers, this book offers the latest and up-to-date information on medication administration. This information will help apply medication administration principles in the clinical setting.

Nursing is challenging enough; med math shouldn't have to be! As a nursing instructor and educator, I know that students learn in different ways. A 'one size fits all' approach doesn't work for all, which is why this book provides different which is why this book provides different approaches for being successful in solving med math calculations. The incredibly easy step-by-step instructions, hints, tips, illustrations, and advice from experts will help you remember and use the information you have learned.

Whether you love or dread med math or dosage calculations, this book is for you!

Kimberly Giddings, MSN, RN, PCCN
Registered Nurse

Contents

Part I

Math basics

Chapter 1

Fractions

Just the facts

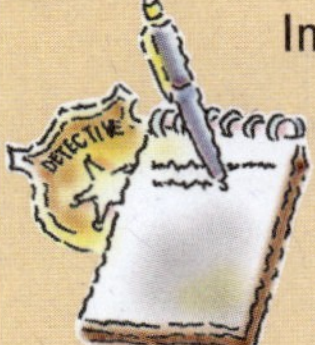

In this chapter, you'll learn how to:

- define a fraction and its different types
- convert fractions, reduce them to their lowest terms, and find the lowest common denominator
- add, subtract, multiply, and divide fractions

A look at fractions

A fraction represents the division of one number by another number. It's a mathematical expression for parts of a whole. (See *Parts of a whole.*)

Parts of a whole

In any fraction, the numerator (top number) and the denominator (bottom number) represent the parts of a whole. The denominator describes the total number of equal parts in the whole; the numerator describes the number of parts being considered.

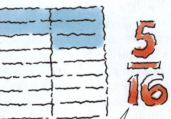

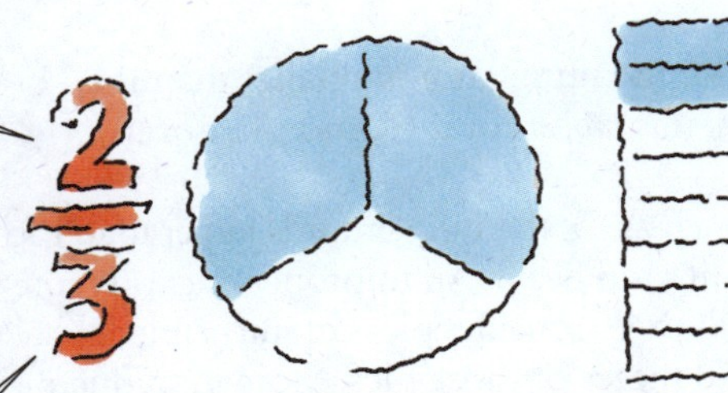
The numerator is on the top.
2/3
The denominator is on the bottom.
5/16
The numerator 5 over the denominator 16 shows that we're considering 5 parts out of 16.

Getting to the bottom of it

The bottom number, or *denominator*, represents the total number of equal parts in the whole. The larger the denominator, the greater the number of equal parts. For example, in the fraction $\frac{3}{5}$, the denominator 5 indicates that the whole has been divided into 5 equal parts. Consider a pie cut into 5 equal pieces.

In the fraction $\frac{7}{12}$, the denominator 12 indicates that the whole has been divided into 12 equal parts. Consider a pie cut into 12 equal pieces.

In addition, the illustrations show that as the denominator becomes larger, the size of the parts becomes smaller.

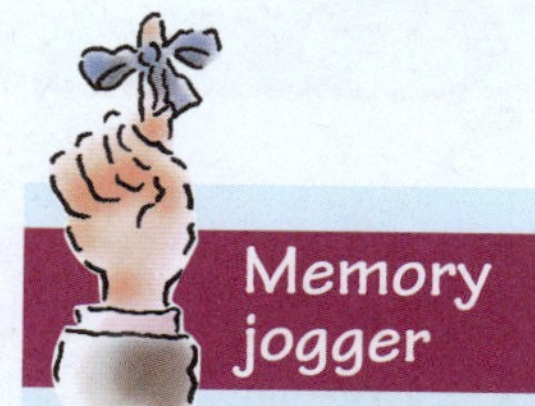

Memory jogger

To remember which number is the numerator and which one is the denominator in a fraction, think of:

Nursing

Diagnosis

The **N**umerator is on the top; the **D**enominator is on the bottom.

Staying on top of it

The top number, or *numerator*, signifies the number of parts of the whole being considered.

In the fraction $\frac{3}{5}$, only 3 of the 5 equal parts are being considered. In other words, 3 equal pieces of pie are being considered.

In the fraction $\frac{7}{12}$, only 7 of the 12 equal parts are being considered. In other words, 7 equal pieces of pie are being considered.

Types of fractions

There are four types of fractions:

- Proper
- Improper
- Common
- Complex

Proper and improper

In a proper fraction, such as $\frac{1}{4}$, the numerator is smaller than the denominator. In other words, it is *proper* for the denominator to *dominate* the fraction.

In an improper fraction, such as $\frac{8}{7}$, the numerator is larger than the denominator. In other words, it's top heavy. An improper fraction represents a number that's greater than 1. Consider pies cut into 7 pieces.

The fraction $\frac{8}{7}$ illustrates 8 pieces of those pies. More than one pie is needed to illustrate the fraction.

An improper fraction can also be expressed as a *mixed number*—a whole number and a fraction. Therefore, $\frac{8}{7}$ can be rewritten as $1\frac{1}{7}$.

Common and complex

In a common fraction, both the numerator and the denominator are whole numbers. For example:

$$\frac{2}{3}$$

In a complex fraction, the numerator and the denominator are fractions. For example:

$$\frac{2/7}{5/16}$$

Working with fractions

Fractions can be manipulated in three ways, including:

- converting mixed numbers to improper fractions and the other way around
- reducing fractions to their lowest terms
- finding a common denominator

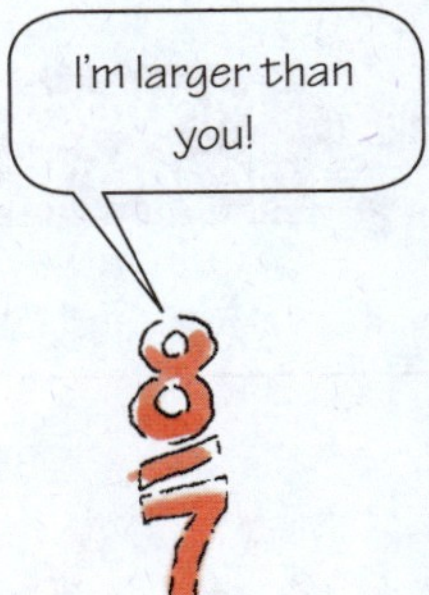

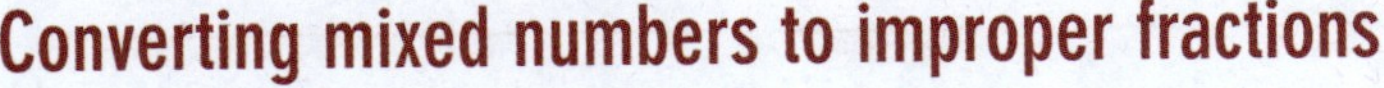

Converting mixed numbers to improper fractions

To convert a mixed number to an improper fraction, follow these incredibly easy steps:

Three incredibly easy steps

Step 1: Multiply the denominator by the whole number. The answer is called the *product*.

Step 2: Add the product from the first step to the numerator. This gives a new numerator.

Step 3: Leave the denominator as it is. When converting mixed numbers to improper fractions, the purpose is to find the number of equal pieces of the whole. The size of the equal pieces is not being changed, which is why the denominator remains the same!

For example, to convert the mixed number $5\,1/3$ to an improper fraction:

Step 1: Multiply the denominator 3 by the whole number 5, to get the product of 15.

Step 2: Add 15 to the numerator 1, for a new numerator of 16.

Step 3: Leave the denominator as it is. The improper fraction is $16/3$.

$$5\,1/3 \text{ is } \frac{16}{3}$$

The illustration shows how the mixed number and the improper fraction are the same. The mixed number simply expresses the 5 *whole* pies (cut into 3 equal parts each) plus the additional piece of pie. The improper fraction illustrates 16 pieces of pie cut into 3 equal parts. When converting the mixed number to an improper fraction, the denominator does not change just like the size of the pieces of the pies that does not change.

Encore!

Here's another example! To convert the mixed number 8 ⅘ to an improper fraction:

Step 1: Multiply the denominator 5 by the whole number 8, to get the product, 40.

Step 2: Add 40 to the numerator 4, for a new numerator of 44.

Step 3: Leave the denominator as it is. The improper fraction is $^{44}/_{5}$.

$$8\tfrac{4}{5} \text{ is } \frac{44}{5}$$

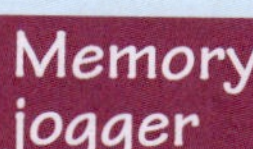

Memory jogger

Here's a way to remember how to convert mixed numbers to improper fractions. Think MAST: "Multiply, Add, and Stack on Top."

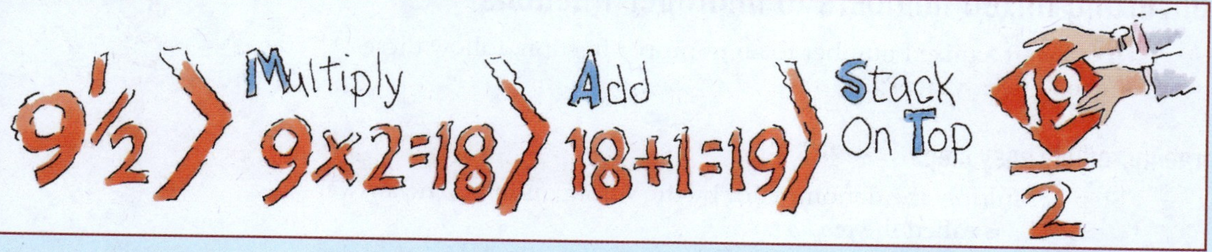

9½
Multiply
9×2=18
Add
18+1=19
Stack On Top
19
2

Putting it in reverse

At times, it might be necessary to convert improper fractions to mixed numbers. To convert the improper fraction $^{16}/_{3}$ to a mixed number:

Step 1: Divide the numerator 16 by the denominator 3. The result is 5 with 1 left over.

Step 2: The 1 becomes the new numerator, and the denominator stays the same.

Step 3: The mixed number is 5 ⅓.

$$\frac{16}{3} \text{ is } 5\tfrac{1}{3}$$

One more time

To convert the improper fraction $^{44}/_{5}$ to a mixed number:

Step 1: Divide the numerator 44 by the denominator 5. The answer is 8 with 4 left over.

Step 2: Place the 4 over the 5.

Step 3: The mixed number is 8 ⅘.

$$\frac{44}{5} \text{ is } 8\tfrac{4}{5}$$

Reducing fractions to their lowest terms

For simplicity's sake, a fraction should usually be reduced to its lowest terms. In other words, fractions should be simplified to the smallest numerator and the smallest denominator. Remember to reduce both the numerator and the denominator equally. To simplify a fraction, follow these incredibly easy steps:

Step 1: Determine the largest common divisor of the numerator and the denominator—the largest number by which both can be divided equally (into whole numbers).

Step 2: Divide both the numerator and the denominator by that number, separately, to reduce the fraction to its lowest terms without changing its value.

Let's try it

To reduce the fraction $\frac{8}{10}$ to its lowest terms:

Step 1: Determine the largest common divisor of 8 and 10: 2.

Step 2: Divide *both* the numerator and the denominator by 2 to reduce the fraction to its lowest terms, or $\frac{4}{5}$.

$$\frac{8}{10} \text{ is } \frac{8 \div 2}{10 \div 2} \text{ is } \frac{4}{5}$$

Only the *terms* (or numbers) used in the numerator and the denominator change; the *value* does not change.

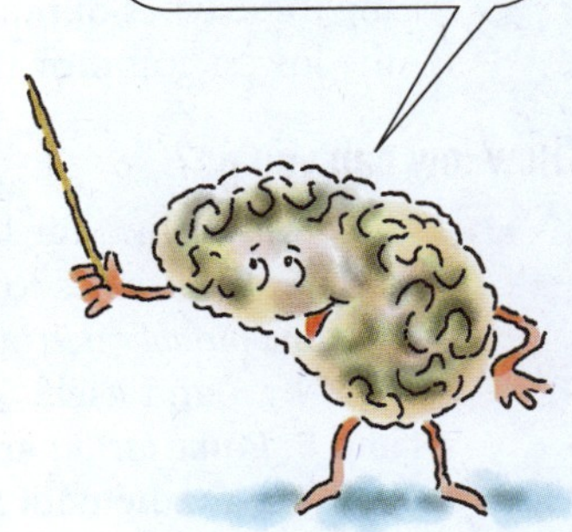
Simply put, find the largest number that can be divided evenly into the numerator and the denominator.

Missed it? Watch again!

To reduce the fraction $\frac{7}{14}$ to its lowest terms:

Step 1: Determine that the number 7 is the largest divisor of the numerator and the denominator. Both numbers 7 and 14 can be divided into whole numbers by the number 7.

Step 2: Divide the numerator and the denominator by 7 to reduce the fraction to its lowest terms, or $\frac{1}{2}$. This fraction can't be reduced further.

$$\frac{7}{14} \text{ is } \frac{7 \div 7}{14 \div 7} \text{ is } \frac{1}{2}$$

One more time

To reduce the fraction $\frac{2}{10}$ to its lowest terms:

Step 1: Determine that the number 2 is the largest divisor that 2 and 10 have in common.

Step 2: Divide the numerator and the denominator by 2 to reduce the fraction to its lowest terms, or $\frac{1}{5}$.

$$\frac{2}{10} \text{ is } \frac{2 \div 2}{10 \div 2} \text{ is } \frac{1}{5}$$

Finding a common denominator

One way to find a common denominator for a set of fractions is to multiply all the denominators. For example, to find a common denominator for the fractions $\frac{2}{5}$ and $\frac{7}{10}$, multiply the denominators 5 and 10 to get the multiplied common denominator 50.

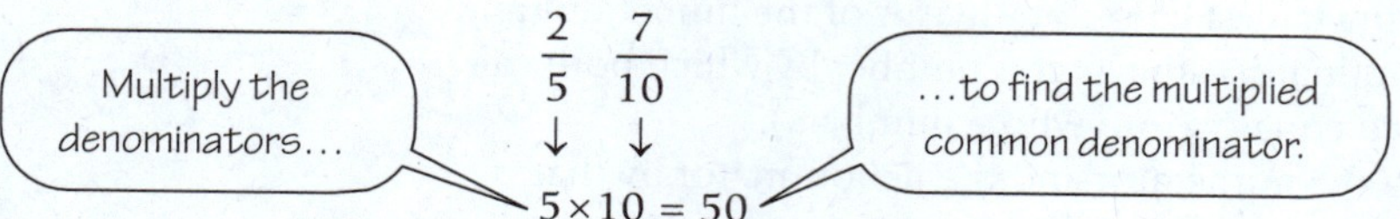
Multiply the denominators...
$\frac{2}{5}$ $\frac{7}{10}$
↓ ↓
$5 \times 10 = 50$
...to find the multiplied common denominator.

To find the multiplied common denominator of the set of fractions $\frac{1}{8}$, $\frac{1}{4}$, and $\frac{1}{5}$, simply multiply all the denominators together to get the common denominator 160.

$$8 \times 4 \times 5 = 160$$

Lowest common denominator

Unfortunately, multiplying all the denominators of a set of fractions won't always give the lowest common denominator. The *lowest common denominator* or *least common multiple*—the smallest number that's a multiple of all the denominators in a set of fractions—is an important tool for working with fractions. Practicing these types of problems will make it easier to find the lowest common denominator!

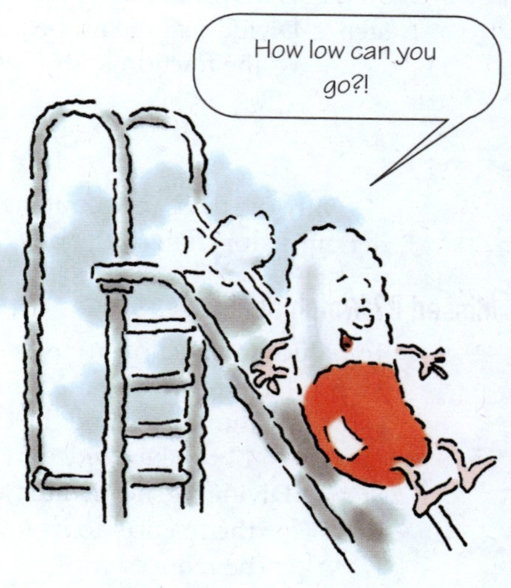
How low can you go?!

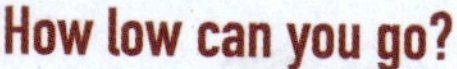

How low can you go?

One way to find the lowest common denominator of a set of fractions is to work with its prime numbers. A *prime number* is a number that's evenly divisible only by 1 and itself. Some prime numbers are 2, 3, 5, and 7. *Prime factors* are prime numbers that can be divided into some part of a mathematical expression; in this case, the denominators in a set of fractions.

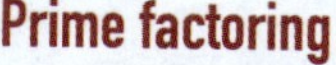

Prime factoring

Let's find the lowest common denominator for $\frac{1}{8}$, $\frac{1}{4}$, and $\frac{1}{5}$. Here's a useful technique, called *prime factoring*:

Step 1: Make a table with two headings: "Prime factors" and "Denominators."

Step 2: Write the denominators 8, 4, and 5 over the top right columns.

Prime factors	Denominators		
	8	4	5

Step 3: Divide the three denominators by the prime factors for each, starting with the smallest prime factor by which one of the denominators can be divided—in this case, 2.

Step 4: Write 2 in the left-hand column and divide the denominators by it. Divide the denominator 8 by the prime factor 2 and write the answer, 4, in the column under the denominator 8.

Step 5: Divide the denominator 4 by the prime factor 2 and write the answer, 2, in the column under the denominator 4.

Step 6: Bring down the numbers in the right-side column that aren't evenly divisible by the prime factor in the left-side column. (In this case, the denominator 5 isn't divisible by the prime factor 2; so just bring the 5 down.)

Prime factors	Denominators		
÷	8	4	5
2 =	4	2	5

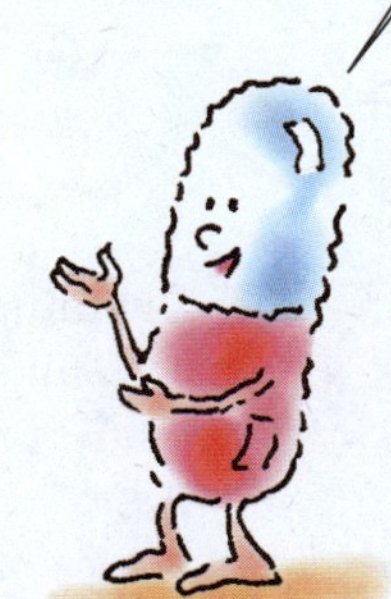

Prime numbers cannot be reduced any further. Examples are 2, 3, 5, 7, and 11.

Step 7: Repeat this process until the numbers in the bottom row can't be divided further.

Prime factors	Denominators		
	8	4	5
2	4	2	5
2	2	1	5
2	1	1	5

Step 8: Multiply the prime factors in the left column by the numbers in the bottom row. Like this:

$$2 \times 2 \times 2 \times 1 \times 1 \times 5 = 40$$

- The lowest common denominator for this set of fractions is 40.

Wow! Show me that again!

OK. Let's use prime factoring to find the lowest common denominator for $\frac{3}{8}$ and $\frac{5}{6}$. Create a table that lists the denominators horizontally; then find the prime factors.

Step 1: Set up a table like this:

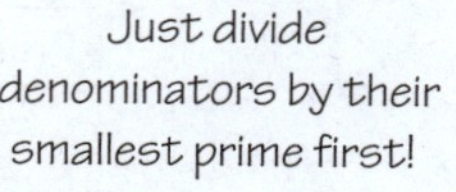

Just divide denominators by their smallest prime first!

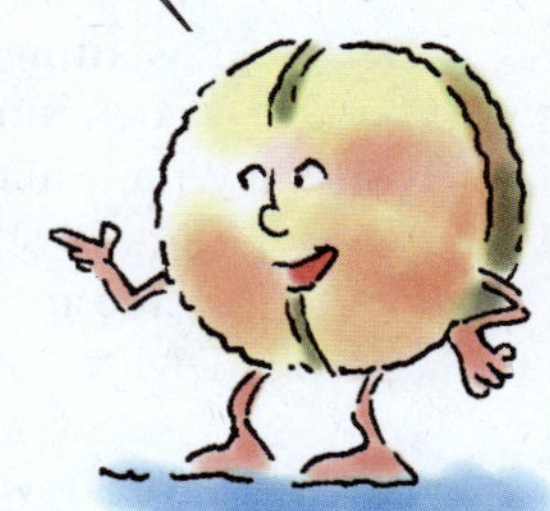

Prime factors	Denominators	
	8	6
2	4	3
2	2	3
2	1	3

Step 2: Multiply the prime factors in the left column by the numbers in the bottom row.

$$2 \times 2 \times 2 \times 1 \times 3 = 24$$

Lowest common denominator

Once more, please

Now, use prime factoring to find the lowest common denominator for $\frac{1}{3}$, $\frac{1}{4}$, and $\frac{1}{2}$.
Step 1: Set up the table:

Prime factors	Denominators		
	3	4	2
2	3	2	1
2	3	1	1

Step 2: Multiply the prime factors in the left column by the numbers in the bottom row:

$$2 \times 2 \times 3 \times 1 \times 1 = 12$$

Lowest common denominator

Converting fractions

When the lowest common denominator of a set of fractions is known, *convert* the fractions so they'll all have the same denominator—the *lowest common denominator*.

One way to convert a set of fractions is to multiply each fraction by 1 in the form of a fraction—that is, a fraction with the same number in the numerator and the denominator. This fraction can be found by taking the lowest common denominator and dividing it by the original denominator.

Here's what the formula looks like:

This is how you convert a fraction using 1 in the form of a fraction.

$$\text{original fraction} \times \frac{\text{lowest common denominator} \div \text{original denominator}}{\text{lowest common denominator} \div \text{original denominator}}$$

Conversion excursion

Convert the set of fractions $\frac{1}{8}$, $\frac{1}{4}$, and $\frac{1}{5}$ so that each has the lowest common denominator. We already know that the lowest common denominator for this set of fractions is 40.

- Here's the conversion of the first fraction, $\frac{1}{8}$, to $\frac{5}{40}$:

$$\frac{1}{8} = \frac{1}{8} \times \frac{40 \div 8}{40 \div 8} = \frac{1}{8} \times \frac{5}{5} = \frac{1 \times 5}{8 \times 5} = \frac{5}{40}$$

- Convert the next fraction, $\frac{1}{4}$, to $\frac{10}{40}$:

$$\frac{1}{4} = \frac{1}{4} \times \frac{40 \div 4}{40 \div 4} = \frac{1}{4} \times \frac{10}{10} = \frac{1 \times 10}{4 \times 10} = \frac{10}{40}$$

- Convert the last fraction in the set, $\frac{1}{5}$, to $\frac{8}{40}$:

$$\frac{1}{5} = \frac{1}{5} \times \frac{40 \div 5}{40 \div 5} = \frac{1}{5} \times \frac{8}{8} = \frac{1 \times 8}{5 \times 8} = \frac{8}{40}$$

Do it again

This is how to convert $\frac{3}{8}$ and $\frac{5}{6}$ to fractions with the lowest common denominator, which is 24.

- Convert the first fraction, $\frac{3}{8}$, to $\frac{9}{24}$:

$$\frac{3}{8} = \frac{3}{8} \times \frac{24 \div 8}{24 \div 8} = \frac{3}{8} \times \frac{3}{3} = \frac{3 \times 3}{8 \times 3} = \frac{9}{24}$$

- Convert the other fraction, $\frac{5}{6}$, to $\frac{20}{24}$:

$$\frac{5}{6} = \frac{5}{6} \times \frac{24 \div 6}{24 \div 6} = \frac{5}{6} \times \frac{4}{4} = \frac{5 \times 4}{6 \times 4} = \frac{20}{24}$$

Once more

OK. Now convert $\frac{1}{3}$, $\frac{1}{4}$, and $\frac{1}{2}$ to fractions with the lowest common denominator, which is 12.

- Convert $\frac{1}{3}$ to $\frac{4}{12}$:

$$\frac{1}{3} = \frac{1}{3} \times \frac{12 \div 3}{12 \div 3} = \frac{1}{3} \times \frac{4}{4} = \frac{1 \times 4}{3 \times 4} = \frac{4}{12}$$

- Convert $\frac{1}{4}$ to $\frac{3}{12}$:

$$\frac{1}{4} = \frac{1}{4} \times \frac{12 \div 4}{12 \div 4} = \frac{1}{4} \times \frac{3}{3} = \frac{1 \times 3}{4 \times 3} = \frac{3}{12}$$

- Convert the last fraction, $\frac{1}{2}$ to $\frac{6}{12}$:

$$\frac{1}{2} = \frac{1}{2} \times \frac{12 \div 2}{12 \div 2} = \frac{1}{2} \times \frac{6}{6} = \frac{1 \times 6}{2 \times 6} = \frac{6}{12}$$

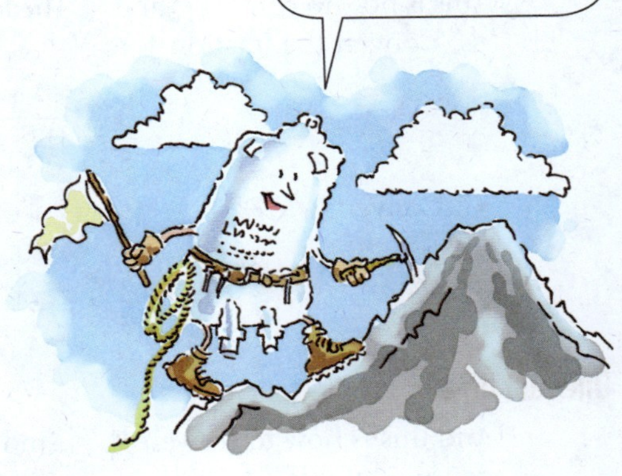

Keep up the good work! Practice makes perfect!

Divide and conquer

Convert a set of fractions by using long division. To convert each fraction, follow these steps:

Step 1: Divide the lowest common denominator by the original denominator. The answer will be the quotient.

Step 2: Multiply the *quotient* by the original numerator to determine the new numerator.

Step 3: Place the new numerator over the lowest common denominator.

Here's how to set up the conversion for each fraction:

$$\text{original denominator}\overset{\text{quotient}}{\overline{\big)\text{lowest common denominator}}} \times \text{original numerator} = \frac{\text{new numerator}}{\text{lowest common denominator}}$$

Set 'em up

This is how to convert $\frac{3}{8}$, $\frac{1}{4}$, and $\frac{2}{5}$. The lowest common denominator is 40.

- Convert the first fraction in the set, $\frac{3}{8}$, to $\frac{15}{40}$:

$$\frac{3}{8} = 8\overset{5}{\overline{\big)40}} \times 3 = \frac{15}{40}$$

- Convert $\frac{1}{4}$ to $\frac{10}{40}$:

$$\frac{1}{4} = 4\overset{10}{\overline{\big)40}} \times 1 = \frac{10}{40}$$

- Convert $\frac{2}{5}$ to $\frac{16}{40}$:

$$\frac{2}{5} = 5\overset{8}{\overline{\big)40}} \times 2 = \frac{16}{40}$$

Amazing! Let's see that again

This is how to convert $\frac{3}{8}$ and $\frac{5}{6}$. The lowest common denominator is 24.

- Convert the fraction $\frac{3}{8}$ to $\frac{9}{24}$:

$$\frac{3}{8} = 8\overset{3}{\overline{\big)24}} \times 3 = \frac{9}{24}$$

- Convert $\frac{5}{6}$ to $\frac{20}{24}$:

$$\frac{5}{6} = 6\overset{4}{\overline{\big)24}} \times 5 = \frac{20}{24}$$

One last time

And this is how to convert $\frac{1}{3}$, $\frac{1}{4}$, and $\frac{1}{2}$. The lowest common denominator is 12.

- Convert $\frac{1}{3}$ to $\frac{4}{12}$:

$$\frac{1}{3} = 3\overset{4}{\overline{)12}} \times 1 = \frac{4}{12}$$

- Convert $\frac{1}{4}$ to $\frac{3}{12}$:

$$\frac{1}{4} = 4\overset{3}{\overline{)12}} \times 1 = \frac{3}{12}$$

- Convert $\frac{1}{2}$ to $\frac{6}{12}$:

$$\frac{1}{2} = 2\overset{6}{\overline{)12}} \times 1 = \frac{6}{12}$$

For math phobics only

Denominators can be deceptive

Would a hungry person rather have 1 slice from a pie that was cut into 4 slices, 8 slices, or 16 slices? Of course, they would choose 4 because the slices would be bigger. The size of fractions can be compared in the same way. When the fractions all have the same numerators—in this case, $\frac{1}{4}$, $\frac{1}{8}$, and $\frac{1}{16}$—the fraction with the lowest denominator is the biggest one. Don't fall into the trap of thinking that the bigger the denominator, the bigger the fraction. Think in terms of a pie, as shown below.

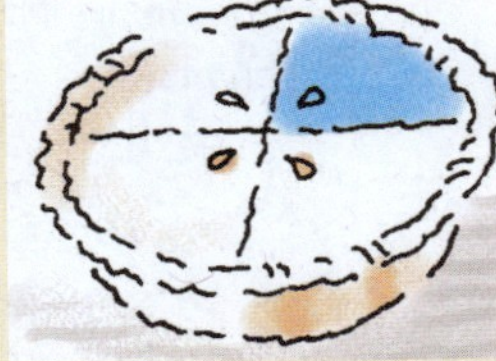
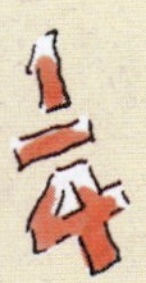

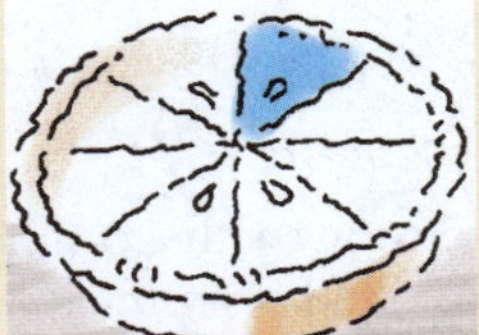
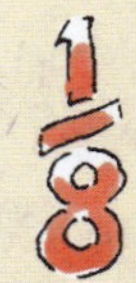

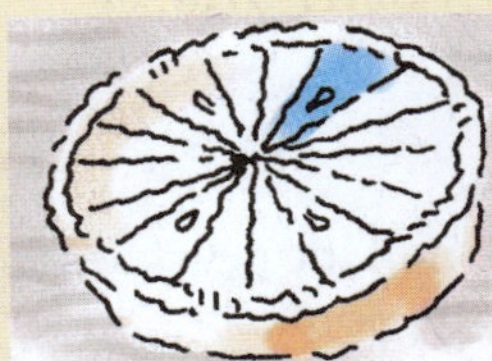
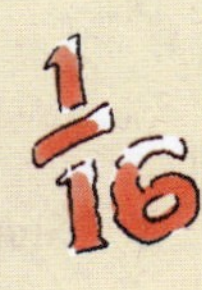

Adding fractions

To add fractions, first convert them to fractions with common denominators. (See *Comparing apples to apples*, p. 14.)

It all adds up

Here's an example of adding fractions. Follow these incredibly easy steps below to add the fractions $\frac{1}{7}$ and $\frac{1}{3}$.

Step 1: Find the lowest common denominator. Because the denominators in $\frac{1}{7}$ and $\frac{1}{3}$ are both prime numbers, multiply 7 by 3 to find the lowest common denominator, 21.

Comparing apples to apples

When adding or subtracting fractions, don't forget to convert them to fractions with common denominators. That way, you'll be comparing apples to apples.

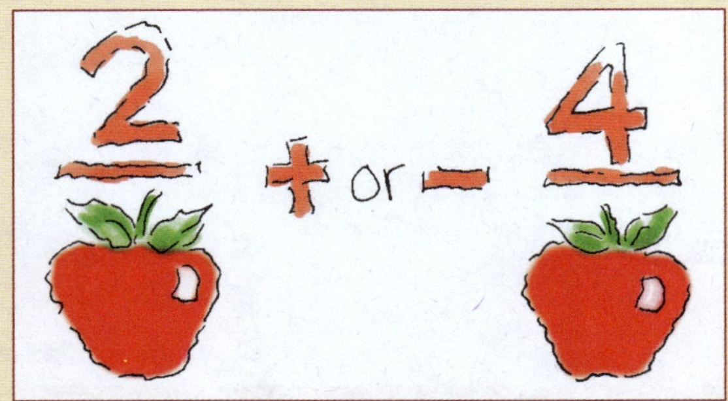

Step 2: Convert the fractions by multiplying each by 1 (in the form of a fraction) to yield fractions with the lowest common denominator.

Step 3: Start by converting $\frac{1}{7}$ to $\frac{3}{21}$:

$$\frac{1}{7} = \frac{1}{7} \times \frac{21 \div 7}{21 \div 7} = \frac{1}{7} \times \frac{3}{3} = \frac{1 \times 3}{7 \times 3} = \frac{3}{21}$$

Step 4: Convert $\frac{1}{3}$ to $\frac{7}{21}$

$$\frac{1}{3} = \frac{1}{3} \times \frac{21 \div 3}{21 \div 3} = \frac{1}{3} \times \frac{7}{7} = \frac{1 \times 7}{3 \times 7} = \frac{7}{21}$$

Step 5: Add the new fractions. To add fractions with a common denominator, add the numerators and place the result over the common denominator. The resulting fraction is the answer. (Reduce it to its lowest terms, if possible.)

$$\frac{3}{21} + \frac{7}{21} = \frac{3+7}{21} = \frac{10}{21}$$

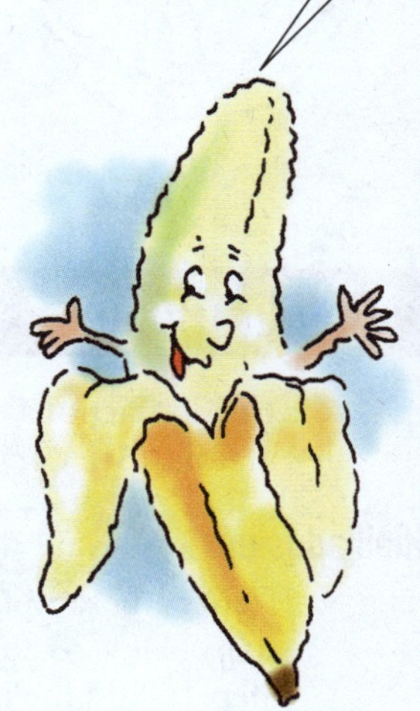

Find the common denominator to make sure that apples are not being compared to bananas.

Additional addition

To add $\frac{1}{2}$ and $\frac{1}{5}$, follow these incredibly easy steps:

Step 1: Find the lowest common denominator. In this case, because the denominators 2 and 5 are both prime numbers, multiply 2 by 5 to find the lowest common denominator, 10.

Step 2: Convert the fractions by multiplying each by 1 (in the form of a fraction) to yield fractions with the lowest common denominator.

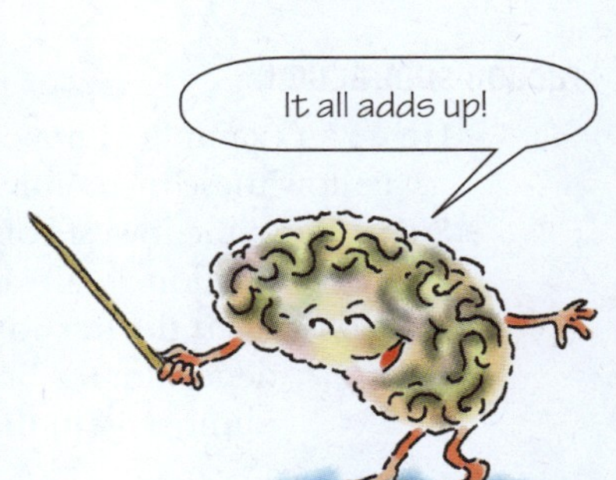

Step 3: Convert the fraction ½ to 5⁄10:

$$\frac{1}{2}=\frac{1}{2}\times\frac{10\div 2}{10\div 2}=\frac{1}{2}\times\frac{5}{5}=\frac{1\times 5}{2\times 5}=\frac{5}{10}$$

Step 4: Convert ⅕ to 2⁄10:

$$\frac{1}{5}=\frac{1}{5}\times\frac{10\div 5}{10\div 5}=\frac{1}{5}\times\frac{2}{2}=\frac{1\times 2}{5\times 2}=\frac{2}{10}$$

Step 5: Add the converted fractions. To do this, add the numerators and place the result over the common denominator:

$$\frac{5}{10}+\frac{2}{10}=\frac{5+2}{10}=\frac{7}{10}$$

Another additional addition

To add ⅗ and ⅔, follow these incredibly easy steps below:

Step 1: Find the lowest common denominator—in this case, 15.

Step 2: Convert the fractions by multiplying each by 1 (in the form of a fraction) to yield fractions with the lowest common denominator.

Step 3: Convert the fraction ⅗ to 9⁄15:

$$\frac{3}{5}=\frac{3}{5}\times\frac{15\div 5}{15\div 5}=\frac{3}{5}\times\frac{3}{3}=\frac{3\times 3}{5\times 3}=\frac{9}{15}$$

Step 4: Convert ⅔ to 10⁄15:

$$\frac{2}{3}=\frac{2}{3}\times\frac{15\div 3}{15\div 3}=\frac{2}{3}\times\frac{5}{5}=\frac{2\times 5}{3\times 5}=\frac{10}{15}$$

Step 5: Add the converted fractions. Do this by adding the new numerators and place the result over the common denominator:

$$\frac{9}{15}+\frac{10}{15}=\frac{9+10}{15}=\frac{19}{15}$$

Step 6: Reduce the fraction to its lowest terms:

$$\frac{19}{15}=1\frac{4}{15}$$

Subtracting fractions

Like addition, subtraction requires converting fractions to terms with common denominators.

Fraction subtraction

Here's an example of how to subtract one fraction from another.

Follow these incredibly easy steps below to subtract $\frac{1}{6}$ from $\frac{5}{12}$.

Step 1: Find the lowest common denominator—in this case, 12. The fraction $\frac{5}{12}$ already has the lowest common denominator.

Step 2: Convert the fraction $\frac{1}{6}$ to a fraction with the lowest common denominator. To do this, multiply the fraction by the number 1 (in the form of a fraction).

$$\frac{1}{6} = \frac{1}{6} \times \frac{12 \div 6}{12 \div 6} = \frac{1}{6} \times \frac{2}{2} = \frac{1 \times 2}{6 \times 2} = \frac{2}{12}$$

Step 3: Subtract the numerators and place the result over the common denominator:

$$\frac{5}{12} - \frac{2}{12} = \frac{5-2}{12} = \frac{3}{12}$$

Step 4: Reduce the fraction to its lowest terms, if possible. The resulting fraction is the answer:

$$\frac{3}{12} = \frac{1}{4}$$

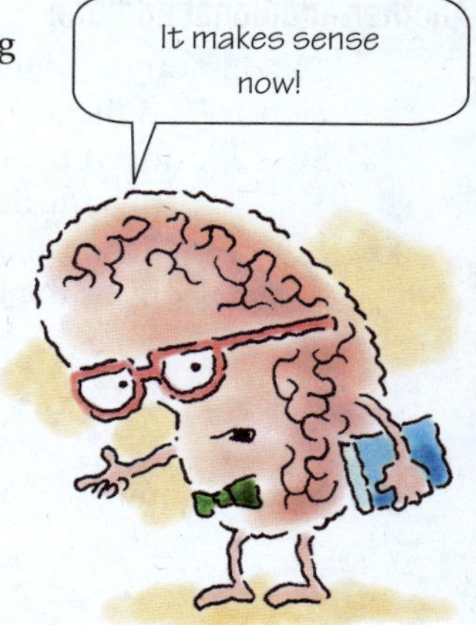

A second subtraction

To subtract $\frac{1}{9}$ from $\frac{5}{6}$, follow these incredibly easy steps:

Step 1: Find the lowest common denominator—in this case, 18. (To find the lowest common denominator in this case, try prime factoring.)

Step 2: Convert the fractions to those with the lowest common denominator by multiplying each fraction by the number 1 (in the form of a fraction).

Step 3: Convert $\frac{5}{6}$ to $\frac{15}{18}$:

$$\frac{5}{6} = \frac{5}{6} \times \frac{18 \div 6}{18 \div 6} = \frac{5}{6} \times \frac{3}{3} = \frac{5 \times 3}{6 \times 3} = \frac{15}{18}$$

Step 4: Convert $\frac{1}{9}$ to $\frac{2}{18}$:

$$\frac{1}{9} = \frac{1}{9} \times \frac{18 \div 9}{18 \div 9} = \frac{1}{9} \times \frac{2}{2} = \frac{1 \times 2}{9 \times 2} = \frac{2}{18}$$

Step 5: Subtract the numerators and place the result over the common denominator.

Step 6: Reduce the fraction to its lowest terms, if possible. In this case, the fraction can't be reduced:

$$\frac{15}{18} - \frac{2}{18} = \frac{15-2}{18} = \frac{13}{18}$$

More subtraction action

Step 1: To subtract $\frac{1}{4}$ from $\frac{2}{3}$, follow these incredibly easy steps: find the lowest common denominator—in this case, 12.

Step 2: Convert the fractions to those with the lowest common denominator by multiplying each fraction by the number 1 (in the form of a fraction).

Step 3: Convert $\frac{2}{3}$ to $\frac{8}{12}$:

$$\frac{2}{3} = \frac{2}{3} \times \frac{12 \div 3}{12 \div 3} = \frac{2}{3} \times \frac{4}{4} = \frac{2 \times 4}{3 \times 4} = \frac{8}{12}$$

Step 4: Convert $\frac{1}{4}$ to $\frac{3}{12}$:

$$\frac{1}{4} = \frac{1}{4} \times \frac{12 \div 4}{12 \div 4} = \frac{1}{4} \times \frac{3}{3} = \frac{1 \times 3}{4 \times 3} = \frac{3}{12}$$

Step 5: Subtract the numerators and place the result over the common denominator:

$$\frac{8}{12} - \frac{3}{12} = \frac{8-3}{12} = \frac{5}{12}$$

Multiplying fractions

Good news! There's no need to convert to common denominators when multiplying fractions. Simply multiply the numerators and the denominators in turn to find the product.

For example, to multiply $\frac{4}{7}$ by $\frac{5}{8}$, multiply the numerators 4 and 5 and the denominators 7 and 8 to get a new fraction. Here's the calculation.

Step 1: Set up the equation:

$$\frac{4}{7} \times \frac{5}{8}$$

Step 2: Multiply the numerators and multiply the denominators:

$$\frac{4 \times 5}{7 \times 8} = \frac{20}{56}$$

Step 3: Reduce the answer to its lowest terms:

$$\frac{5}{14}$$

Let's see it again!

To multiply $\frac{5}{6}$ by $\frac{1}{3}$, multiply the numerators 5 and 1 and the denominators 6 and 3 to get the answer:

$$\frac{5}{6} \times \frac{1}{3} = \frac{5 \times 1}{6 \times 3} = \frac{5}{18}$$

A whole other matter

To multiply a fraction by a whole number, for example 1/9 by 4, follow these incredibly easy steps:

- First, convert the whole number 4 to the fraction 4/1.
- Then multiply the numerators and denominators. The complete calculation looks like this:

$$\frac{1}{9} \times 4 = \frac{1}{9} \times \frac{4}{1} = \frac{1 \times 4}{9 \times 1} = \frac{4}{9}$$

Dividing fractions

In division (as in multiplication), the fractions do not need to be converted. Division problems are usually written as two fractions separated by a division sign. The first fraction is the number to be divided (the *dividend*), and the second fraction is the number doing the dividing (the *divisor*); the answer is the quotient. (See *Divvying up the problem* for a quick review.)

To divide 5/7 by 2/3, first set up the problem:

$$\frac{5}{7} \div \frac{2}{3}$$

This fraction is the dividend.

This fraction is the divisor.

To divide fractions, multiply the dividend by the divisor's *reciprocal*, or the inverted divisor.

- To divide 5/7 by 2/3 (the divisor), first multiply 5/7 (the dividend) by 3/2 (the divisor's reciprocal):

$$\frac{5}{7} \div \frac{2}{3} = \frac{5}{7} \times \frac{3}{2}$$

Here's the divisor's reciprocal.

- Then complete the calculation and reduce the answer (the quotient) to its lowest terms:

$$\frac{5 \times 3}{7 \times 2} = \frac{15}{14} = 1\frac{1}{14}$$

A part divided by a whole

To divide a fraction by a whole number, use the same principle.

- To divide 3/5 by 2, first convert the whole number 2 to the fraction 2/1.

$$\frac{3}{5} \div 2 = \frac{3}{5} \div \frac{2}{1}$$

Divvying up the problem

Before numbers can be divided, the nurse must know what each part of a division problem is called. The division problem below can be written in two different ways, but the terms remain the same.

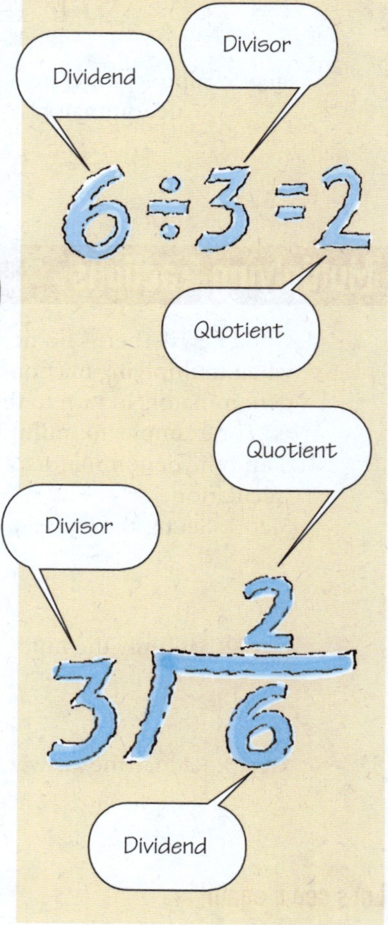

- Then multiply the dividend ($\frac{3}{5}$) by the reciprocal of the divisor ($\frac{1}{2}$). Reduce the answer to its lowest terms:

$$\frac{3}{5} \times \frac{1}{2} =$$
$$\frac{3 \times 1}{5 \times 2} =$$
$$\frac{3}{10}$$

In this case, the answer can't be further reduced.

Making things less complex

In complex fractions, the numerators and denominators are fractions themselves. Complex fractions can be simplified by following the rules for division of fractions. Think of the line separating the two fractions as a division sign. For example, follow the incredibly easy steps below to simplify the complex fraction:

$$\frac{\frac{1}{3}}{\frac{5}{8}}$$

Step 1: First, rewrite the complex fraction as a division problem:

$$\frac{\frac{1}{3}}{\frac{5}{8}} = \frac{1}{3} \div \frac{5}{8}$$

Step 2: Multiply the dividend ($\frac{1}{3}$) by the reciprocal of the divisor ($\frac{8}{5}$):

$$\frac{1}{3} \times \frac{8}{5}$$

Step 3: Complete the calculation:

$$\frac{1 \times 8}{3 \times 5} = \frac{8}{15}$$

Real-world problem

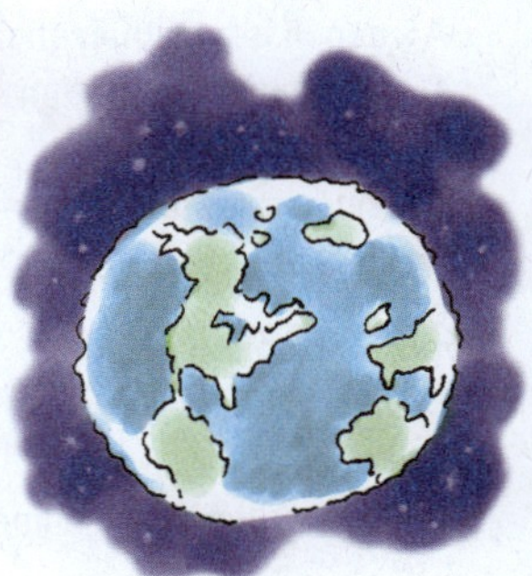

The nurse needs to add the total amount of fluid a patient drank during an 8-hour shift. During the shift, the patient drank $\frac{1}{2}$ cup broth, $\frac{2}{3}$ cup ginger ale, and $\frac{3}{4}$ cup water. How many cups of fluid has the patient had to drink?

Adding for a liquid solution

To solve this problem, add the fractions.

Step 1: Find the lowest common denominator for $\frac{1}{2}$, $\frac{2}{3}$, and $\frac{3}{4}$—in this case, 12.

Step 2: Convert each fraction by multiplying each by 1 (in the form of a fraction) to yield fractions with the lowest common denominator:

$$\frac{1}{2} = \frac{1}{2} \times \frac{12 \div 2}{12 \div 2} = \frac{1}{2} \times \frac{6}{6} = \frac{1 \times 6}{2 \times 6} = \frac{6}{12}$$

$$\frac{2}{3} = \frac{2}{3} \times \frac{12 \div 3}{12 \div 3} = \frac{2}{3} \times \frac{4}{4} = \frac{2 \times 4}{3 \times 4} = \frac{8}{12}$$

$$\frac{3}{4} = \frac{3}{4} \times \frac{12 \div 4}{12 \div 4} = \frac{3}{4} \times \frac{3}{3} = \frac{3 \times 3}{4 \times 3} = \frac{9}{12}$$

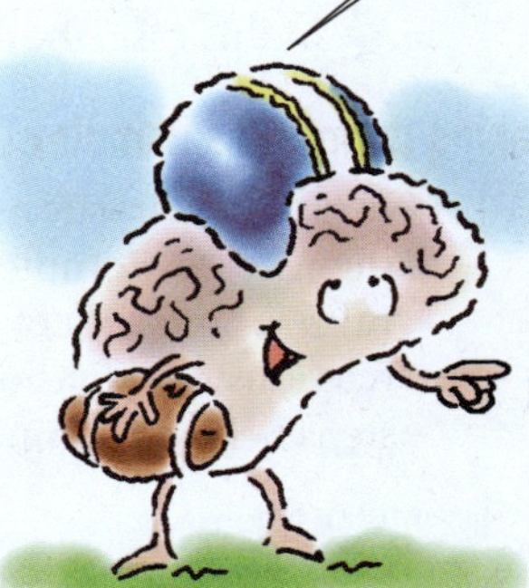

In the real world, nurses don't get three tries to get it right. So now is the time to practice, practice, and practice!

Step 3: Lastly, add the converted fractions, and reduce to the lowest terms:

$$\frac{6}{12} + \frac{8}{12} + \frac{9}{12} = \frac{6+8+9}{12} = \frac{23}{12} = 1\frac{11}{12}$$

- The patient has had $1^{11}/_{12}$ cups of fluid to drink during the 8-hour shift. In most facilities, the metric system is utilized to calculate a patient's fluid intake. This requires converting cups to mL. Since 1 cup equals 240 mL, how many mL did this patient have for intake? Take a look back at *multiplying fractions* if help is needed!

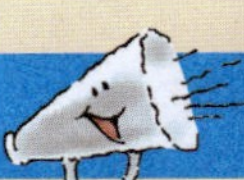

That's a wrap!

Fractions review

Here are some important facts about fractions that nurses need to remember.

Fraction basics

- A fraction is a mathematical expression for parts of a whole.
- The denominator (bottom number) represents the total number of equal parts in the whole.
- The numerator (top number) represents the number of parts of the whole being considered.

Types of fractions

- *Common fraction:* both the numerator and the denominator are whole numbers (such as $^2/_3$).
- *Complex fraction:* the numerator and the denominator are fractions (such as $\frac{^2/_7}{^5/_8}$).
- *Proper fraction:* the numerator is smaller than the denominator (such as $^1/_4$).
- *Improper fraction:* the numerator is larger than the denominator (such as $^8/_3$).

Fractions review (*continued*)

Converting to improper fractions

- Multiply the denominator by the whole number.
- Add the product to the numerator.
- The resulting sum is the new numerator.
- Leave the denominator as it is.

Reducing fractions

- Determine the largest common divisor.
- Divide the numerator and the denominator by that number.

Common denominators

- Multiply all the denominators in a set of fractions to find the common denominator.
- The smallest multiple of the denominators is the lowest common denominator.
- Use prime factoring to determine the lowest common denominator.
- Adding and subtracting fractions. Always convert to fractions with common denominators first, then add or subtract the numerators and keep the denominator as it is.

Multiplying fractions

- Don't convert fractions to common denominators.
- Multiply the numerators and the denominators in turn.

Dividing fractions

- Don't convert fractions to common denominators.
- Write them as two fractions separated by a division sign.
- Invert the divisor.
- Multiply the dividend by the inverted divisor (reciprocal).

Don't forget!

- Always reduce the final answer to its lowest terms.
- If the fraction is improper, convert to a mixed number.

Quick quiz

1. What is the product of $\frac{2}{3} \times \frac{5}{7}$?
   A. $\frac{14}{15}$
   B. $\frac{10}{21}$
   C. $\frac{7}{5}$
   D. $\frac{1}{21}$

Answer: B. To multiply two common fractions, multiply the numerators and then the denominators. The calculation looks like this:

$$\frac{2}{3} \times \frac{5}{7} = \frac{2 \times 5}{3 \times 7} = \frac{10}{21}$$

2. In the fraction $\frac{4}{5}$, what is the denominator?
   A. $\frac{5}{4}$
   B. $1\frac{1}{5}$
   C. 4
   D. 5

Answer: D. The denominator is the bottom number of a fraction. The numerator is the top number.

3. When reducing the fraction $\frac{8}{24}$ to its lowest terms, which answer is correct?
   A. $\frac{2}{6}$
   B. $\frac{3}{4}$
   C. $\frac{1}{3}$
   D. $\frac{1}{8}$

Answer: C. Both the numerator and the denominator are divisible by 8, leaving the reduced fraction $\frac{1}{3}$.

4. Which of the following is an improper fraction?
   A. $\frac{9}{17}$
   B. $\frac{11}{2}$
   C. $\frac{1}{3}$
   D. $\frac{3}{4}$

Answer: B. An improper fraction has a numerator that's larger than the denominator.

5. When adding the fractions $\frac{1}{3}$ and $\frac{1}{2}$, which one is the correct answer?
   A. $\frac{2}{5}$
   B. $\frac{5}{6}$
   C. $\frac{3}{6}$
   D. $\frac{5}{20}$

Answer: B. To add $\frac{1}{2}$ and $\frac{1}{3}$, first find the common denominator, which is 6. Convert the fractions to $\frac{3}{6}$ and $\frac{2}{6}$. The calculation looks like this. Then add the numerators and place the result over the common denominator.

$$\frac{1}{2}+\frac{1}{3}=\frac{3}{6}+\frac{2}{6}=\frac{3+2}{6}=\frac{5}{6}$$

6. Which one is a prime number?
   A. 4
   B. 5
   C. 6
   D. 8

Answer: B. The number 5 is a prime number because it can be divided only by itself and 1.

Scoring

☆☆☆ If you answered all six items correctly, wow! You're a number 1 math whiz (which is the same as a $^2/_2$, a $^3/_3$, or a $^6/_6$ math whiz).

☆☆ If you answered four or five items correctly, fantastic! You're a freewheeling fraction fiend.

☆ If you answered fewer than four items correctly, stick with it! You're showing great promise in working with fractions!

Chapter 2

Decimals and percentages

Just the facts

In this chapter, you'll learn how to:

- define decimals and percentages
- add, subtract, multiply, divide, and round off decimal numbers
- convert common fractions to decimal numbers and the other way around
- convert percentages to decimal numbers and common fractions and the other way around
- solve percentage problems

A look at decimals and percentages

The teacher told us that 35% of the class received A's on the last exam. Since there are 20 of us in the class, what is the chance that I got an A?

People use decimals and percentages as part of their everyday life. For most people, decimals and percentages are a part of everyday life. Figuring a tip at a restaurant, balancing a checkbook, and interpreting the results of an election or a survey are just a few ways people use decimals and percentages.

Nurses encounter decimals and percentages every day at work. The metric system, the most common system for measuring medications, is based on decimal numbers. Decimals and percentages are used when administering solutions, such as 0.9% sodium chloride solution, and medications, such as a 2.5% cream.

In the know

To administer medications accurately and efficiently, nurses must understand decimals and percentages. Understanding how to work with them in common calculations will help ensure safe medication administration throughout a nurse's career. In addition, nurses need to know how to convert from percentages to decimal numbers and common fractions and then back to percentages. This chapter will sharpen your calculation skills and help you build confidence. Practice will go a long way. Take advantage of the *Quick quiz* at the end of this chapter.

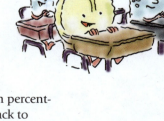

Deciphering decimals

A *decimal fraction* is a proper fraction in which the denominator is a power of 10, signified by a decimal point placed at the left of the numerator. An example of a decimal fraction is 0.2, which is the same as $\frac{2}{10}$.

In a *decimal number*—for example, 2.25—the decimal point separates the whole number from the decimal fraction. To simplify this lesson, the term "decimal number" will refer to either decimal fractions or decimal numbers.

Look to the left . . .

Each number or place to the left of the decimal point represents a whole number that's a power of 10, starting with ones and working up to tens, hundreds, thousands, ten thousands, and so on.

. . . and then to the right

Each place to the right of the decimal point signifies a fraction whose denominator is a power of 10, starting with tenths and working up to hundredths, thousandths, ten thousandths, and so on. Nurses rarely encounter decimal numbers extending beyond the thousandths place. (See *Know your places.*)

Know your places

Based on its position relative to the decimal point, each decimal place represents a power of 10 or a fraction with a denominator that's a power of 10, as shown here:

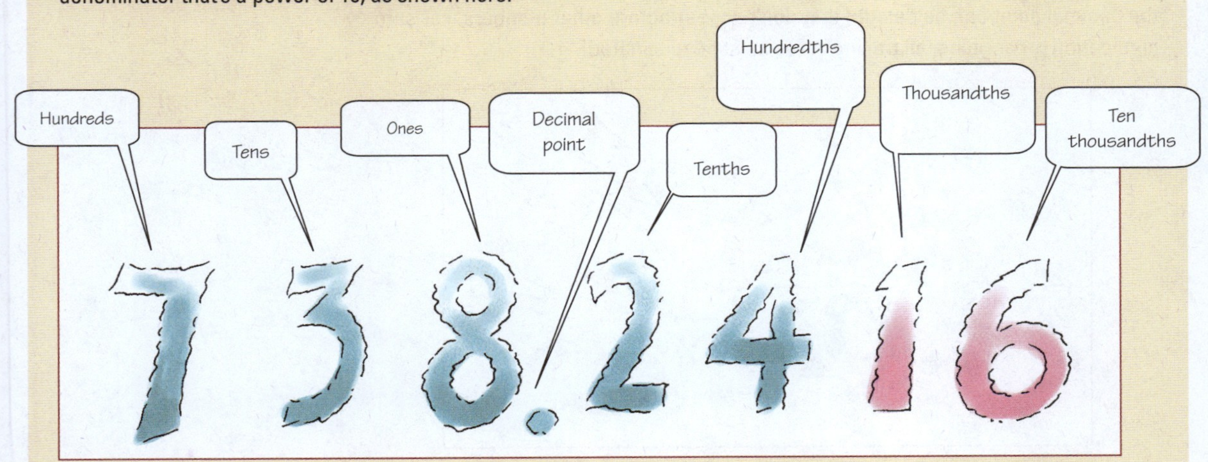

Getting to the point

When discussing money, people use the word *and* to signify the decimal point. For example, people say $5.20 as "5 dollars and 20 cents." However, when discussing decimal numbers in dosage calculations, nurses use the word *point* to signify the decimal point. For example, nurses say the number 5.2 as "5 point 2."

Zeroing in on zeros

Now that we have reviewed the basic terms used with decimals, let's review the decimal calculations most often performed by nurses. But first, review these two important rules:

- After performing mathematical functions with decimal numbers, nurses are encouraged to remove zeros to the right of the decimal point that don't appear before other numbers. (See *Zap those zeros*.) In other cases, when working with fractions, nurses may wish to *add* zeros at the end for a placeholder. Deleting or adding zeros at the end of a decimal number doesn't change the value of the number, but can prevent potential medication errors.
- When writing answers to mathematical calculations and specifying medication dosages, always put a zero to the left of the decimal point if no other number appears there. This helps prevent errors. (See *Disappearing decimal alert*, p. 27.)

Zap those zeros

Solving a problem with decimal numbers? In most cases, the zeros to the right of the decimal point can be deleted that don't appear before other numbers. For safe medication prescribing, all trailing zeros must be eliminated!

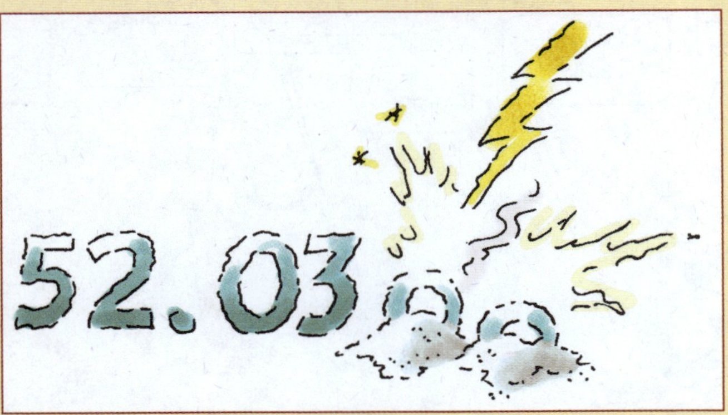

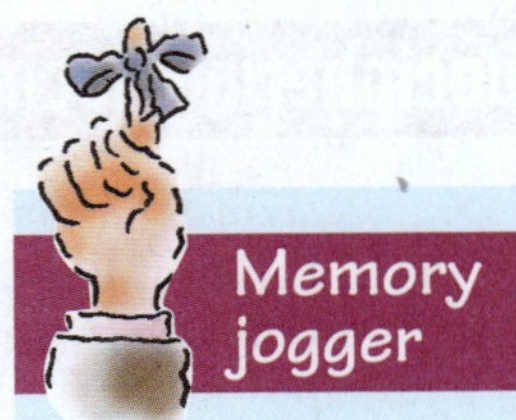

Memory jogger

To remember which zeros can be safely eliminated in a decimal number, think of the letters "l" and "r" in the words *left* and *right*:

- ***Leave*** a zero to the **left** of the decimal point if no other number appears there and a placeholder is needed (as in 0.5 mL). This is referred to as a ***Leading Zero***! This ensures safe medication administration. (See *Disappearing decimal alert*, p. 27.)
- ***Remove*** any trailing zeros to the **right** of the decimal point if no other number follows and a placeholder is not needed (as in 7.50 mg). This is referred to as ***Trailing Zeros***!

Before you give that medication!

Disappearing decimal alert

Decimal points and zeros may be small items, but they're big deals in medication orders and administration records. Medication orders should be reviewed carefully. If a dose doesn't sound right, maybe a decimal point was left out or incorrectly placed.

For instance, an order that calls for ".5 mg lorazepam IV" may be mistaken for "5 mg of lorazepam IV." The correct way to write this order is to use a zero as a placeholder before the decimal point. The order would then become "0.5 mg lorazepam IV." Remember to look for missing leading zeros!

Adding and subtracting decimal numbers

Before adding and subtracting decimal numbers, align the decimal points vertically to help keep track of the decimal positions.

Placeholders, take your place

To maintain column alignment, add a zero as a placeholder in decimal numbers.

Here's how to use zeros to align the decimal numbers 2.61, 0.315, and 4.8 before adding:

$$\begin{array}{r} 2.610 \\ 0.315 \\ +4.800 \\ \hline 7.725 \end{array}$$

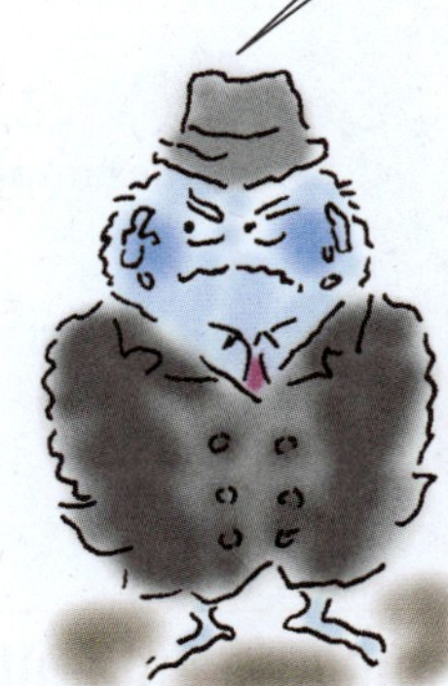

One sneaky decimal point can make a good dosage go bad!

Working it out

Here are two more examples of adding and subtracting decimal numbers.

- First, add 0.017, 4.8, and 1.22:

$$\begin{array}{r} 0.017 \\ 4.800 \\ +1.220 \\ \hline 6.037 \end{array}$$

- Next, subtract 0.05 from 4.726:

$$\begin{array}{r} 4.726 \\ -0.050 \\ \hline 4.676 \end{array}$$

Multiplying decimal numbers

Aligning the decimal points isn't necessary before doing a multiplication problem with decimals. Just leave the decimal points in their original positions and multiply the factors to find the product.

To determine where to place the decimal point in the final product:

- First, add together the number of decimal places in both factors being multiplied.
- Then, count out the same total number of places in the answer, starting from the right and moving to the left, and place the decimal point just to the left of the last place counted.
- Here's how to multiply 2.7 and 0.81:

$$\begin{array}{r} 2.70 \\ \times\, 0.81 \\ \hline 2.1870 \end{array}$$

The decimal point goes here because there are three decimal places in the factors

All decimal points, please line up at your proper places... All decimal points, please line up...

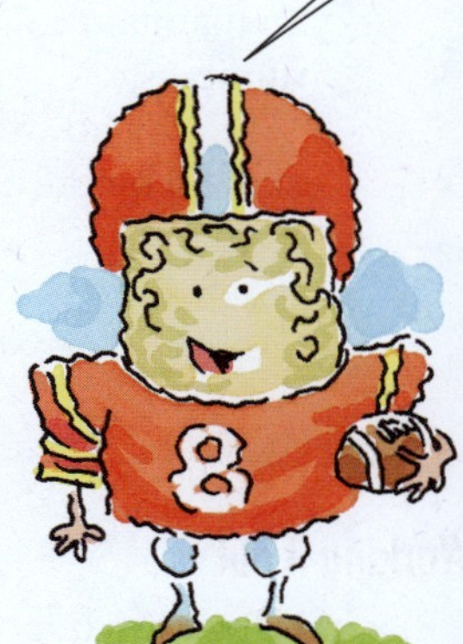

Multiple multiplications

Here are two more examples of multiplying decimal numbers.

- First example, multiply 1.423 and 8.59:

$$\begin{array}{r} 1.423 \\ \times\, 8.59 \\ \hline 12.22357 \end{array}$$

- Next example, multiply 42.1 and 0.376:

$$\begin{array}{r} 42.1 \\ \times\, 0.376 \\ \hline 15.8296 \end{array}$$

Dividing decimal numbers

When dividing decimal numbers, align the decimal points but don't add zeros as placeholders. *Remember:* the number to be divided is the *dividend,* the number that does the dividing is the *divisor,* and the answer is the *quotient.*

Whole-number divisors

Decimal point placement is easiest when the divisor is a whole number. Just place the decimal point in the quotient directly above the decimal point in the dividend and then work the problem. For example, here's how to divide 4.68 by 2:

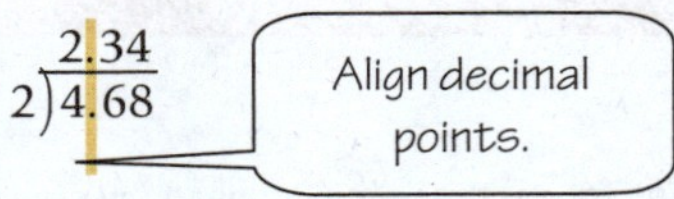

Revisiting decimal division

Here are two more examples of decimal point placement when the divisor is a whole number.

- First example, divide 44.02 by 10:

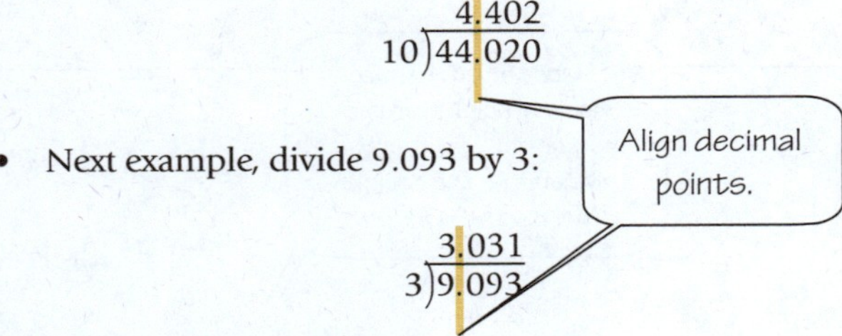

- Next example, divide 9.093 by 3:

$$3\overline{)9.093} = 3.031$$

Decimal-number divisors

Of course, not every divisor is a whole number—some contain decimals. Dividing one decimal number *into* another requires moving the decimal points in both the divisor and the dividend. (See *Dividing decimal numbers,* p. 28.)

Rounding off decimal numbers

Most of the instruments and measuring devices a nurse uses measure accurately only to a tenth or, at most, to a hundredth. Therefore, nurses need to know how to correctly round off decimal numbers—that is, convert long numbers to those with fewer decimal places. (See *Remember rounding,* p. 31.)

Whittling decimals down

To round off a decimal number, follow these incredibly easy steps:

Let's round off the decimal number 0.4293.

Step 1: Decide how many places to the right of the decimal point that needs to be kept. If the number needs to be rounded off to the hundredths, keep two places to the right of the decimal point and delete the rest (the 9 and the 3).

Step 2: Look at the first number that has been deleted. Is this number 5 or greater than 5? If so, add 1 to the number in the hundredths place—that is, to the number 2. The rounded-off number is now 0.43.

For math phobics only

Dividing decimal numbers

When dividing one decimal number by another, follow these incredibly easy steps:

Step 1: Move the divisor's decimal point all the way to the right to convert it to a whole number.

Step 2: Move the dividend's decimal point the same number of places to the right.

Step 3: After completing the division problem, place the quotient's decimal point directly above the new decimal point in the dividend.

The example here shows how to divide 10.45 by 2.6. The quotient is rounded to the nearest hundredth place.

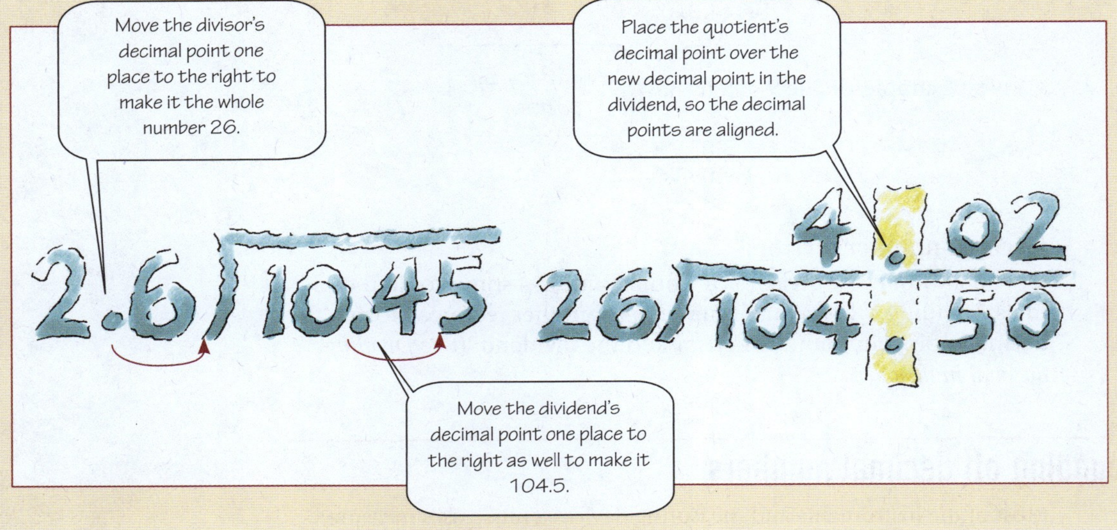

Move the divisor's decimal point one place to the right to make it the whole number 26.
Place the quotient's decimal point over the new decimal point in the dividend, so the decimal points are aligned.
2.6)10.45
4.02
26)104.50
Move the dividend's decimal point one place to the right as well to make it 104.5.

Step 3: Suppose the number that was deleted is less than 5. If this is the case, don't add 1 to the number on the left. For example, to round off 1.9085 to the nearest tenth, identify the number in the tenths position (9) and delete all the numbers to the right of it (0, 8, and 5). Since the number directly to the right of 9—the 0—is less than 5, the number 9 stays the same. The number 1.9085 rounded off to the nearest tenth is 1.9.

A practice round

Try rounding off 14.723 to the nearest hundredth:

- First, decide what number is in the hundredths place (2) and delete all the numbers to the right of it (only the number 3).
- Since 3 is lower than 5, don't add 1 to the 2. So, the rounded-off number is 14.72.

WAIT!
Now let's round 14.723 to the nearest tenth. Since 7 is in the tenths place, and 2 is directly to the right of it (and is less than 5), do not add 1 to 7. So, the rounded-off number would now be 14.7.

ONE MORE TIME!

Now, round the *same* number 14.723 to a *whole number*. What number is directly to the right of 4 in the whole number 14? Since 7 is greater than 5, add 1 to 14, making the new rounded-off *whole* number 15.

See the differences in the answers depending on how the numbers are rounded? It's *crazy*!

Now, round off 0.9875 to the nearest thousandth:

- The number in the thousandth place is 7. All numbers to the right of the 7—the 5—will be deleted.
- Since the number to be deleted is 5, the 7 is rounded *up* to 8 (7 + 1). The rounded-off number is therefore 0.988.

Again, try to round this same number 0.9875 to the nearest hundredths, tenths, and whole number. Look back at the last example if you get stuck! You *can* do this!

Remember rounding

When rounding, remember that 5 is the magic number. Check the number to the right of the decimal place that will be rounded off. If that number is 5 or greater, then add 1 to the place. If it's less than 5, leave the number alone.

For example, round off the following numbers to the nearest hundredths place:

- 6.447
- 2.992
- 4.119

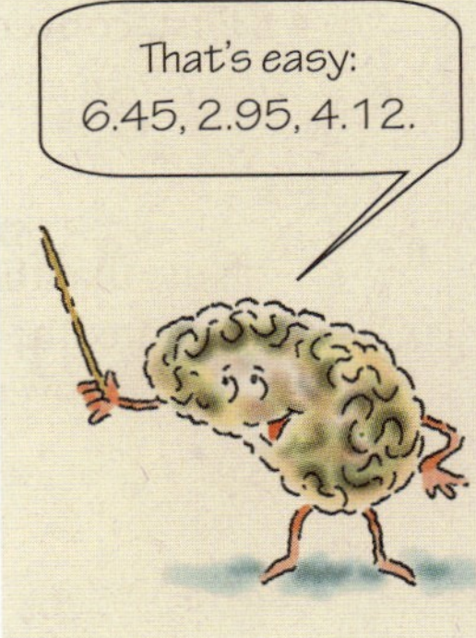

Converting fractions

Many measuring devices have metric calibrations; therefore, common fractions often need to be converted to a decimal number. At times, decimal numbers may need to be converted back to common fractions.

Converting common fractions to decimals

Changing a common, proper fraction into a decimal number is simple. Just divide the numerator by the denominator. Add a zero as a placeholder to the left of the decimal point.

Commence converting

For example, here's how to convert $\frac{4}{10}$ to a decimal number:

$$\frac{4}{10} = 4 \div 10 = 10\overline{)4.0}\ \ (0.4)$$

Keep on converting

Here are two more examples.

- First, convert $\frac{2}{5}$ to a decimal number:

$$\frac{2}{5} = 2 \div 5 = 5\overline{)2.0}\ \ (0.4)$$

- Next, convert $\frac{3}{8}$ to a decimal number:

$$\tfrac{3}{8} = 3 \div 8 = 8\overline{)3.000}\quad 0.375$$

Converting mixed numbers to decimals

Need to convert a mixed number to a decimal number? First, convert it to an improper fraction and then divide the numerator by the denominator, as shown earlier.

Mixing it up

Here's an example. To convert $4\frac{3}{4}$ to a decimal number:

- First, convert the mixed number $4\frac{3}{4}$ to the improper fraction $\frac{19}{4}$.
- Then, divide 19 by 4 to find the decimal number:

$$4\tfrac{3}{4} = \tfrac{19}{4} = 19 \div 4 = 4\overline{)19.00}\quad 4.75$$

Let's see that again

Here are two more calculations to try.

- First, convert $10\frac{7}{8}$ to a decimal number:

$$10\tfrac{7}{8} = \tfrac{87}{8} = 87 \div 8 = 8\overline{)87.00}\quad 10.88$$

  Note that the quotient above has been rounded off to the nearest hundredth.

- Next, convert $1\frac{2}{9}$ to a decimal number:

$$1\tfrac{2}{9} = \tfrac{11}{9} = 11 \div 9 = 9\overline{)11.00}\quad 1.22$$

Converting decimals to common fractions

To convert a decimal number to a common fraction, count the number of decimal places in the decimal number. This number reflects the number of zeros in the denominator of the common fraction.

For example, to convert the decimal number 0.33 into a common fraction, follow these incredibly easy steps:

Step 1: Count the number of decimal places in 0.33. There are two decimal places; therefore, the denominator of its common fraction is 100 because 100 has two zeros.

Step 2: Remove the decimal point from 0.33 and use this number as the numerator. Reduce the fraction, if possible.

The calculation looks like this:

$$0.33 = \frac{33}{100}$$

This fraction can't be reduced further.

Practice, practice, practice

Try two more calculations.

- First example, convert 0.413 to a common fraction. Here, the denominator is 1,000 because the decimal number 0.413 has three places after the decimal point.
- The calculation looks like this:

$$0.413 = \frac{413}{1{,}000}$$

- This fraction can't be reduced further.
- Second example, convert 0.65 to a common fraction. The denominator is 100 because this decimal number has two places after the decimal point.
- The calculation looks like this:

$$0.65 = \frac{65}{100} = \frac{13}{20}$$

Note that this fraction has been reduced to its lowest terms.

Converting decimals to mixed numbers

Use the same method as described previously to convert a decimal number to a mixed number (or to an improper fraction).

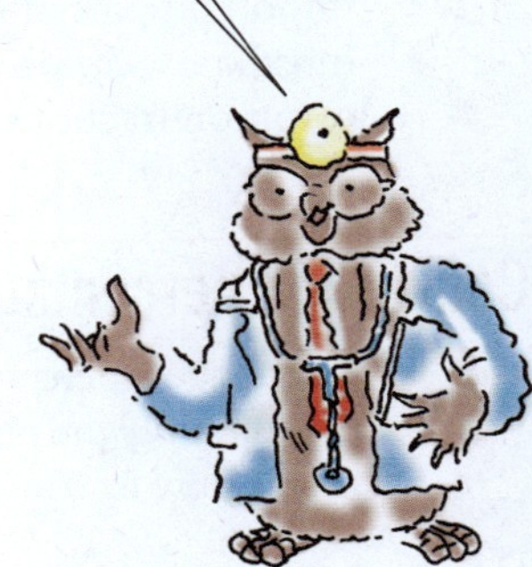

You mean figuring out the denominator is just a matter of counting decimal places?

Mixed up but methodical

Here's an example.

- Convert 5.75 to a fraction using 100 as the denominator since 5.75 has two decimal places. Then convert the fraction to a mixed number.
- The calculation looks like this:

$$5.75 = \frac{575}{100} = 5\,{}^{75}\!/_{100} = 5\,{}^{3}\!/_{4}$$

Note that this mixed number has been reduced to its lowest terms.

That was beautiful! Do it again!

Here are two more sample calculations.

- Convert 3.25 to a fraction. Use 100 as the denominator since 3.25 has two decimal places. Then convert the fraction to a mixed number.
- The calculation looks like this:

$$3.25 = \frac{325}{100} = 3\,{}^{25}\!/_{100} = 3\,{}^{1}\!/_{4}$$

Note that this mixed number has been reduced.

Once more and you got it!

- Convert 1.9 to a fraction. Use 10 as the denominator since 1.9 has only one decimal place. Then convert the fraction to a mixed number.
- The calculation looks like this:

$$1.9 = \frac{19}{10} = 1\,{}^{9}\!/_{10}$$

Note that this mixed number can't be further reduced.

A point about percents

When you see the percent symbol, %, think "for every hundred." Why? Percentage means any quantity stated as parts per hundred. In other words, 75% is actually $^{75}\!/_{100}$ since the percent sign takes the place of the denominator 100.

Understanding percentages

Percentages are another way to express fractions and numerical relationships. The percent symbol may be used with a whole number (such as 21%), a mixed number (such as $34^{1}/_{2}$%), a decimal number (such as 0.9%), or a fraction (such as $^{1}/_{8}$%). (See *A point about percents.*)

From discounts to medication doses

Percentages are used in everyday life such as figuring out how much money 40% off of a sale item would be or when leaving a 20% tip at a restaurant. Nurses also use them in nursing when calculating solutions and medication doses. Working with percentages is an important part of medication administration. Respectively, nurses must know how to easily convert from percentages to decimals and common fractions and the other way around.

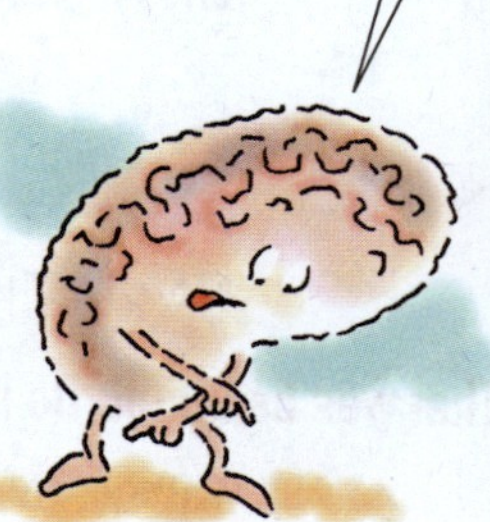

Be careful to watch which direction the decimal point is shifted!

Converting percentages to decimals

To change a percentage to a decimal number, remove the % symbol and multiply the number in the percentage by $^{1}\!/_{100}$, or 0.01. For example, this is how to convert 84% and 35% to decimal numbers:

$$84 \times 0.01 = 0.84$$
$$35 \times 0.01 = 0.35$$

For math phobics only

From percentages to decimals (and back again)

Although it seems like a harmless dot, a misplaced decimal point can lead to a serious medication error. Study the following examples to see how to perform conversions quickly and accurately.

Jump to the left

To convert from a percentage to a decimal, remove the percent sign and move the decimal point two places to the *left*. Here's how:

$$97\% = 0.97$$

Remove the percent sign and move the decimal point two places to the left.

Jump to the right

To convert a decimal to a percentage, reverse the process. Move the decimal point two places to the *right*; add a zero as a placeholder, if necessary; and then add a percent sign. If the resulting percentage is a whole number, remove the decimal because it's understood. Here's what the calculation looks like:

$$0.20 = 20\%$$

Move the decimal point two places to the right and add a percent sign.

Watch that decimal point!

Make sure that the decimals points are shifted in the right direction (to the left, when converting a percentage to a decimal); otherwise, a medication dose could be calculated incorrectly. (See *From percentages to decimals [and back again]*.)

Converting percentages to common fractions

Suppose that 50% needs to be converted to a common fraction. To convert a percentage to a common fraction, follow these incredibly easy steps:

Step 1: Remove the percent sign and put the decimal point two places to the left, creating the decimal number 0.50:

$$50\% = 0.50$$

Step 2: Convert 0.50 to a common fraction with a denominator that's a factor of 10. The result is $^{50}/_{100}$ since 0.50 has two decimal places:

$$0.50 = \frac{50}{100}$$

Step 3: Reduce the fraction to its lowest terms:

$$\frac{50}{100} = \frac{1}{2}$$

Therefore,

$$50\% = \frac{1}{2}$$

Incredible! Do it again!

Here's another example. Convert 32.7% to a common fraction.

Step 1: Remove the percent sign and put the decimal point two places to the left, creating the decimal number 0.327.

Step 2: Convert 0.327 to a common fraction using 1,000 as the denominator since 0.327 has three decimal places:

$$32.7\% = 0.327 = \frac{327}{1{,}000}$$

The result is $^{327}\!/_{1{,}000}$, a fraction that's already reduced to its lowest terms.

Again?

Alright, here's one last example. Convert 20.05% to a common fraction.

Step 1: Remove the percent sign and put the decimal point two places to the left, creating the decimal number 0.2005.

Step 2: Use 10,000 as the denominator because 0.2005 has four decimal places:

$$20.05\% = 0.2005 = \frac{2{,}005}{10{,}000} = \frac{401}{2{,}000}$$

The result is $^{2{,}005}\!/_{10{,}000}$, which becomes $^{401}\!/_{2{,}000}$ when reduced.

Converting common fractions to percentages

Converting a common fraction to a percentage involves two incredibly easy steps. Convert $^{2}\!/_{5}$ to a percentage.

Step 1: Convert a decimal number by dividing the numerator, 2, by the denominator, 5. This can be done by hand or with a calculator. (See *Thank heaven for calculators,* p. 37.)

The calculation looks like this:

$$\frac{2}{5} = 2 \div 5 = 5\overline{)2.0}^{\;0.4}$$

Thank heaven for calculators

A calculator can simplify converting a common fraction to a decimal number. For example, to convert a mixed number like $2\frac{4}{5}$ to a decimal number, first convert it to the improper fraction $\frac{14}{5}$. Then follow these steps on the calculator:

1. Enter the numerator, 14.
2. Press ÷.
3. Enter the denominator, 5.
4. Press = to obtain the converted number, 2.8.

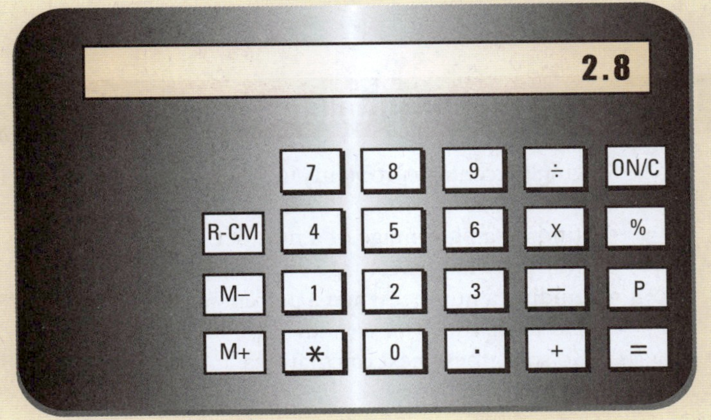

Step 2: Convert the decimal number to a percentage by moving the decimal point two places to the right (add a 0 as a placeholder) and then add the percent sign.

Here's what the calculation looks like:

$$0.40 = 40\%$$

More practice to make you proficient

Here's a second example. Convert $\frac{1}{3}$ to a percentage.

Step 1: Create a decimal number by dividing 1 by 3. Round off the quotient to two decimal places:

$$\frac{1}{3} = 1 \div 3 = 0.333 = 0.33$$

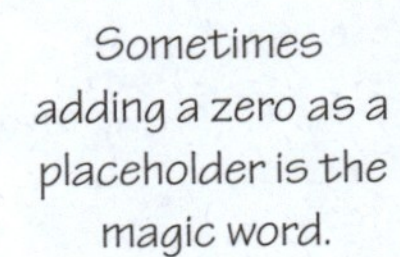

Sometimes adding a zero as a placeholder is the magic word.

Step 2: Convert the decimal number to a percentage by moving the decimal point two places to the right and add the percent sign:

$$0.33 = 33\%$$

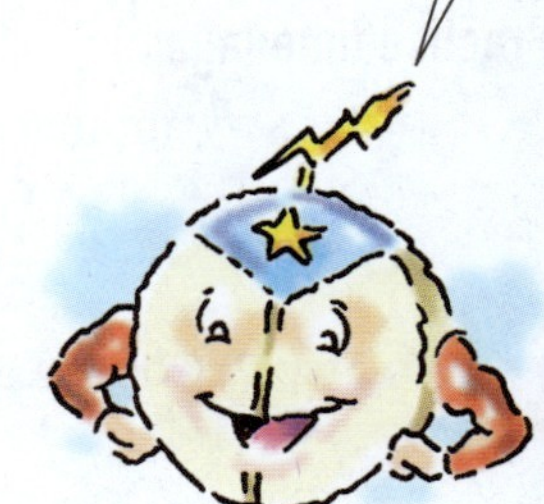

Once more to make sure

Here's a third example. Convert $\frac{3}{8}$ to a percentage.

Step 1: Create a decimal number by dividing 3 by 8:

$$\frac{3}{8} = 3 \div 8 = 0.375$$

Step 2: Convert the decimal number to a percentage by moving the decimal point two places to the right and add the percent sign.

The result is:

$$0.375 = 37.5\%$$

Solving percentage problems

Solving percentage problems involves three types of calculations. They are:

- finding a percentage of a number
- finding what percentage one number is of another
- finding a number when a percentage of it is known. (See *Percentage problems: Watch the wording.*)

To solve these next calculations, follow these incredibly easy guidelines.

Finding a percentage of a number

The question "What is 40% of 200?" is an example of the first type of calculation. To solve it, change the word *of* to a multiplication sign. This looks like:

$$40\% \times 200 = ?$$

- Next, convert 40% to a decimal number by removing the percent sign and moving the decimal point two places to the left:

$$40\% = 0.40$$

- Now, multiply the two numbers to get the answer:

$$0.40 \times 200 = 80$$

Therefore, 80 is 40% of 200.

Practice time (again)

Let's try another problem. Solve for: "What is 5% of 150?"
Step 1: Restate it as a multiplication problem:

$$5\% \times 150 = ?$$

Step 2: Convert 5% to the decimal number 0.05:

$$5\% = 0.05$$

Step 3: Multiply the two numbers to arrive at the answer:

$$0.05 \times 150 = 7.5$$

Therefore, 7.5 is 5% of 150.

Percentage problems: Watch the wording

When a percentage problem is worded as "What is 25% of 80?", mentally change the *of* to a multiplication sign so the problem becomes "What is 25% (or, using a decimal number, 0.25) × 80?" Then continue with the calculation. (The answer is 20.)

If a problem is worded as "25 is what percentage of 80?", treat the *what* as a division sign so the problem becomes $^{25}/_{80}$. Then continue with the calculation. (The answer is 0.3125, or 31.25%.)

More practice (and you thought the piano was rough)

Here's one more example: "What is 7% of 300?"

Step 1: Restate the question as a multiplication problem:

$$7\% \times 300 = ?$$

Step 2: Convert 7% to the decimal number 0.07:

$$7\% = 0.07$$

Step 3: Multiply the two numbers to arrive at the answer:

$$0.07 \times 300 = 21$$

Therefore, 21 is 7% of 300.

Finding what percentage one number is of another

Solve the question "10 is what percentage of 200?"

Step 1: Restate the question as a division problem, with the number 10 as the dividend and the number 200 as the divisor. Here's how the calculation looks so far:

$$200\overline{)10.00} = 0.05$$

Step 2: Move the decimal point in the quotient two places to the right and add a percent sign:

$$0.05 = 5\%$$

Therefore, 10 is 5% of 200.

Again (with a twist)

This type of problem can also be expressed in this way: "What percentage of 28 is 14?" Use the following incredibly easy steps to solve this problem.

Step 1: Restate the question as a division problem by making 28 the divisor and 14 the dividend:

$$28\overline{)14.00} = 0.50$$

Step 2: Move the decimal point two places to the right and add a percent sign:

$$0.50 = 50\%$$

Therefore, 14 is 50% of 28.

One more time

Here's one last problem: "What percentage of 30 is 6?"

Step 1: Restate the question as a division problem by making 30 the divisor and 6 the dividend:

$$30\overline{)6.00} = 0.20$$

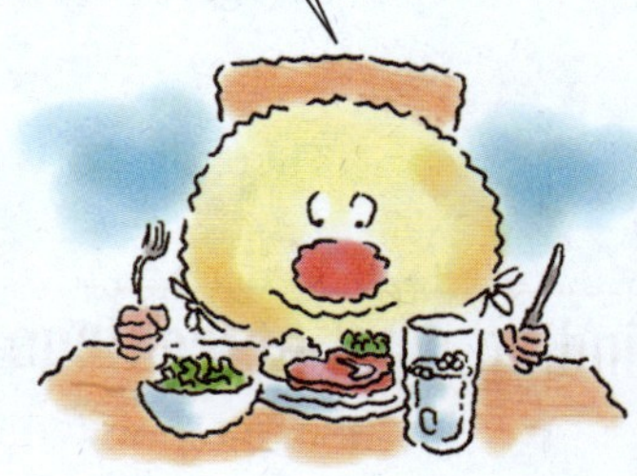
What to do
with leftovers is
always a challenge.
In percentages, just
make a common
fraction.

Step 2: Move the decimal point two places to the right and add a percent sign:

$$0.20 = 20\%$$

Therefore, 6 is 20% of 30.

What to do with the remainder

Sometimes, when determining what percentage one number is of another number, the divisor won't divide exactly into the dividend. In these cases, state the quotient as a mixed number by turning the remainder—the undivided part of the quotient—into a common fraction.

Here's how to do this using the problem "3 is what percentage of 11?"

Step 1: Restate the question as a division problem, making 11 the divisor and 3 the dividend. Work out the quotient to two places; then take the remainder, 3, and make it the numerator of a fraction with the divisor, 11, as the denominator.

Here's what the calculation looks like:

$$\begin{array}{r} 0.27 \\ 11\overline{)3.00} \\ \underline{22} \\ 80 \\ \underline{77} \\ 3 \end{array}$$

The remainder as a common fraction is $\frac{3}{11}$.

Step 2: Move the decimal point in the quotient two places to the right and add a percent sign. (The remaining fraction, $\frac{3}{11}$, is placed to the left of the percent sign.)

$$0.27 \text{ and } \tfrac{3}{11} = 27\tfrac{3}{11}\%$$

Therefore, 3 is 27% of 11.

Back to practice

Let's try a second problem: "5 is what percent of 22?"

Step 1: Restate the question as a division problem, leaving the remainder after two places as a common fraction:

$$\begin{array}{r} 0.22 \\ 22\overline{)5.00} \\ \underline{44} \\ 60 \\ \underline{44} \\ 16 \end{array}$$

The remainder as a common fraction is $\frac{16}{22}$ (reduce to $\frac{8}{11}$).

Step 2: Move the decimal point in the quotient two places to the right and add a percent sign:

$$0.22\tfrac{8}{11} = 22\tfrac{8}{11}\%$$

Therefore, 5 is 22% of 22.

Just can't get enough of those mixed number quotients

Here's the last example: "13 is what percentage of 45?"

Step 1: Restate the question as a division problem, leaving the remainder after two places as a common fraction:

$$\begin{array}{r} 0.28 \\ 45\overline{)13.00} \\ \underline{90} \\ 400 \\ \underline{360} \\ 40 \end{array}$$

The remainder as a common fraction is $\frac{40}{45}$ (reduce to $\frac{8}{9}$).

Step 2: Move the decimal point in the quotient two places to the right and add a percent sign:

$$0.28\tfrac{8}{9} = 28\tfrac{8}{9}\%$$

Therefore, 13 is 28% of 45.

Finding a number when a percentage of it is known

The third type of problem, finding a number when a percentage of it is known or given, also requires division. For example, consider the following question: "70% of what number is 7?" Here's how to do this calculation.

Step 1: Convert 70% into a decimal number by removing the percent sign and moving the decimal point two places to the left:

$$70\% = 0.70$$

Step 2: Divide 7 by 0.70. Move the decimal point two places to the right in both the divisor (to make it a whole number) and the dividend. The quotient (answer) is 10:

$$0.70\overline{)7.00\ 0}\quad 10.0$$

Therefore, 70% of 10 is 7.

Do you feel perfect yet?

Now solve the problem "30% of what number is 90?"

Step 1: Convert 30% to a decimal number by removing the percent sign and moving the decimal point two places to the left:

$$30\% = 0.30$$

Step 2: Divide 90 by 0.30. Move the decimal point two places to the right in both the divisor (to make it a whole number) and the dividend. The quotient is 300.

$$0.30\overline{)90.000}\quad 300.0$$

Therefore, 30% of 300 is 90.

Now you're getting the hang of it!

Here's a third example: "70% of what number is 28?"

Step 1: Convert 70% to a decimal number by removing the percent sign and moving the decimal point two places to the left:

$$70\% = 0.70$$

Step 2: Divide 28 by 0.70. Move the decimal point two places to the right in both the divisor (to make it a whole number) and the dividend. The quotient is 40:

$$0.70\overline{)28.00\ 0}\quad 40.0$$

Therefore, 70% of 40 is 28.

Real-world problem

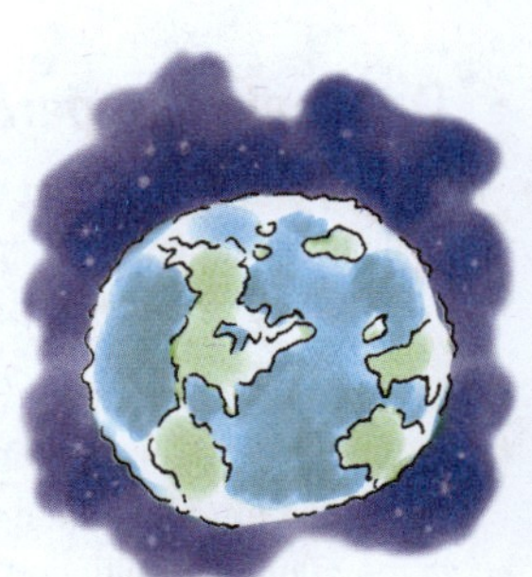

The patient received 600 mL of IV fluid out of 1,000 mL that was ordered. What percentage of IV fluid did the patient receive?

Devising the division

What the nurse really needs to know in this problem is "600 is what percentage of 1,000?"

Step 1: Restate it as a division problem, with 600 as the dividend and 1,000 as the divisor:

$$\begin{array}{r} 0.60 \\ 1000\overline{)600.00} \\ \underline{6000} \\ 00 \end{array}$$

Step 2: Move the decimal point in the quotient two places to the right and add a percent sign:

$$0.60 = 60\%$$

Therefore, 600 is 60% of 1,000. The patient received 60% of the IV fluid.

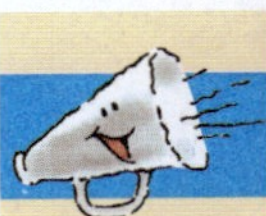

That's a wrap!

Decimals and percentages review

Keep in mind these important facts when working with decimals and percentages.

Decimals and percentages

- Each number or place to the left of the decimal point represents a whole number that's a power of 10.
- Each place to the right of the decimal point represents a fraction whose denominator is a power of 10.
- A percentage is any quantity stated as parts per hundred (the percent sign takes the place of the denominator 100).

Writing decimals

- Eliminate any trailing zeroes.
  – Remove zeros to the right of the decimal point that don't appear before other numbers.
- Always use leading zeros.
  – Always place a zero to the left of the decimal point if no other number appears there.

(continued)

Decimals and percentages review (*continued*)

Adding and subtracting decimals
- Align the decimal points vertically.
- Use zeros to maintain column alignment.

Multiplying decimals
- Don't move decimal points when multiplying.
- The number of decimal places in the product equals the sum of the decimal places in the numbers multiplied.

Dividing decimals
- When a whole number is the divisor, place the quotient's decimal point directly above the dividend's decimal point.
- When a decimal number is the divisor:
  - First, move the divisor's decimal point to the right to convert to a whole number.
  - Then move the dividend's decimal point the same number of places to the right.
  - Finally, place the quotient's decimal point directly above the dividend's decimal point.

Rounding off decimals
- Remember, when rounding, to pay attention to which place the decimal needs to go.
  - If rounding to the tenths, only one number will be to the right of the decimal.
  - If rounding to the hundredths, you can expect two numbers to the right of the decimal.
- Check the number to the right of the decimal place that will be rounded off.
  - If that number is less than 5, leave the number in the decimal place alone and delete the number less than 5.
  - If that number is 5 or greater, add 1 to the decimal place and delete the number greater than 5.

Converting percentages to decimals
- Multiply the percentage number by $\frac{1}{100}$ (or 0.01).
- Another option is to shift the decimal two places to the left.

Converting decimals to percentages
- Divide the decimal number by $\frac{1}{100}$ (or 0.01).
- Another option is to shift the decimal two places to the right.

Converting percentages to common fractions

Step 1: Remove the percent sign.

Step 2: Move the decimal point two places to the left.

Step 3: Convert to a common fraction with a denominator that's a factor of 10.

Converting common fractions to percentages

Step 1: Divide the numerator by the denominator.

Step 2: Convert to a percentage by moving the decimal point two places to the right.

Finding a percentage of a number

Step 1: Restate as a multiplication problem by changing the word of to a multiplication sign.

Decimals and percentages review (*continued*)

Step 2: Convert the percentage to a decimal number.
Step 3: Multiply the two numbers.

Finding what percentage one number is of another
Step 1: Restate as a division problem.
Step 2: Convert the quotient to a percentage.
Step 3: If there's a remainder from the division problem, state the quotient as a mixed number by turning the remainder into a common fraction.

Finding a number when you know a percentage of it
Step 1: Convert the percentage into a decimal number.
Step 2: Divide the number by the decimal number.

Quick quiz

1. What is 16% of 79?
   A. 0.20
   B. 4.16
   C. 4.93
   D. 12.64

Answer: D. To solve this, restate the question as a multiplication problem. Convert 16% to a decimal number by removing the percent sign and moving the decimal point two places to the left. The decimal number is 0.16. Then multiply 0.16 by 79.

2. In the decimal number 1.2058, which number represents the tenths place?
   A. 2
   B. 0
   C. 1
   D. 5

Answer: A. The tenths place is to the immediate right of the decimal point.

3. Convert 3% to a decimal number. Which one is correct?
   A. 3.0
   B. 0.30
   C. 0.03
   D. 0.33

Answer: C. Remove the percent sign and move the decimal point two places to the left.

4. Converting the common fraction $\frac{1}{8}$ to a percentage yields which correct answer?

A. 12.5%
B. 8%
C. $\frac{1}{8}$%
D. 0.125%

Answer: A. To obtain 12.5, divide 1 by 8; then convert the answer to a percentage by moving the decimal point two places to the right and add the percent sign.

5. The decimal number 1.9 divided by 3.2 yields which number?

A. 1.5
B. 0.59
C. 6.08
D. 10.55

Answer: B. To solve this, move the decimal points of both the divisor and the dividend one place to the right before dividing. Place the quotient's decimal point over the new decimal point in the dividend.

6. Multiplying 4.9 by 10.203 yields which product (answer)?

A. 49.9947
B. 49994.7
C. 0.499947
D. 499.947

Answer: A. When multiplying, the number of decimal places in the final product equals the sum of the decimal places in the numbers being multiplied. Count the decimal places starting from the right and place the decimal point there.

7. Round 4.6729 to the nearest tenth place.

A. 4.67
B. 4.7
C. 4.673
D. 4.6

Answer: B. The tenths place is the number 6 in this problem. When rounding to the nearest tenth, look to the number to the right of the tenths place (7). Since it is larger than 5, add 1 to the tenths place, making the answer 4.7.

8. Round 4.6729 to the nearest hundredth place.

A. 4.7
B. 4.68
C. 4.67
D. 4.673

Answer: C. The hundredths place in this problem is the number 7. Look to the right of the hundredths place at the 2. Since it is smaller than 5, do not add 1 to the hundredths place. This makes the answer 4.67.

9. Round 4.6729 to the nearest thousandth place.
   A. 4.673
   B. 4.672
   C. 4.6729
   D. 4.67

Answer: A. The thousandths place in this problem is the number 2. Noting that the place to the right of the thousandths place is 9, which is greater than 5, add 1 to the thousandths place (2). The answer becomes 4.673.

Scoring

☆☆☆ If you answered all nine items correctly, that's 100% (or $\frac{9}{9}$ or, if you prefer decimal number, 1.00).

☆☆ If you answered seven or eight items correctly, excellent! As they say, $\frac{7}{9}$ to $\frac{8}{9}$ isn't bad.

☆ If you answered fewer than six items correctly, here's what to do: subtract the number you got right from 6 and add the result back to your score. Now you've got 100%. Reward yourself with a new calculator! But really, keep practicing! The incredibly easy steps in this chapter take practice to remember!

Chapter 3

Ratios, fractions, proportions, and solving for *X*

Just the facts

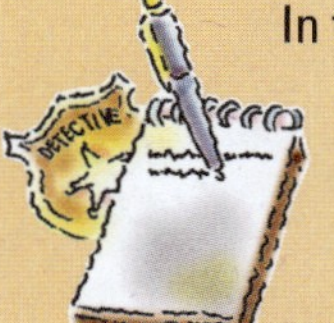

In this chapter, you'll learn how to:

- define ratios and proportions
- set up proportions using ratios and fractions
- solve for *X* in an equation
- relate ratios, proportions, and solving for *X* to dosage calculations

A look at numerical relationships

Ratios, fractions, and proportions describe relationships between numbers. Ratios use a colon between the numbers in the relationship, as in 4:9. Fractions use a slash between numbers in the relationship, as in $\frac{4}{9}$. Ratios are like fractions that have fallen over.

Proportions are statements of equality between two ratios. For example, to show that 4:9 is equal to 8:18, write:

$$4:9::8:18$$

or

$$\frac{4}{9} = \frac{8}{18}$$

Three major problem solvers

When calculating dosages, nurses can use several different formats to solve math problems. One common format is using ratios, fractions, and proportions. Nurses use them to perform many related tasks, such as calculating intravenous (IV) infusion rates and converting weights between systems of measurement. In specialty settings, these formats can be used to perform oxygenation and hemodynamic calculations. However, before ratios, fractions, and proportions can be used, nurses must know how to develop and express them appropriately.

Ratios and fractions

Ratios and fractions are numerical ways to compare items.

Dare to compare

If 100 syringes come in 1 box, then the number of syringes compared to the number of boxes is 100 to 1. This can be written as the ratio 100:1 or as the fraction $^{100}/_{1}$.

Conversely, the number of boxes to syringes would be 1:100 or the fraction $^{1}/_{100}$; so pay attention to which item is mentioned first. This ratio reflects 1 box with 100 syringes inside.

Twice more, with feeling

Here are two more examples.

If a hospital's critical care area requires 1 registered nurse for every 2 patients, then the relationship of registered nurses to patients is 1 to 2. This can be expressed with the ratio 1:2 or with the fraction $^{1}/_{2}$. On the other hand, the ratio of patients to registered nurses is 2:1 or $^{2}/_{1}$.

Suppose a vial contains 8 mg (milligrams) of medication in 1 mL (milliliter) of solution. By using a ratio, this can be expressed as 8 mg:1 mL. By using a fraction, it can be written as: $^{8\ \text{mg}}/_{1\ \text{mL}}$. What would be the ratio of mL to mg? You *know* this!

Proportions

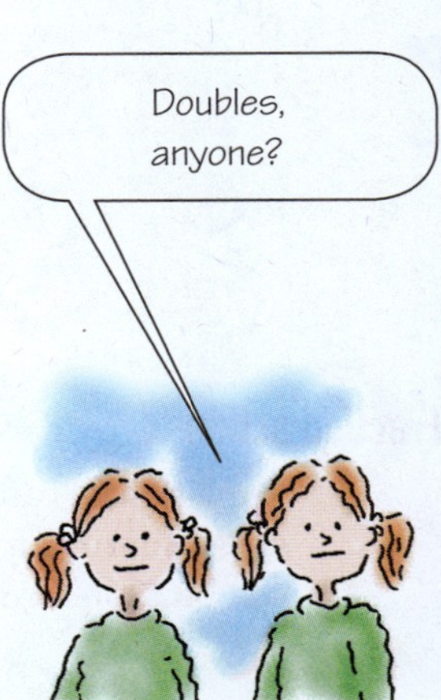

Any proportion that's expressed as two ratios can also be expressed as two fractions.

Using ratios in proportions

When using ratios in a proportion, separate them with double colons. Double colons represent equality between the two ratios.

For example, if the ratio of syringes to boxes is 100:1, then 200 syringes are provided in 2 boxes. This proportion can be written as:

100 syringes:1 box::200 syringes:2 boxes

or

100:1::200:2

Proportion practice

Here's another example. If the critical care area has 1 nurse for every 2 patients, it can be expressed as the ratio 1:2. Subsequently, this also equals a ratio of 3 nurses for every 6 patients. In a proportion, this relationship can be expressed as:

1 nurse:2 patients::3 nurses:6 patients

or

1:2::3:6

Another portion of proportions

Now, suppose a vial contains 8 mg of medication in 1 mL of a solution. This can be stated as the ratio 8 mg:1 mL, which equals 16 mg:2 mL. This proportion can be expressed with ratios as follows:

8 mg:1 mL::16 mg:2 mL

or

8:1::16:2

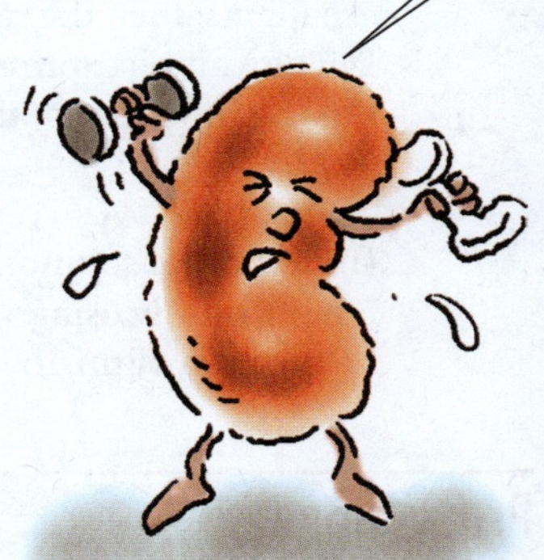

Working out ratios, fractions, and proportions puts you in good shape for dosage calculations.

Using fractions in proportions

Any proportion that can be expressed with ratios can also be expressed with fractions. Here's how to do this using the previous examples.

If 100 syringes come in 1 box, this means that 200 syringes come in 2 boxes. Using fractions, this proportion can be written as follows:

$$\frac{100 \text{ syringes}}{1 \text{ box}} = \frac{200 \text{ syringes}}{2 \text{ boxes}}$$

or

$$\frac{100}{1} = \frac{200}{2}$$

Fraction action

If the critical care area has 1 nurse for every 2 patients, this means that it has 3 nurses for every 6 patients. Using fractions, this relationship can be expressed as:

$$\frac{1 \text{ nurse}}{2 \text{ patients}} = \frac{3 \text{ nurses}}{6 \text{ patients}}$$

or

$$\frac{1}{2} = \frac{3}{6}$$

How would the fraction be written if the ratio was expressed as patient to nurses? *Upside down*!

Vial trial run

If there are 8 mg of medication in 1 mL, this means there are 16 mg in 2 mL. This proportion can be expressed with fractions as:

$$\frac{8 \text{ mg}}{1 \text{ mL}} = \frac{16 \text{ mg}}{2 \text{ mL}}$$

or

$$\frac{8}{1} = \frac{16}{2}$$

Practice! How would the fraction be written if the ratio was expressed as mL to mg?

Solving for *X*

We know that a proportion is a set of two equal ratios or fractions, but what if one ratio or fraction is incomplete? In this case, the unknown part of the ratio or fraction is represented by *X*. Solve for *X* to determine the value of the unknown quantity.

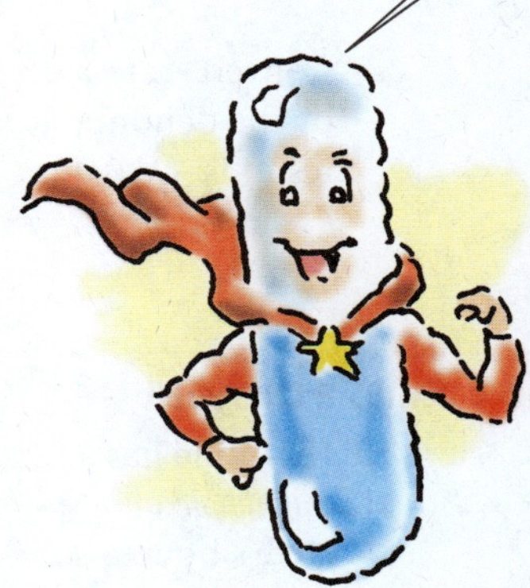

You don't need to be a superhero to solve for X. Just use your brain power and follow these incredibly easy steps!

Solving common-fraction equations

The method used to solve common-fraction equations forms the basis for solving other types of simple equations to find the value of *X*. For example, here's how to solve the common-fraction equation:

$$X = \frac{1}{5} \times \frac{3}{9}$$

1. Multiply the numerators:

$$1 \times 3 = 3$$

2. Multiply the denominators:

$$5 \times 9 = 45$$

3. Restate the equation with this new information:

$$X = \frac{1 \times 3}{5 \times 9} = \frac{3}{45}$$

4. Reduce the fraction by dividing the numerator and denominator by the lowest common denominator (3), to find that $X = \frac{1}{15}$.

$$X = \frac{3 \div 3}{45 \div 3} = \frac{1}{15}$$

5. Most dosage calculations require answers to be expressed in decimal form, so convert $\frac{1}{15}$ to a decimal fraction by dividing the numerator by the denominator. Round the answer off to the nearest hundredth. The final result is $X = 0.07$.

$$X = \frac{1}{15} = 1 \div 15 = 0.07$$

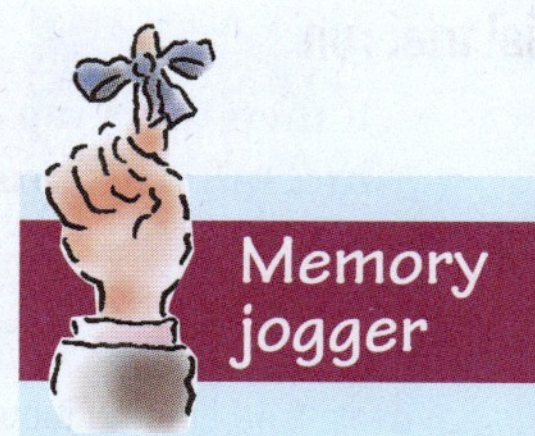
Memory
jogger

The term *X-factor* is commonly used to describe a person or event that could cause unexpected, or *unknown*, outcomes. Keep this in mind and remember that *X* represents the unknown part of a ratio or fraction.

Try this X-ample

Now, solve for *X* in the equation:

$$X = \frac{2}{3} \times \frac{5}{8}$$

1. Multiply the numerators:

$$2 \times 5 = 10$$

2. Multiply the denominators:

$$3 \times 8 = 24$$

3. Restate the equation with this new information:

$$X = \frac{2 \times 5}{3 \times 8} = \frac{10}{24}$$

4. Reduce the fraction by dividing the numerator and denominator by the lowest common denominator (2), to find that $X = \frac{5}{12}$.

$$X = \frac{10 \div 2}{24 \div 2} = \frac{5}{12}$$

5. Convert $\frac{5}{12}$ to a decimal fraction by dividing the numerator by the denominator and then rounding it off. The final result is $X = 0.42$.

$$X = \frac{5}{12} = 5 \div 12 = 0.42$$

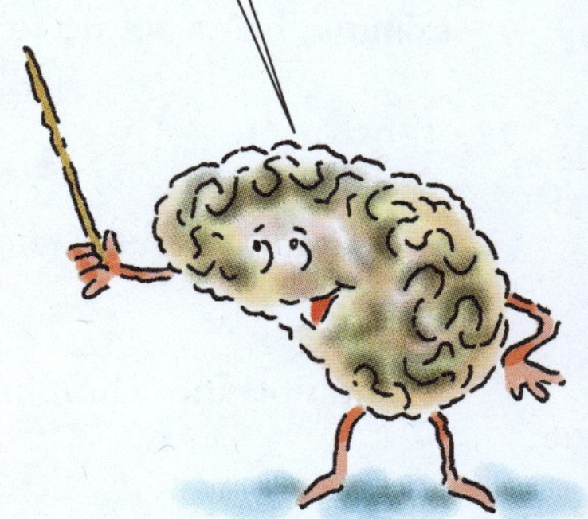
Multiply, multiply,
restate, reduce,
convert...

Here comes a curveball

This example has a twist—the whole number 3 is involved. (See *Making whole numbers fractions*, p. 53.)

Here's how to solve for *X* in an equation with a whole number:

$$X = \frac{125}{500} \times 3$$

1. Convert the whole number 3 into the fraction $\frac{3}{1}$. The equation becomes:

$$X = \frac{125}{500} \times \frac{3}{1}$$

For math phobics only

Making whole numbers fractions

Whole numbers can be changed into a fraction by making the whole number the numerator and placing it over a 1, which is the denominator. The value of the number doesn't change.

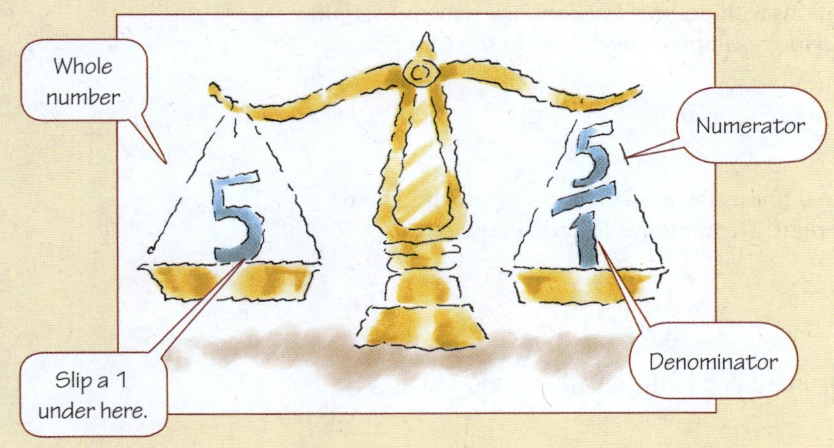

2. Reduce $^{125}/_{500}$ by dividing the numerator and denominator by the lowest common denominator (125) to get $^{1}/_{4}$. The equation becomes:

$$X = \frac{125 \div 125}{500 \div 125} \times \frac{3}{1}$$

or

$$X = \frac{1}{4} \times \frac{3}{1}$$

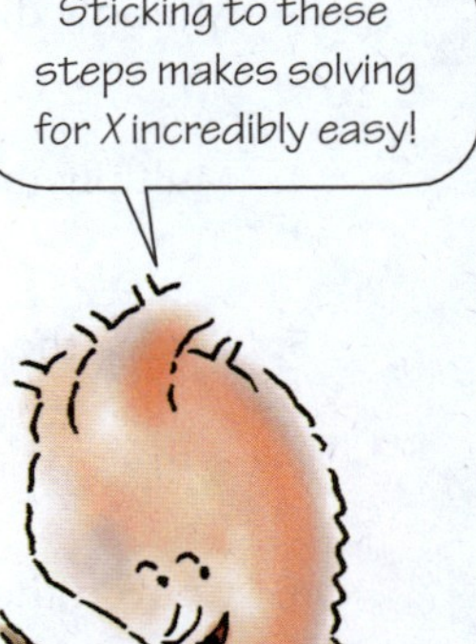

Sticking to these steps makes solving for *X* incredibly easy!

Then proceed as usual.

1. Multiply the numerators:

$$1 \times 3 = 3$$

2. Multiply the denominators:

$$4 \times 1 = 4$$

3. Restate the equation with this new information:

$$X = \frac{1 \times 3}{4 \times 1} = \frac{3}{4}$$

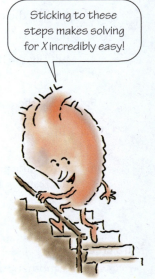

4. The fraction $\frac{3}{4}$ can't be reduced. Convert it to a decimal fraction by dividing the numerator by the denominator. The final result is $X = 0.75$.

$$X = \frac{3}{4} = 3 \div 4 = 0.75$$

Solving decimal-fraction equations

To solve for X in equations with decimal fractions, use a method similar to that used in the previous examples. Here's how to solve for X in the equation:

$$X = \frac{0.05}{0.02} \times 3$$

1. Remove the decimal points from the fraction by moving them two spaces to the right. Then remove the zeros. The equation becomes:

$$X = \frac{5}{2} \times 3$$

2. Convert the whole number 3 to the fraction $\frac{3}{1}$. The equation becomes:

$$X = \frac{5}{2} \times \frac{3}{1}$$

3. Multiply the numerators:

$$5 \times 3 = 15$$

4. Multiply the denominators:

$$2 \times 1 = 2$$

5. Restate the equation with this new information:

$$X = \frac{5 \times 3}{2 \times 1} = \frac{15}{2}$$

6. Convert the answer to decimal form by dividing 15 by 2. The final result is $X = 7.5$.

$$X = \frac{15}{2} = 15 \div 2 = 7.5$$

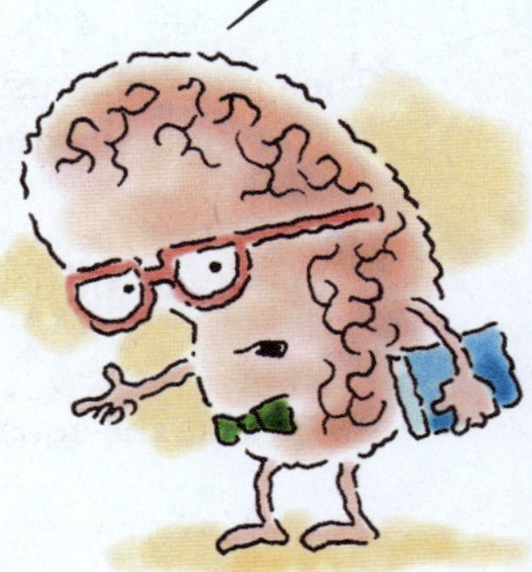

Don't be decimated by decimal-fraction equations by allowing decimal-fractions fracture your ambition!

X-tra credit

Here's another practice problem:

$$X = \frac{0.33}{0.11} \times 0.6$$

1. Remove the decimal points from the fraction by moving them two spaces to the right. Then remove the zeros.

$$X = \frac{33}{11} \times 0.6$$

2. Convert the number 0.6 into the fraction $^{0.6}/_{1}$. The equation becomes:

$$X = \frac{33}{11} \times \frac{0.6}{1}$$

3. Multiply the numerators:

$$33 \times 0.6 = 19.8$$

4. Multiply the denominators:

$$11 \times 1 = 11$$

5. Restate the equation with this new information:

$$X = \frac{33 \times 0.6}{11 \times 1} = \frac{19.8}{11}$$

6. Convert the answer to decimal form by dividing 19.8 by 11. The final result is $X = 1.8$.

$$X = \frac{19.8}{11} = 19.8 \div 11 = 1.8$$

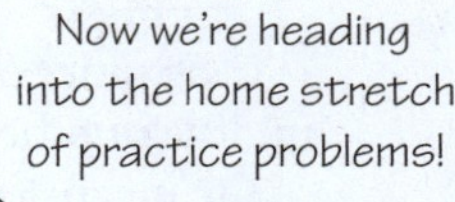

Now we're heading into the home stretch of practice problems!

X-tra, X-tra credit

Here's the last problem:

$$X = \frac{0.04}{0.05} \times 4$$

1. Remove the decimal points from the fraction by moving them two places to the right. Then delete the zeros. The equation becomes:

$$X = \frac{4}{5} \times 4$$

2. Turn 4 into the fraction $^{4}/_{1}$. The equation becomes:

$$X = \frac{4}{5} \times \frac{4}{1}$$

3. Multiply the numerators:

$$4 \times 4 = 16$$

4. Multiply the denominators:

$$5 \times 1 = 5$$

5. Restate the equation with this new information:

$$X = \frac{4 \times 4}{5 \times 1} = \frac{16}{5}$$

6. Convert the answer to decimal form by dividing 16 by 5. The final answer is $X = 3.2$.

$$X = \frac{16}{5} = 16 \div 5 = 3.2$$

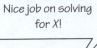

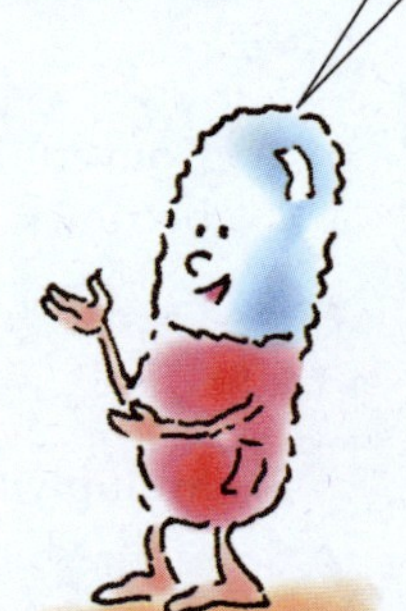
Nice job on solving for X!

Solving proportion problems with ratios

A proportion can be written with ratios, as in:

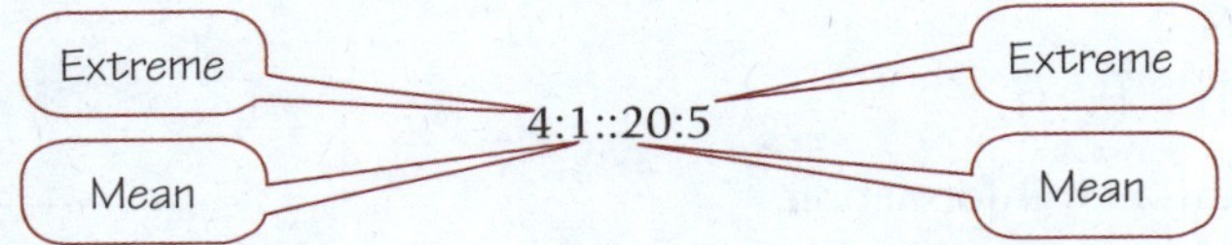
Extreme
Extreme
4:1::20:5
Mean
Mean

The outer or end numbers are called the *extremes*, and the inner or middle numbers are called the *means*. In such a proportion, the product of the means equals the product of the extremes. In this case,

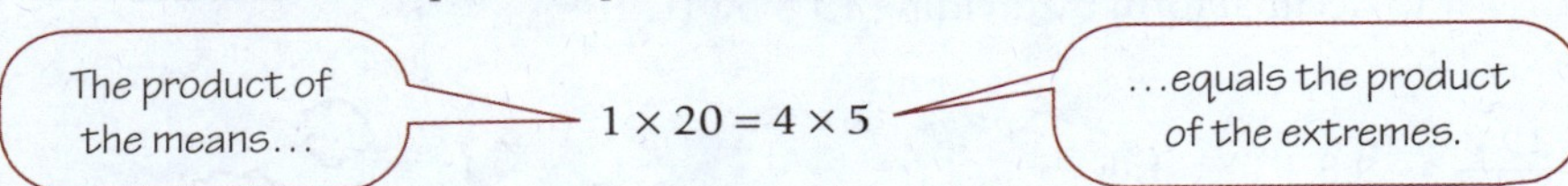
The product of the means...
1 × 20 = 4 × 5
...equals the product of the extremes.

This principle lets nurses solve for any of four unknown parts in a proportion.

X marks another spot

Here's an example. Solve for *X* in the proportion:

$$4:8::8:X$$

Follow these incredibly easy steps:

1. Rewrite the problem so that the means and the extremes are multiplied:

$$8 \times 8 = 4 \times X$$

2. Obtain the products of the means and extremes and put them into an equation:

$$64 = 4X$$

3. Solve for *X* by dividing both sides by 4. Cancel the number (4) that appears in both the numerator and denominator. This isolates *X* on one side of the equation.

$$\frac{64}{4} = \frac{\cancel{4}X}{\cancel{4}}$$

4. Find X:

$$64 \div 4 = X$$

or

$$X = 16$$

5. Replace X with 16 and restate the proportion in ratios:

$$4:8::8:16$$

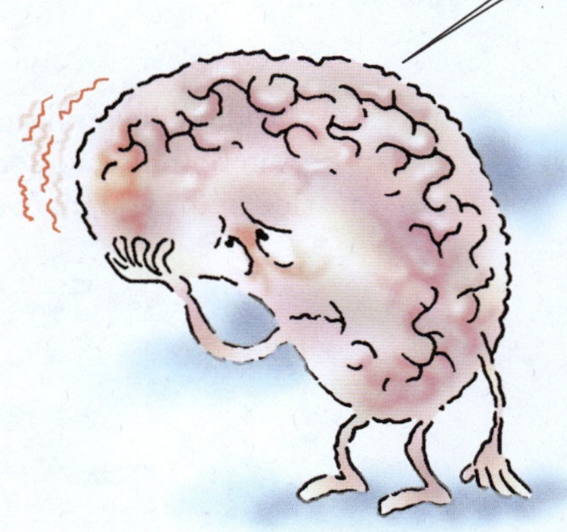

Arrrgh! That darn X keeps moving around!

X moves back to the front

Solve for X in the proportion:

$$X:12::6:24$$

Follow these incredibly easy steps:

1. Rewrite the problem so that the means and the extremes are multiplied:

$$12 \times 6 = X \times 24$$

2. Obtain the products of the means and extremes and put them into an equation:

$$72 = 24X$$

3. Solve for X by dividing both sides by 24. Cancel the number (24) that appears in both the numerator and denominator. This isolates X on one side of the equation:

$$\frac{72}{24} = \frac{\cancel{24}X}{\cancel{24}}$$

4. Find X:

$$72 \div 24 = X$$

or

$$X = 3$$

5. Replace X with 3 and restate the proportion in ratios:

$$3:12::6:24$$

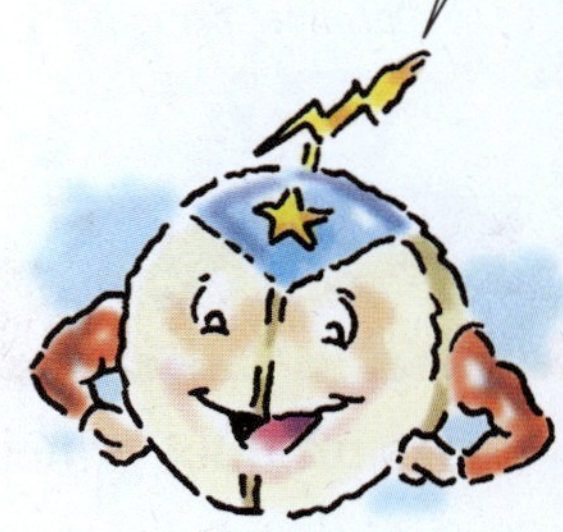

Practicing solving for X helps limber up mathematical muscles for the real world of dosage calculations.

Another X-treme shift

Try one last problem, using this proportion:

$$10:20::X:40$$

1. Rewrite the problem so that the means and the extremes are multiplied:

$$20 \times X = 10 \times 40$$

2. Obtain the products of the means and extremes and put them into an equation:

$$20X = 400$$

3. Solve for *X* by dividing both sides by 20. Cancel the number (20) that appears in both the numerator and denominator. This isolates *X* on one side of the equation:

$$\frac{\cancel{20}X}{\cancel{20}} = \frac{400}{20}$$

4. Find *X*:

$$X = \frac{400}{20}$$

or

$$X = 20$$

5. Replace *X* with 20 and restate the original proportion in ratios:

$$10{:}20{::}20{:}40$$

Solving proportion problems with fractions

Proportion problems may also be set up with fractions. In a proportion expressed as a fraction, cross products are equal—just as the means and extremes are equal in a proportion with ratios. (See *Cross product principle*.)

For math phobics only

Cross product principle

In a proportion expressed as fractions, cross products are equal. In other words, the numerator on the equation's left side multiplied by the denominator on the equation's right side equals the denominator on the equation's left side multiplied by the numerator on the equation's right side.

The above statement has a lot of words. The same meaning is communicated more simply in the illustration to the left below.

Cross product principle (*continued*)

Applies to ratios as well.
Note that the same principle applies to ratios. In a proportion expressed as ratios, the product of the means (numbers in the middle) equals the product of the extremes (numbers on the ends). Consider the illustration to the right below.

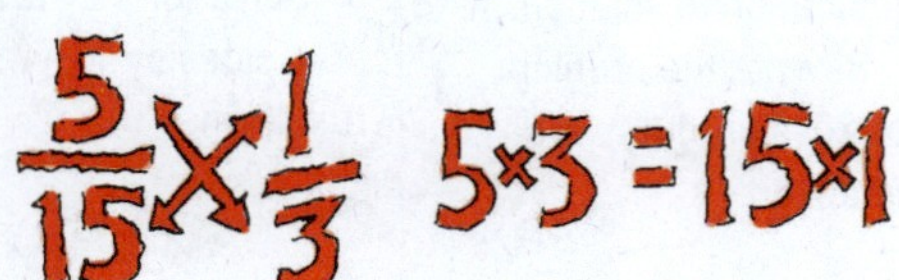

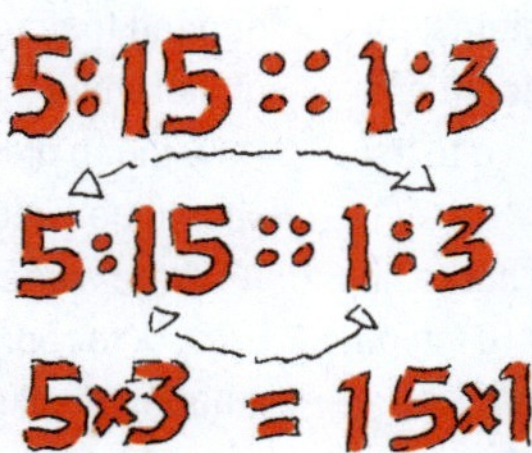

Using the cross products of a proportion, any of the four unknown parts can be solved. Once again, the position of the *X* doesn't matter because the cross products of a proportion are always equal. (See *Cross products to the rescue*, p. 60.)

Keeping things in proportion

After studying the example in *Cross products to the rescue*, practice solving for *X* using this proportion:

$$\frac{3}{4} \times \frac{9}{X}$$

Follow these incredibly easy steps:

1. Rewrite the problem so the cross products are multiplied:

$$3 \times X = 4 \times 9$$

2. Obtain the cross products and put them into an equation:

$$3X = 36$$

3. Solve for *X* by dividing both sides by 3. Cancel the number (3) that appears in both the numerator and denominator. This isolates *X* on one side of the equation:

$$\frac{\cancel{3}X}{\cancel{3}} = \frac{36}{3}$$

4. Find *X*:

$$X = \frac{36}{3}$$

For math phobics only

Cross products to the rescue

Fractions can be used to describe the relative proportion of ingredients; for example, the amount of a medication relative to its solution.

Suppose the nurse has a vial containing 10 mg/mL of morphine. The nurse would write this fraction to describe it:

Amount of drug

$$\frac{10 \text{ mg}}{1 \text{ mL}}$$

Amount of solution

The plot thickens

Now suppose the nurse needed to administer 8 mg of morphine to a patient. How much of the solution should be used?

1. Write a second fraction using *X* to represent the amount of solution:

An unknown quantity

$$\frac{8 \text{ mg}}{X \text{ mL}}$$

2. Set up the equation. Keep the fractions in the same relative proportion of medication to solution.

3. Rewrite the problem so cross products are multiplied:

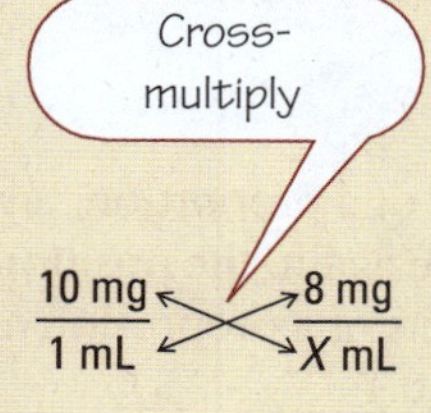

4. This results in:

$$10X = 8$$

5. Solve for *X* by dividing both sides by 10, which results in:

$$X = \frac{8}{10}$$

6. Convert this to a decimal fraction because nurses must draw up the medication expressed as decimals.

$$X = 0.8 \text{ mL}$$

The answer!

This is how much of the morphine should be used.

or

$$X = 12$$

5. Replace the *X* with 12 and restate the proportion in fractions:

$$\frac{3}{4} = \frac{9}{12}$$

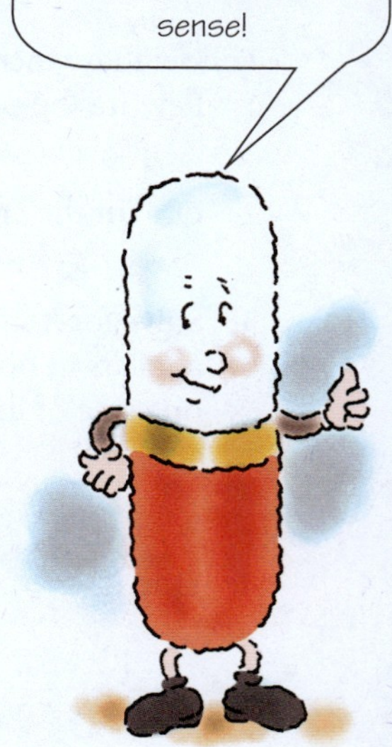

Final practice problem (Yippee!)

Solve one more problem:

$$\frac{12}{25} = \frac{X}{50}$$

1. Rewrite the problem so the cross products are multiplied:

$$12 \times 50 = 25 \times X$$

2. Obtain the cross products and put them into an equation:

$$600 = 25X$$

3. Solve for *X* by dividing both sides by 25:

$$\frac{600}{25} = \frac{\cancel{25}X}{\cancel{25}}$$

4. Find *X*:

$$X = 24$$

5. Replace *X* with 24 and restate the proportion in fractions:

$$\frac{12}{25} = \frac{24}{50}$$

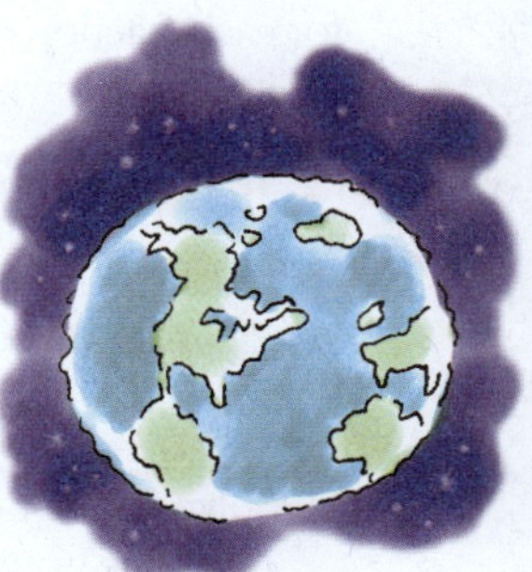

Real-world problems

Next, let's review three practical examples of proportions in everyday nursing practice.

How should a nurse set up a proportion to solve a real-world problem? Just place the known ratio on one side of the double colon and the unknown ratio on the other side. Make sure that the units of measure in each ratio are in the same positions on both sides of the proportion. (See *Write it down*.)

> **Advice from the experts**
>
> **Write it down**
>
> When calculating dosages, nurses may be able to figure out some problems in their head. For instance, 4 mg in 2 mL has the same proportion as 2 mg in 1 mL. If stumped, don't be shy about writing the proportion down on paper. Taking the time to see the numbers will help avoid confusion and solve for *X* more quickly and accurately. If the answer makes no sense at all, it is quicker and more accurate to see the steps on paper.

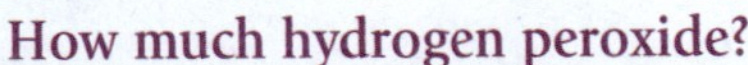

How much hydrogen peroxide?

Set up a proportion to find out how much hydrogen peroxide (H_2O_2) should be added to 1,000 mL of water (H_2O) to make a solution that contains 50 mL of H_2O_2 for every 100 mL of H_2O.

The ratio approach

To solve this problem using ratios, follow these incredibly easy steps:

1. Decide what part of the ratio is *X*. In this case, it's the amount of H_2O_2 in 1,000 mL of H_2O.
2. Set up the proportion so that similar parts of each ratio are in the same position:

$$X{:}1{,}000 \text{ mL } H_2O{::}50 \text{ mL } H_2O_2{:}100 \text{ mL } H_2O$$

3. Multiply the means and the extremes and restate the problem as an equation:

$$1{,}000 \text{ mL } H_2O \times 50 \text{ mL } H_2O_2 = X \text{ mL } H_2O_2 \times 100 \text{ mL } H_2O$$

4. Solve for *X* by dividing both sides of the equation by 100 mL H_2O and canceling units that appear in both the numerator and denominator:

$$\frac{1{,}000 \cancel{\text{ mL } H_2O} \times 50 \text{ mL } H_2O_2}{100 \cancel{\text{ mL } H_2O}} = \frac{X \text{ mL } H_2O_2 \times \cancel{100 \text{ mL } H_2O}}{\cancel{100 \text{ mL } H_2O}}$$

5. Find *X*:

$$\frac{50{,}000 \text{ mL } H_2O_2}{100} = X$$

or

$$X = 500 \text{ mL } H_2O_2$$

The fraction approach

If the proportion is set up with fractions, place similar units of measure for each fraction in the same position. Here's what the previous example looks like in fraction form:

$$\frac{X}{1{,}000 \text{ mL } H_2O} = \frac{50 \text{ mL } H_2O_2}{100 \text{ mL } H_2O}$$

1. Rewrite the equation by cross-multiplying the fractions:

$$X \times 100 \text{ mL } H_2O = 1{,}000 \text{ mL } H_2O \times 50 \text{ mL } H_2O_2$$

2. Solve for *X* by dividing both sides of the equation by 100 mL H_2O and canceling units that appear in both the numerator and denominator:

$$\frac{X \times 100 \cancel{\text{ mL } H_2O}}{100 \cancel{\text{ mL } H_2O}} = \frac{1{,}000 \cancel{\text{ mL } H_2O} \times 50 \text{ mL } H_2O_2}{100 \cancel{\text{ mL } H_2O}}$$

3. Find *X*:

$$X = \frac{50{,}000 \text{ mL } H_2O_2}{100}$$

$$X = 500 \text{ mL } H_2O_2$$

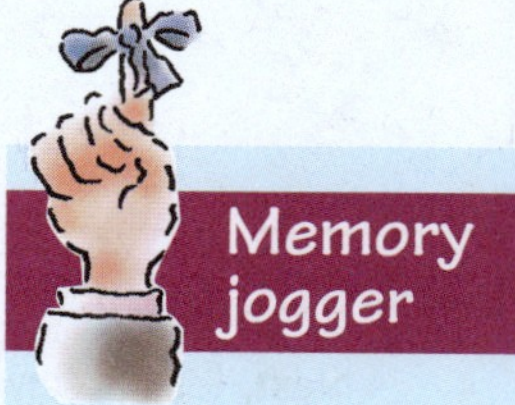

When working with ratios, the product of the ***means*** always equals the product of the ***extremes***. To differentiate these terms, remember:

means (**m**iddle numbers)

extremes (**e**nd numbers)

How many clinical instructors?

Set up another proportion problem with both ratios and fractions. If a school of nursing requires 1 clinical instructor for every 8 students, how many instructors are needed for a class of 24 students?

Resolving it with ratios

Use ratios first. Follow these incredibly easy steps:

1. Decide what part of the proportion is *X*. In this case, it's the number of instructors for 24 students.
2. Set up the proportion so that the units of measure (instructors and students) in each ratio are in the same position:

1 instructor:8 students::*X*:24 students

3. Multiply the means and the extremes and set up the equation:

$$8 \text{ students} \times X = 1 \text{ instructor} \times 24 \text{ students}$$

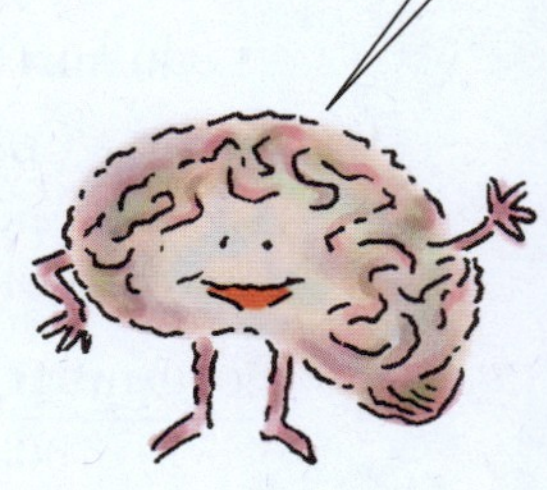

Fractions and ratios can be very helpful in everyday situations!

4. Solve for *X* by dividing both sides of the equation by 8 students and canceling units that appear in both the numerator and denominator:

$$\frac{\cancel{8\ \text{students}} \times X}{\cancel{8\ \text{students}}} = \frac{1\ \text{instructor} \times 24\ \cancel{\text{students}}}{8\ \cancel{\text{students}}}$$

$$X = \frac{24}{8}$$

5. Find *X*:

$$X = 3\ \text{instructors}$$

Figuring it out with fractions

If the preference is to solve the previous problem using fractions, follow these incredibly easy steps:

1. Set up the proportion so that the units of measure are in the same position in each fraction. Here's what the problem looks like in fraction form:

$$\frac{1\ \text{instructor}}{8\ \text{students}} = \frac{X}{24\ \text{students}}$$

2. Rewrite the equation by cross-multiplying the fractions:

$$1\ \text{instructor} \times 24\ \text{students} = X\ \text{instructors} \times 8\ \text{students}$$

3. Solve for *X* by dividing both sides of the equation by 8 students and canceling units that appear in both the numerator and denominator:

$$\frac{1\ \text{instructor} \times 24\ \cancel{\text{students}}}{8\ \cancel{\text{students}}} = \frac{X \times \cancel{8\ \text{students}}}{\cancel{8\ \text{students}}}$$

or

$$24 \div 8 = X\ \text{instructors}$$

4. Find *X*:

$$X = 3\ \text{instructors}$$

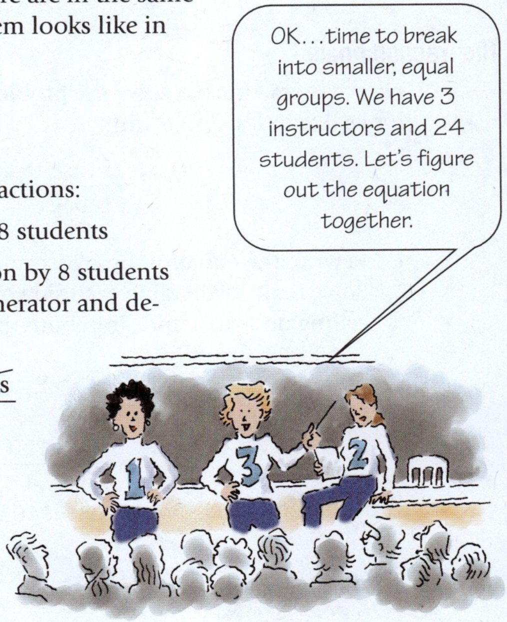

OK. . .time to break into smaller, equal groups. We have 3 instructors and 24 students. Let's figure out the equation together.

How many bags of IV fluid?

Here's one more problem. One case of IV fluid holds 20 bags. If a home care agency receives 6 cases, how many bags of IV fluid does it have?

The ratio rally

Solve this problem using ratios first. Follow these incredibly easy steps:

1. Decide what part of the ratio is *X*. In this case, it's the number of bags of IV fluid in 6 cases.

2. Set up the proportion so that the units of measure in each ratio are in the same position:

$$1\text{ case}:20\text{ bags}::6\text{ cases}:X$$

3. Multiply the means and the extremes and set up the equation:

$$20\text{ bags} \times 6\text{ cases} = X\text{ bags} \times 1\text{ case}$$

4. Solve for X by dividing both sides of the equation by 1 case and canceling units that appear in both the numerator and denominator:

$$\frac{20\text{ bags} \times 6\ \cancel{\text{cases}}}{1\ \cancel{\text{case}}} = \frac{X \times \cancel{1\text{ case}}}{\cancel{1\text{ case}}}$$

5. Find X.

$$120\text{ bags} = X$$

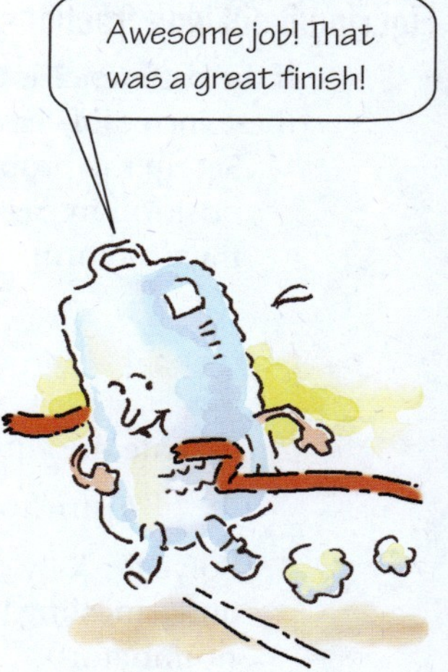
Awesome job! That was a great finish!

The fraction finale

Now, use fractions to solve the problem. Here's what the equation looks like in fraction form:

$$\frac{1\text{ case}}{20\text{ bags}} = \frac{6\text{ cases}}{X}$$

1. Rewrite the equation by cross-multiplying the fractions.
2. Solve for X by dividing each side of the equation by 1 case and cancelling units that appear in both the numerator and denominator:

$$\frac{\cancel{1\text{ case}} \times X}{\cancel{1\text{ case}}} = \frac{6\ \cancel{\text{cases}} \times 20\text{ bags}}{1\ \cancel{\text{case}}}$$

$$X = \frac{120}{1}$$

$$X = 120\text{ bags}$$

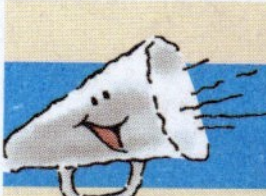

That's a wrap!

Ratios, fractions, proportions, and solving for *X* review

Some important facts about ratios, fractions, proportions, and solving for *X* are outlined below.

Numerical relationship basics

- Ratio: uses a colon between the numbers in a numerical relationship

Ratios, fractions, proportions, and solving for *X* review (*continued*)

- Fraction: uses a slash between numbers in a numerical relationship
- Proportion: a statement of equality between two ratios or two fractions

Solving common-fraction equations

- Multiply numerators
- Multiply denominators
- Restate the equation
- Reduce the fraction
- Convert the fraction to decimal form by dividing the numerator by the denominator

Solving decimal-fraction equations

- Move the decimal points two spaces to the right
- Remove the zeros
- Convert the whole number to a fraction
- Multiply the numerators
- Multiply the denominators
- Restate the equation
- Convert the answer to decimal form by dividing the numerator by the denominator.

Solving proportions with ratios

- Means—middle numbers
- Extremes—end numbers
- Product of the means = product of the extremes
- Isolate *X* on one side of the equation
- Solve for *X*.

Solving proportions with fractions

- Cross products of a proportion are always equal
- Multiply the cross products
- Put the cross products into the equation, and isolate *X* on one side of the equation
- Solve for *X*.

Quick quiz

1. Which is an example of a proportion?
   A. 4:5::8:12
   B. 6:1::18:3
   C. 7:1::14:7
   D. 3:8::2:6

Answer: B. In a proportion, the ratios are equal.

2. The proportion 1:5::2:10 can be restated in which fraction form?
   A. $\frac{1}{5} = \frac{2}{10}$
   B. $\frac{5}{1} = \frac{2}{10}$
   C. $\frac{2}{5} = \frac{1}{10}$
   D. $\frac{5}{2} = \frac{10}{1}$

Answer: A. Make the ratios on both sides into fractions by substituting slashes for colons.

3. If there are 50 mg of medication in 5 mL of solution. What is the amount of medication in 15 mL of solution?

   A. 10 mg
   B. 150 mg
   C. 75 mg
   D. 100 mg

Answer: B. Substitute *X* for the amount of medication in 15 mL of solution and then set up a proportion with ratios or fractions.

4. If ½ (0.5) tsp of salt is added to 8 oz of water to make a solution, how much salt should be added to 32 oz of water to make a solution?

   A. 2 tsp
   B. 4 tsp
   C. 1 tsp
   D. 3 tsp

Answer: A. Substitute *X* for the amount of salt in 32 oz of water and then set up a proportion with ratios or fractions.

5. A licensed practitioner prescribes 0.125 mg of medication. The vial contains 0.25 mg per 1 mL of solution. How many mL of the solution should be administered?

   A. 1 mL
   B. 2 mL
   C. 0.5 mL
   D. 1.5 mL

Answer: C. Substitute *X* for the amount of solution needed to administer 0.125 mg of the medication and then set up a proportion with ratios or fractions.

6. A licensed practitioner prescribes 40 mg of the medication furosemide (Lasix). The vial contains 10 mg per mL of solution. How many mL of solution should be administered?

   A. 1 mL
   B. 2 mL
   C. 3 mL
   D. 4 mL

Answer: D. Substitute *X* for the amount of solution needed to administer 40 mg of the medication and then set up a proportion with ratios or fractions.

Scoring

☆☆☆ If you answered all six items correctly, wow! You're a whiz at relationships (numerical relationships, that is).

☆☆ If you answered four or five items correctly, all right! You have everything in proportion.

☆ If you answered fewer than four items correctly, a quick review will get your numbers back on track!

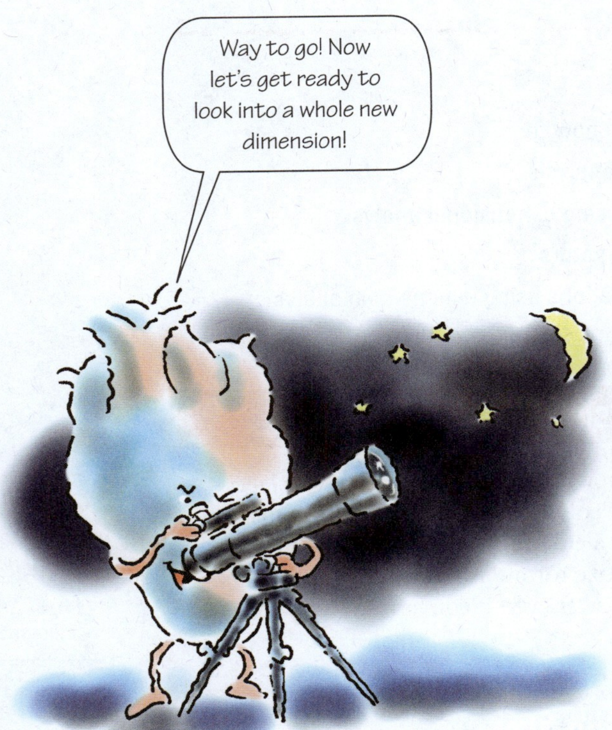

Way to go! Now let's get ready to look into a whole new dimension!

Chapter 4

Dimensional analysis

Just the facts

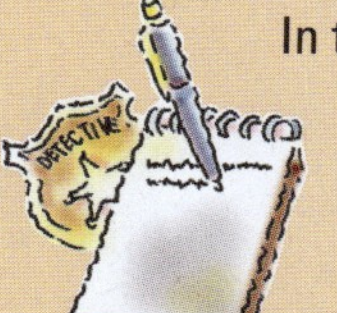

In this chapter, you'll learn how to:

- define dimensional analysis
- set up an equation using dimensional analysis
- identify conversion factors
- solve dosage calculations using dimensional analysis

A look at dimensional analysis

Dimensional analysis, also known as *factor analysis* or *factor labeling,* is an alternative format of solving mathematical problems. It's a basic and easy approach to calculating drug dosages because it eliminates the need to memorize formulas. Only one equation is required to determine each answer even if converting to like units is needed.

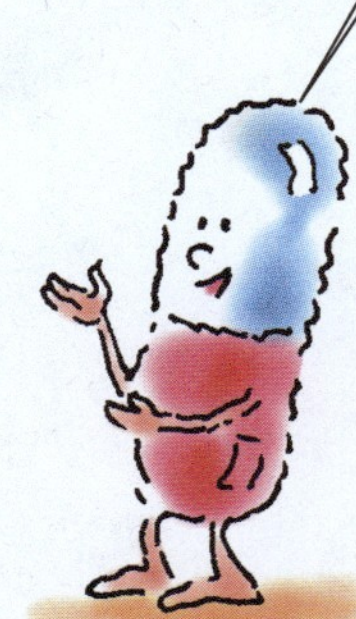
Some people think dimensional analysis is like the Twilight Zone . . . a whole other dimension.

Factors are the main actors

When using dimensional analysis, a series of ratios, called *factors or units,* are arranged in a fractional equation. Each factor, written as a fraction, consists of two quantities of measurement that are related to each other in a given problem. Dimensional analysis uses the same terms as fractions, specifically the terms *numerator* and *denominator.*

Setting the stage

Let's change 48 inches to feet. The problem is written as follows:

$$48 \text{ inches} = X \text{ feet}$$

Some problems contain all of the information needed to identify the factors where only the equation needs to be set up to find the solution. Other problems, such as this one, require a conversion factor.

Conversion factors

Conversion factors are equivalents between two measurement systems or units of measurement. For example, 1 day equals 24 hours. In this case, day and hour are units of measurement and, when stated as 1 day = 24 hours, they're equivalent. This conversion factor can be used to solve problems involving the measure of time. There are many commonly used conversion factors. (See *Common conversion factors*.)

Putting it into practice

In the previous problem of how many feet are in 48 inches, use the conversion factor 12 inches equals 1 foot.

Because the quantities and unit of measurement are equivalent, they can serve as the numerator or denominator. The conversion can be written as:

$$\frac{12}{1}$$

or

$$\frac{1}{12}$$

Setting up the equation

Solving a problem using dimensional analysis is like climbing a staircase—it requires steps. Six incredibly easy steps need to be followed to solve any problem. (See *Following the steps*.)

Advice from the experts

Common conversion factors

Keep this chart handy for quick reference to breeze through problems that call for these common conversions.

1 kg	= 2.2 lb
16 oz	= 1 lb
8 oz	= 1 cup
1 oz	= 30 mL
1 tsp	= 5 mL
1 inch	= 2.5 cm
12 inches	= 1 foot
3 feet	= 1 yard

Advice from the experts

Following the steps

Remember these steps when calculating an equation using dimensional analysis and be on top of a solution in no time!

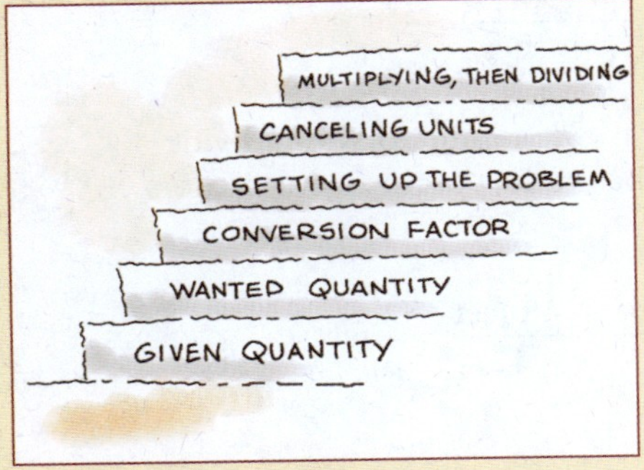

Stepping up to the problem

Let's take it one step at a time:

1. Given quantity—this is the beginning point of the problem. Identify the given quantity in the problem. In this case,

   48 inches

2. Wanted quantity—this is the answer to the problem. Identify the wanted quantity in the problem as an unknown unit. In this problem, it is:

   X feet

3. Conversion factors—again, these are the equivalents that are necessary to convert between systems. The conversion factor for this problem is:

   12 inches = 1 foot

4. Set up the problem using necessary equivalents as conversion factors. When setting up equations, make sure the units needing to be canceled appear in both a numerator and a denominator. However, if an unwanted unit appears in two numerators, they won't be canceled. In this example, after the inches are canceled, the answer is left in the desired unit of feet. To do this, multiply 48 inches by a fraction that has inches in the denominator and feet in the numerator. The problem should be set up as:

$$\frac{48 \text{ inches}}{1} \times \frac{1 \text{ foot}}{12 \text{ inches}}$$

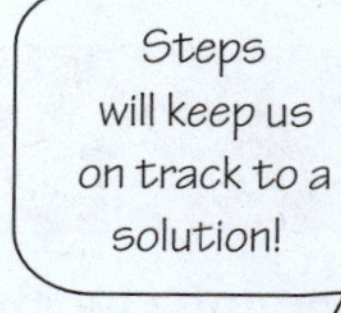

Steps will keep us on track to a solution!

5. Just as with any type of mathematical problem, cancel units that appear in both the numerator and denominator to isolate the desired units. In this case, cancel inches, thereby isolating feet, which is the desired measurement. The step will look like this:

$$\frac{48 \cancel{\text{inches}}}{1} \times \frac{1 \text{ foot}}{12 \cancel{\text{inches}}}$$

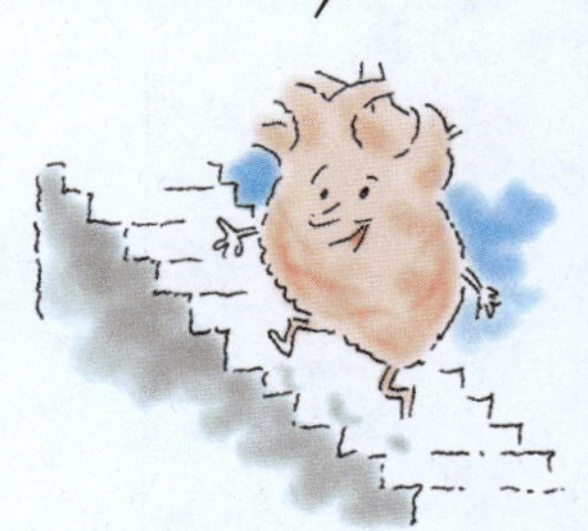

6. Multiply the numerators, multiply the denominators, and divide the product of the numerators by the product of the denominators to reach the wanted quantity.

$$\frac{48}{1} \times \frac{1 \text{ foot}}{12} = \frac{48 \times 1 \text{ foot}}{1 \times 12} = \frac{48 \text{ feet}}{12} = 4 \text{ feet}$$

There are 4 feet in 48 inches.

Let's step into it again!

Now try to solve another problem using dimensional analysis. If a package weighs 38 oz, how many pounds does it weigh?

- Identify the given:

$$38 \text{ oz}$$

- Identify the wanted:

$$X \text{ lb}$$

- Identify the conversion factor:

$$1 \text{ lb} = 16 \text{ oz}$$

- Set up the equation:

$$\frac{38 \text{ oz}}{1} \times \frac{1 \text{ lb}}{16 \text{ oz}}$$

- Cancel units that appear in both the numerator and the denominator:

$$\frac{38 \not{\text{oz}}}{1} \times \frac{1 \text{ lb}}{16 \not{\text{oz}}}$$

- Multiply the numerators and denominators and divide the products:

$$\frac{38 \times 1 \text{ lb}}{1 \times 16} = \frac{38 \text{ lb}}{16} = 2.4 \text{ lb}$$

There are 2.4 lb in 38 oz.

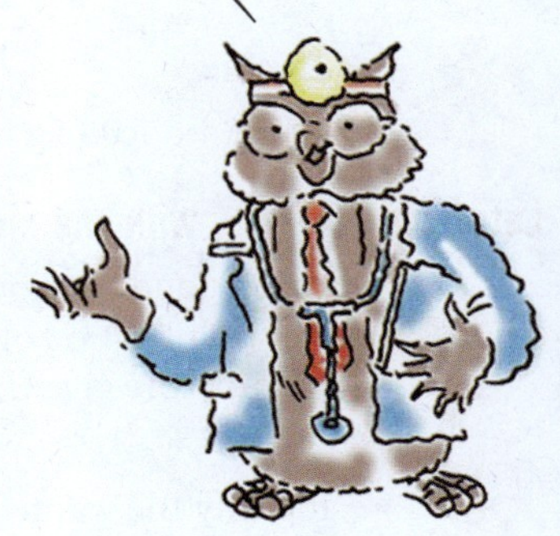
To simplify
this problem, try
converting to
kilograms!

Feel the conversion burn!

Now, let's use dimensional analysis to take this same example a little further. If the same package weighs 38 oz, how much does it weigh in kilograms?

- Identify the given:

$$38 \text{ oz}$$

- Identify the wanted:

$$X \text{ kg}$$

- Identify the conversion factors (in this case, there are two):

$$1 \text{ lb} = 16 \text{ oz}$$

$$1 \text{ kg} = 2.2 \text{ lb}$$

- Set up the equation:

$$\frac{38 \text{ oz}}{1} \times \frac{1 \text{ lb}}{16 \text{ oz}} \times \frac{1 \text{ kg}}{2.2 \text{ lb}}$$

- Cancel units that appear in both the numerator and the denominator:

$$\frac{38\ \cancel{oz}}{1} \times \frac{1\ \cancel{lb}}{16\ \cancel{oz}} \times \frac{1\ kg}{2.2\ \cancel{lb}}$$

- Multiply the numerators and denominators and divide the products:

$$\frac{38 \times 1 \times 1\ kg}{1 \times 16 \times 2.2} = \frac{38\ kg}{35.2} = 1.08\ kg$$

There are 1.08 kg in 38 oz.

Let's cool down . . . with one more rep!

Getting a good workout? Try one more to keep in peak shape. If a patient drank 64 oz of juice, how many cups does this equal?

- Identify the given:

$$64\ oz$$

- Identify the wanted:

$$X\ cups$$

- Identify the conversion factor:

$$8\ oz = 1\ cup$$

- Set up the equation:

$$\frac{64\ oz}{1} \times \frac{1\ cup}{8\ oz}$$

- Cancel units that appear in both the numerator and the denominator:

$$\frac{64\ \cancel{oz}}{1} \times \frac{1\ cup}{8\ \cancel{oz}}$$

- Multiply the numerators and denominators and divide the products:

$$\frac{64 \times 1\ cup}{1 \times 8} = \frac{64\ cups}{8} = 8\ cups$$

There are 8 cups in 64 oz.

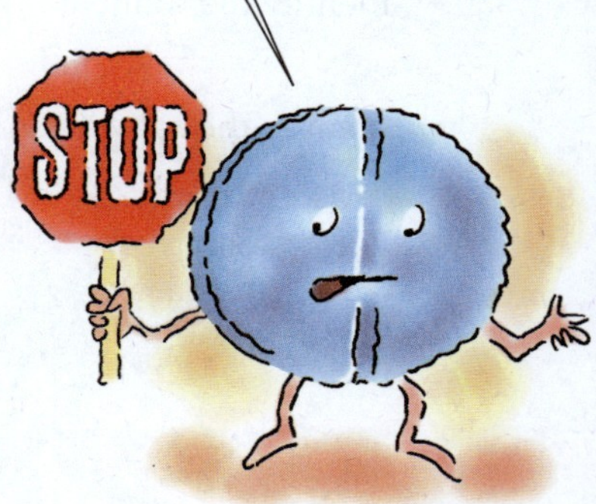

Stop! Review the keys of dimensional analysis.
STOP

Take a breath and let's review

Now that we have made it through the steps again, let's pause to study some key ideas. Dimensional analysis is a method of problem solving that can be used whenever two quantities are directly proportional to each other. One of the quantities can be converted to another unit of measurement by using common equivalents or conversion factors. The problem is treated as an equation using fractions. (See *Quick guide to dimensional analysis*, p. 73.)

Advice from the experts

Quick guide to dimensional analysis

Need to calculate a dosage? Need to figure out a drip rate? Don't panic! Just follow this step-by-step guide to dimensional analysis to come up with the number needed quickly and accurately.

Step 1: Given
Identify the **given** quantity in the problem. This is what the problem already *gives* in the problem! Get it?

Step 2: Wanted
Identify the **wanted** quantity in the problem (the unknown unit, the answer to the problem, or what is ***wanted*** (or ***needed)***.

Step 3: Conversion factor
Write down the equivalents that are necessary to convert between systems. Remember, conversion factors can *convert* to either fraction needed. Depending on what the *wanted* quantity in the numerator is, it can be decided which conversation factor fraction to use.

Step 4: The problem
Set up the fractions so that the units needed to cancel appear as both a numerator and a denominator. Units can't be canceled if they appear only as numerators or only as denominators.

Step 5: Unwanted units
Cancel unwanted units that appear in the numerator and denominator to isolate the unit desired for the answer.

Step 6: Multiply, multiply, and divide
This is where to use math to solve the problem. Multiply the numerators, multiply the denominators, and divide the products.

Fun with dimensional analysis!
Now try this sample problem using the steps identified above.

A licensed practitioner prescribes 75 mg of a medication. The pharmacy stocks a solution containing the medication at a concentration of 100 mg/mL. What dose should be given in mL?

- *Step 1:* Given = 75 mg
- *Step 2:* Wanted = *X* mL
- *Step 3:* Conversion factor: 100 mg = 1 mL
- *Step 4:* Set up the equation (Remember that any unit needing to be canceled should be positioned in both a numerator and a denominator):

$$\frac{75\text{ mg}}{1} \times \frac{1\text{ mL}}{100\text{ mg}}$$

- *Step 5:* Cancel unwanted units:

$$\frac{75\text{ }\cancel{\text{mg}}}{1} \times \frac{1\text{ mL}}{100\text{ }\cancel{\text{mg}}}$$

- *Step 6:* Multiply, multiply, and divide:

$$\frac{75 \times 1\text{ mL}}{1 \times 100} = \frac{75}{100} = 0.75\text{ mL of the solution}$$

More fun!
Here's one more:

The licensed practitioner prescribes 250 mg of amoxicillin (Amoxil), which comes in a suspension of 25 mg/mL. The nurse needs to give the dose in teaspoons (tsp). How many teaspoons of the suspension should be given?

- *Step 1:* Given = 250 mg
- *Step 2:* Wanted = *X* tsp
- *Step 3:* Conversion factors (Remember, some conversion factors should be memorized, such as 1 tsp = 5 mL): 25 mg = 1 mL; 1 tsp = 5 mL
- *Step 4:* Set up the equation:

$$\frac{1\text{ tsp}}{5\text{ mL}} \times \frac{1\text{ mL}}{25\text{ mg}} \times \frac{250\text{ mg}}{1}$$

- *Step 5:* Cancel unwanted units:

$$\frac{1\text{ tsp}}{5\text{ }\cancel{\text{mL}}} \times \frac{1\text{ }\cancel{\text{mL}}}{25\text{ }\cancel{\text{mg}}} \times \frac{250\text{ }\cancel{\text{mg}}}{1}$$

- *Step 6:* Multiply, multiply, and divide:

$$\frac{1\text{ tsp} \times 1 \times 250}{5 \times 25 \times 1} = \frac{250\text{ tsp}}{125} = 2\text{ tsp of the suspension}$$

Now do it again!

Apply the concepts just reviewed above. A patient is recovering from arthroscopic surgery. As part of their rehabilitation, they walk one half of a mile each day. If they walk at a pace of 1.5 miles per hour, how long will it take the patient to complete the walk?

- Identify the given:

$$0.5 \text{ miles}$$

- Identify the wanted:

$$X \text{ hr}$$

- Identify the conversion factor:

$$1.5 \text{ miles} = 1 \text{ hr}$$

- Set up the equation:

$$\frac{0.5 \text{ miles}}{1} \times \frac{1 \text{ hr}}{1.5 \text{ miles}}$$

- Cancel units that appear in both the numerator and the denominator:

$$\frac{0.5 \cancel{\text{miles}}}{1} \times \frac{1 \text{ hr}}{1.5 \cancel{\text{miles}}}$$

- Multiply the numerators and denominators and divide the products:

$$\frac{0.5 \times 1 \text{ hr}}{1 \times 1.5} = \frac{0.5 \text{ hr}}{1.5} = 0.33 \text{ hr}$$

It will take the patient 0.33 hours to complete the walk.

Real-world problems

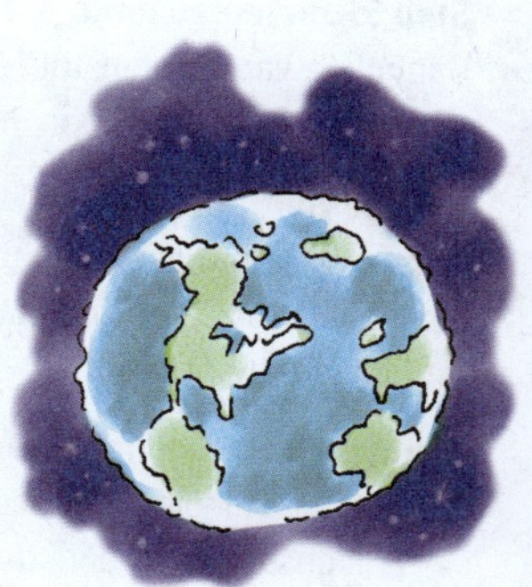

A patient is ordered to receive 70 mg of enoxaparin (Lovenox). It comes available in a prefilled syringe containing 30 mg per 0.3 mL. How much enoxaparin should the patient receive?

- Begin by identifying the given quantity:

$$70 \text{ mg}$$

- Then isolate what is wanted:

$$X \text{ mL}$$

- Know the conversion factor:

$$30 \text{ mg} = 0.3 \text{ mL}$$

- Set up the equation:

$$\frac{70 \text{ mg}}{1} \times \frac{0.3 \text{ mL}}{30 \text{ mg}}$$

- Identify and cancel units that appear in both the numerator and the denominator:

$$\frac{70\ \cancel{mg}}{1} \times \frac{0.3\ mL}{30\ \cancel{mg}}$$

- Finally, multiply the numerators and denominators and divide the products:

$$\frac{70 \times 0.3\ mL}{1 \times 30} = \frac{21\ mL}{30} = 0.7\ mL$$

The patient would receive 0.7 mL of enoxaparin (Lovenox).

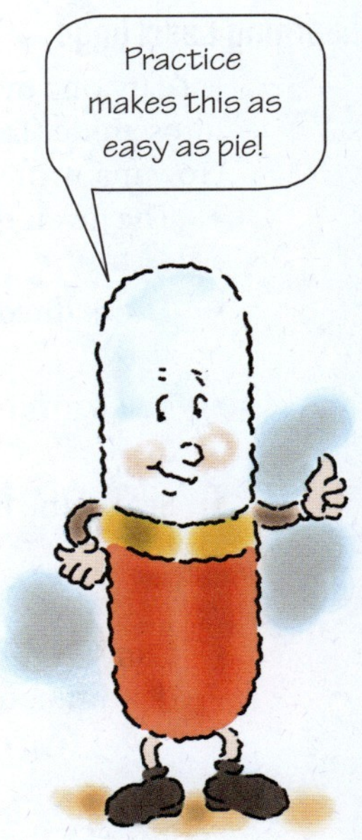

Practice makes this as easy as pie!

Solve for Synthroid

A patient is to receive 50 mcg of levothyroxine (Synthroid). The medication is available as 200 mcg per 5 mL. How many mL should the nurse prepare?

- The given quantity:

$$50\ mcg$$

- The wanted quantity:

$$X\ mL$$

- The conversion factor:

$$200\ mcg = 5\ mL$$

- Set up the equation:

$$\frac{50\ mcg}{1} \times \frac{5\ mL}{200\ mcg}$$

- Cancel units that appear in both the numerator and the denominator:

$$\frac{50\ \cancel{mcg}}{1} \times \frac{5\ mL}{200\ \cancel{mcg}}$$

- Then multiply the numerators and denominators and divide the products:

$$\frac{50 \times 5\ mL}{1 \times 200} = \frac{250\ mL}{200} = 1.3\ mL$$

The nurse should prepare 1.3 mL of levothyroxine (Synthroid).

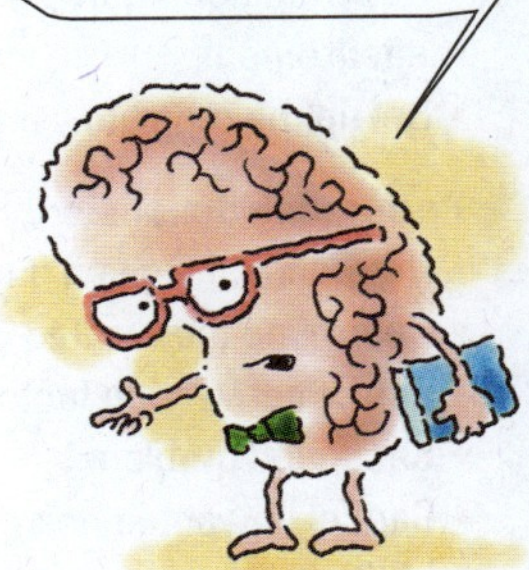

Have a table of common conversion factors to refer to until they are memorized. Don't forget during the problem to cancel out the right units and always double-check your work!

Learning Lasix lingo

Let's try one more problem. A patient has been prescribed 20 mg of furosemide (Lasix) oral solution. The bottle is labeled 40 mg per 5 mL. How many mL will the patient receive?

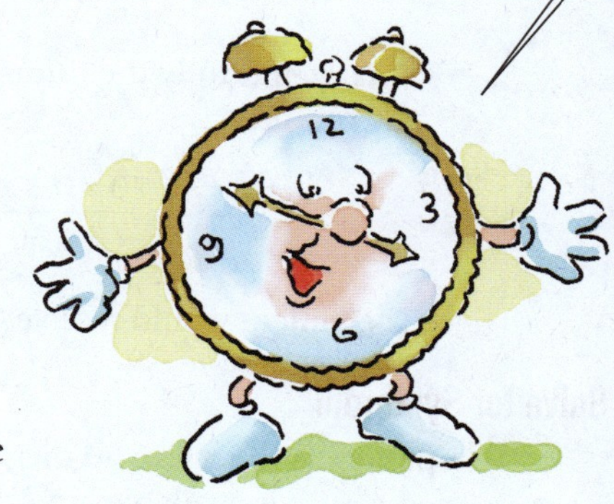

Looks like we have time for one more practice problem.
12
3
9
6

- The given quantity:

$$20 \text{ mg}$$

- The wanted quantity:

$$X \text{ mL}$$

- The conversion factor:

$$40 \text{ mg} = 5 \text{ mL}$$

- Set up the equation:

$$\frac{20 \text{ mg}}{1} \times \frac{5 \text{ mL}}{40 \text{ mg}}$$

- Cancel units that appear in both the numerator and the denominator:

$$\frac{20 \cancel{\text{mg}}}{1} \times \frac{5 \text{ mL}}{40 \cancel{\text{mg}}}$$

- Multiply the numerators and denominators and divide the products:

$$\frac{20 \times 5 \text{ mL}}{1 \times 40} = \frac{100 \text{ mL}}{40} = 2.5 \text{ mL}$$

The patient would receive 2.5 mL of furosemide (Lasix) oral solution.

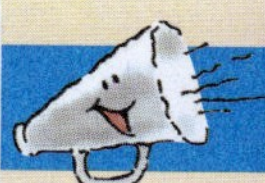

That's a wrap!

Dimensional analysis review

Remember these important facts about dimensional analysis for dosage calculations.

Dimensional analysis basics

- Use whenever two quantities are directly proportional to each other.
- Use common equivalents or conversion factors to convert to the same unit of measurement.
- Set up the problem using fractions.

Performing dimensional analysis—6 steps

- Determine the given quantity.
- Determine the wanted quantity.
- Select conversion factors.
- Set up the problem.
- Cancel unwanted units.
- Multiply the numerators, multiply the denominators, and divide the products.

Quick quiz

1. When using dimensional analysis, how are factors written?
   A. fractions
   B. whole numbers
   C. percentages
   D. ratios

Answer: A. Factors are always written as common fractions. When a problem includes a quantity and its unit of measurement is unrelated to any other factor in the problem, that quantity serves as the numerator of the fraction, and 1 (which is implied) becomes the denominator.

2. Which statement about conversion factors in a dimensional analysis equation is true?
   A. They are identified as the given quantity and the wanted quantity.
   B. They are equivalents necessary to convert between two systems.
   C. They are always placed as numerators.
   D. They are always placed as denominators.

Answer: B. Conversion factors involve equivalent measurements that allow for conversion between different systems.

3. How are dimensional analysis calculations solved?
   A. in three simple steps.
   B. in a single equation.
   C. using formulas that must be memorized.
   D. using common denominators.

Answer: B. Although dimensional analysis uses a step-by-step approach, the problem can be simplified in one single equation.

4. A patient measures 60 inches tall. How tall is this patient in feet?
   A. 6 feet
   B. 6 feet 3 inches
   C. 5 feet
   D. 5 feet 3 inches

Answer: C. Use the conversion factor 12 inches equals 1 foot. Then set up the equation and follow the steps:

$$\frac{60\ \cancel{\text{inches}}}{1} \times \frac{1\ \text{foot}}{12\ \cancel{\text{inches}}}$$

$$\frac{60 \times 1\ \text{foot}}{1 \times 12} = \frac{60\ \text{feet}}{12} = 5\ \text{feet}$$

5. How many pounds are in 48 oz?
   A. 4 lb
   B. 6 lb
   C. 5 lb
   D. 3 lb

Answer: D. Use the conversion factor 16 oz equals 1 lb to solve:

$$\frac{48\ \cancel{oz}}{1} \times \frac{1\ \text{lb}}{16\ \cancel{oz}}$$

$$\frac{48 \times 1\ \text{lb}}{1 \times 16} = \frac{48\ \text{lb}}{16} = 3\ \text{lb}$$

Scoring

☆☆☆ If you answered all five items correctly, congratulations! You've added an impressive dimension to your intellect!

☆☆ If you answered three or four items correctly, label yourself a factor to be reckoned with. Don't convert to lazy ways; keep up the good work!

☆ If you answered fewer than three items correctly, please retrace your steps to discover where you went wrong. You'll soon be the equivalent of an expert!

Suggested Reference

Toney-Butler, T. J., & Wilcox, L. (2023). *Dose Calculation Dimensional Analysis Factor-Label Method.* https://www.ncbi.nlm.nih.gov/books/NBK430724/

Part II

Measurement system

Chapter 5

Metric system

Just the facts

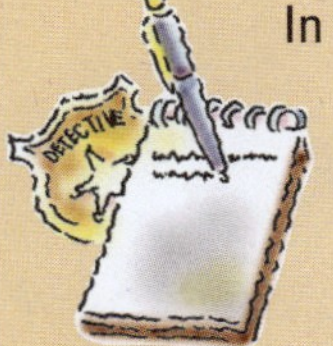

In this chapter, you'll learn how to:

- define metric units of measure
- convert measurements from one metric unit to another
- solve basic arithmetic problems in metric units
- calculate medication dosages using the metric system

A look at the metric system

Today, most nations of the world rely on the metric system of measurement. It's also the most widely used system for measuring medications.

The metric system is a decimal system. That means it's based on the number 10 and multiples, and subdivisions of 10. The metric system offers three advantages over other systems:

- It eliminates common fractions.
- It simplifies the calculation of large and small units.
- It simplifies the calculation of medication doses. (See *Tips for going metric*, p. 82.)

Beginning with the basics

The three basic units of measurement in the metric system (along with the symbol for each) are the meter (m), liter (L), and gram (g):

- The meter is the basic unit of length.
- The liter is the basic unit of volume—it's equivalent to $\frac{1}{10}$ of a cubic meter.
- The gram is the basic unit of weight—it represents the weight of 1 cubic centimeter (cm^3 or cc) of water at 4°C (39.2°F).

What's in a name?

All other units of measure are based on these three major units. When the root word *meter, liter,* or *gram* is used within a measurement, it indicates what is being measured such as length, volume, or weight.

Advice from the experts

Tips for going metric

Remember these tips when using the metric system.

Tip	Example
Use the correct symbol for each unit of measurement. The symbol always follows a number that represents a quantity.	Five kilograms is abbreviated as 5 kg. Five and one-half milligrams is abbreviated as 5.5 mg.
Symbols are case sensitive, so upper and lowercase letters are not interchangeable. In addition, symbols do not indicate the plural form with the use of an "s" at the end.	mL is the milliliter (one-thousandth of a liter), but ML is the megaliter (one million liters). Two milliliters is correctly written as 2 mL, with no "s" at the end of the symbol.
Use decimal fractions to represent a part of a whole.	2.5 mg represents 2 milligrams plus five out of ten parts of 1 milligram.
Place a zero before the decimal point for amounts that are less than 1 to reduce reading errors.	0.5 mg, 0.2 mL, and 0.65 mcg are less than 1.
Eliminate extra zeros so they aren't misread. (See Chapter 2: *Zeroing in on zeros*, p. 26.)	Use 5 mg (not 5.0 mg) and 0.5 mL (not 0.500 mL).

For example, centi*meter* (cm) and milli*meter* (mm) are units of length, centi*liter* (cL) and milli*liter* (mL) are units of volume, and kilo*gram* (kg) and milli*gram* (mg) are units of weight.

Measure for measure

Three devices—the metric ruler, the metric graduate, and metric weights—are used to measure meters, liters, and grams. (See *Measuring meters, liters, and grams*, p. 83.)

Building on the basics

Multiples and subdivisions of meters, liters, and grams are indicated by using a prefix before the basic unit. Each prefix that's used in the metric system represents a multiple or subdivision of 10.

Consider the gram. The most common multiple of a gram is the *kilo*gram, which is 1,000 times greater than the gram. The most common subdivision of a gram is the *milli*gram, which represents one thousandth of a gram, or 0.001 g.

Measuring meters, liters, and grams

What tools are needed to measure meters, liters, and grams? Well, the appropriate measuring devices, of course! A metric ruler, which resembles a yardstick, is used to measure length. A metric graduate can be used to measure the volume of a fluid in liters. (An enclosed chamber, such as a cylinder with a tight-fitting lid, is needed to measure a volume of gas.) A set of metric weights can be used with a metric balance to measure weight in grams.

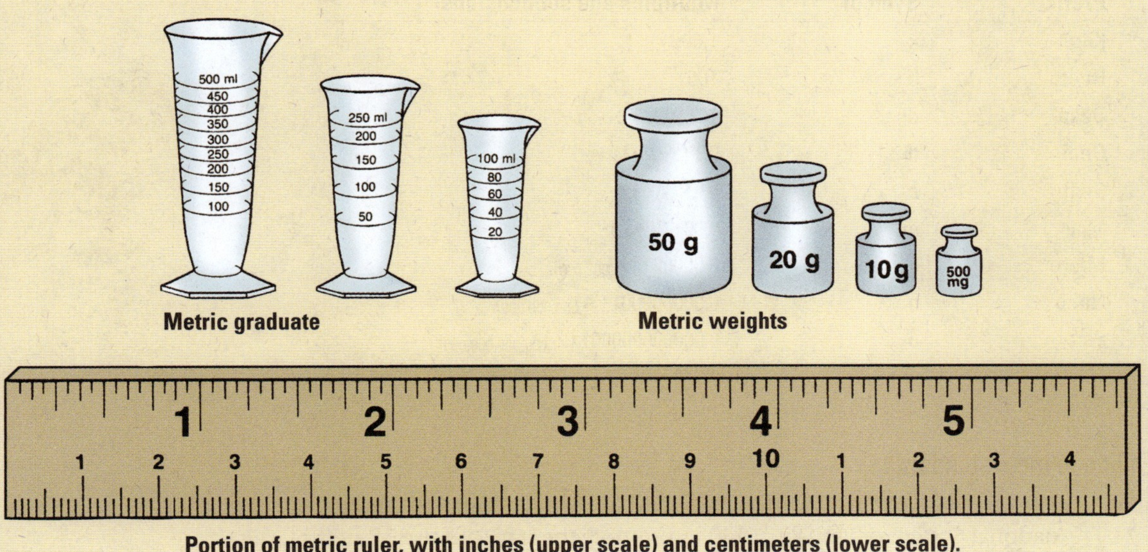

Portion of metric ruler, with inches (upper scale) and centimeters (lower scale).

Keeping it brief

Any metric measurement can be represented by a number and a symbol that represents the unit of measure. The symbol stands for the basic unit of measure—gram (g), meter (m), liter (L)—and the prefix, such as kilo (k), centi (c), and milli (m). For example, *kg* stands for kilogram, *cm* for centimeter, and *mL* for milliliter. (See *What a little prefix can do*, p. 84.)

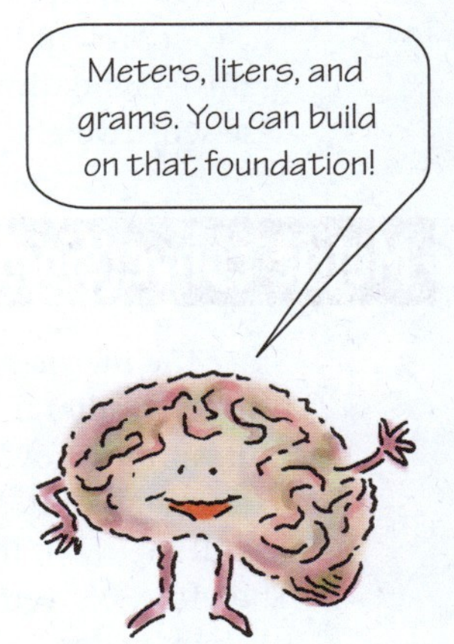
Meters, liters, and grams. You can build on that foundation!

A cubic curiosity

The metric system also includes one unusual unit of volume—the cubic centimeter. The cubic centimeter occupies the same space as 1 mL of liquid; therefore, the two units of volume are considered equal and are sometimes used interchangeably. However, the symbol *cc* can contribute to medication errors and is not recommended for use.

What a little prefix can do

In the metric system, the addition of a prefix to one of the basic units of measure indicates a multiple or subdivision of that unit. Here's a list of prefixes, symbols, and multiples and subdivisions of each unit.

Prefix	Symbol	Multiples and subdivisions
Kilo	k	1,000
Hecto	h	100
Deka	dk	10
Deci	d	0.1 (1/10)
Centi	c	0.01 (1/100)
Milli	m	0.001 (1/1,000)
Micro	mc	0.000001 (1/1,000,000)
Nano	n	0.000000001 (1/1,000,000,000)
Pico	p	0.000000000001 (1/1,000,000,000,000)

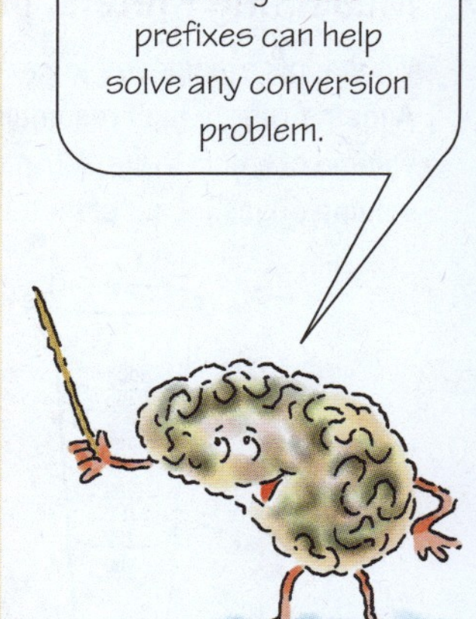

Knowing these prefixes can help solve any conversion problem.

Failing to meet standards

The International Bureau of Weights and Measures adopted the International System of Units in 1960 to promote the standard use of metric symbols and prevent errors in medication transcriptions. Unfortunately, some health care providers still use the old abbreviations.

As a result, nurses must stay alert for nonstandard abbreviations, especially with the use of the letter "l" instead of the approved symbol "L" to represent liters, and "gm" or "GM" instead of "g" to represent grams. As mentioned in the *Tips for going metric*, p. 82, symbols are case sensitive and can have different meanings.

Metric conversions

Since the metric system is decimal based, converting from one metric unit to another is incredibly easy. To convert a smaller unit to a larger unit, simply move the decimal point to the left. To convert a larger unit to a smaller unit, simply move the decimal point to the right.

All metric units are multiples or subdivisions of the major units. Therefore, converting a smaller unit to a larger unit can be accomplished by dividing the appropriate multiple or multiplying by the appropriate subdivision. To convert a larger unit to a smaller unit, multiply by the appropriate multiple or divide by the appropriate subdivision.

Insta-metric conversion table

Want an incredibly easy way to jump back and forth between different metric measures? Just use the fantastic "insta-metric" table below. Make a copy and keep it on hand for an easy reference. Always remember, a milliliter is to a liter as a microgram is to a milligram.

Liquids	Solids
1 mL = 1 cm^3 (or cc)	1,000 mcg = 1 mg
1,000 mL = 1 L	1,000 mg = 1 g
100 cL = 1 L	100 cg = 1 g
10 dL = 1 L	10 dg = 1 g
10 L = 1 dkL	10 g = 1 dkg
100 L = 1 hL	100 g = 1 hg
1,000 L = 1 kL	1,000 g = 1 kg

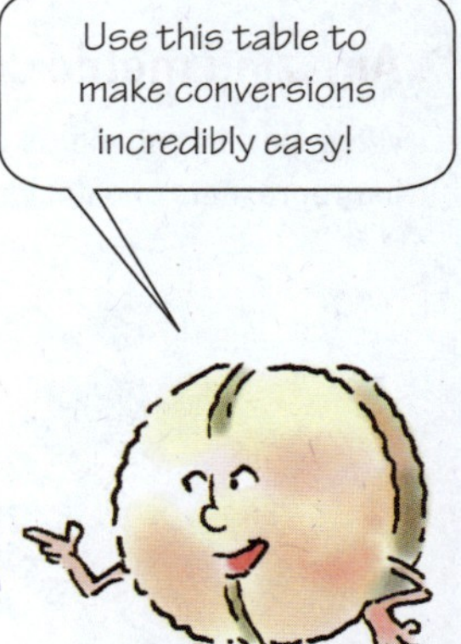

Use this table to make conversions incredibly easy!

Turning the tables on measurements

Luckily, there are tables available to turn to for help in quickly converting measurements. (See *Insta-metric conversion table*, and *Amazing metric decimal place finder*, p. 86.)

Converting meters to kilometers

Let's convert 15 meters (m) to kilometers (km). There are two ways to accomplish this!

Dancing decimal

Using the *Amazing metric decimal place finder*, p. 86, follow these incredibly easy steps:

Step 1: Count the number of places to the right or left of *meters* it takes to reach *kilo*. Referring to the scale, note that *kilo* is *three* places to the left, indicating that a kilometer is 1,000 times larger than a meter (note the three zeros in 1,000).

Step 2: Move the decimal point in 15.0 three places to the *left*, creating the number 0.015. Therefore, 15 m = 0.015 km. *Remember to place a zero in front of the decimal point to draw attention to the decimal point's presence. This will help prevent medication errors!*

Amazing metric decimal place finder

When performing metric conversions, use the following scale as an incredibly easy guide to decimal placement. Each bar represents one decimal place.

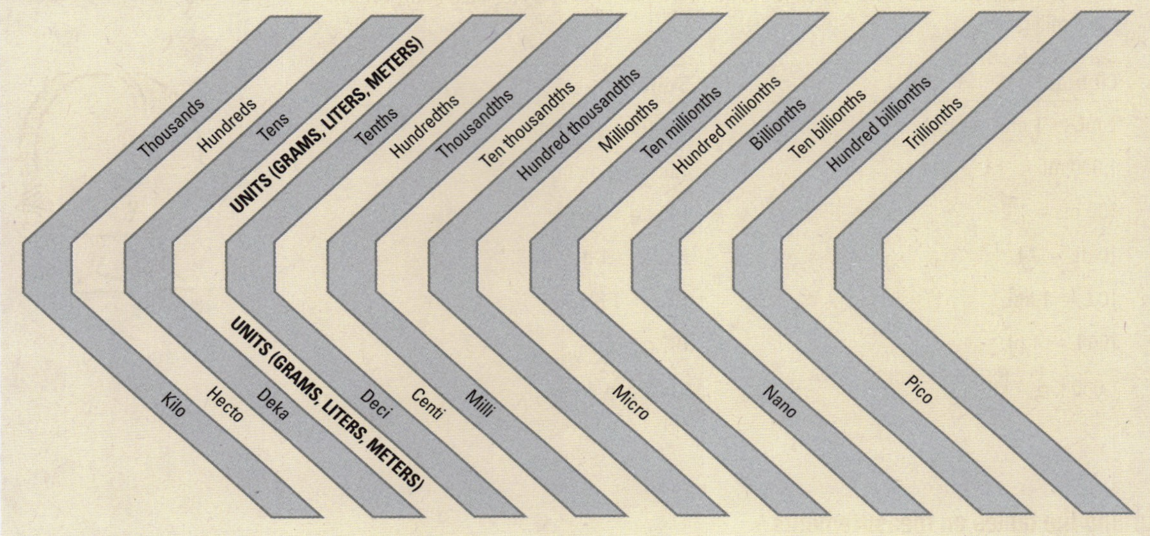

On another road to conversion

Another way to complete this conversion is to use the chart in *What a little prefix can do*, p. 84.

- First, find *kilo*. Notice that it indicates a multiple of 1,000. When using this chart to go from smaller units to larger units (as with meters to kilometers), divide by the multiple.

Here's why: 1 m multiplied by 1,000 equals 1 km. Think about driving in Europe or Canada where road distance is measured in kilometers. A car that is driven 1 m of a 1-km road is already $\frac{1}{1,000}$ of the way there. Therefore, 1 m equals $\frac{1}{1,000}$ km.

To convert 15 m to kilometers, divide by 1,000. Setting up a simple equation might be helpful.

$$X = \frac{15 \text{ m}}{1,000}$$

$$X = 0.015 \text{ km}$$

Therefore, 15 m = 0.015 km, or 15 thousandths of a kilometer.

Converting grams to milligrams

Now, let's convert 5 g to milligrams. Again, use one of two methods.

Decimal dances again

Using the *Amazing metric decimal place finder*, p. 86 follow these incredibly easy steps:

Step 1: Count the number of places to the right or left of *grams* it takes to reach *milli*. Notice that *milli* is three places to the right, indicating that a milligram is 1,000 times smaller than a gram (note the three zeros in 1,000).

Step 2: Move the decimal point in 5.0 three places to the right, creating the number 5,000.

Therefore, 5 g = 5,000 mg.

The multiplying subdivision

Let's use the chart in *What a little prefix can do*, p. 84, to help complete the conversion.

- This time, find *milli*. Note that its subdivision is 0.001, or $\frac{1}{1{,}000}$. When using this table to go from a larger unit to a smaller unit (such as grams to milligrams), divide by the subdivision.

Here's why: 1 milligram is $\frac{1}{1{,}000}$ of a gram. Therefore, 1 g equals 1,000 mg. Dividing 1 g by the subdivision ($\frac{1}{1{,}000}$), results in 1,000 mg. Know why? When a denominator happens to be a fraction, invert the fraction and multiply the two numbers. Dividing by $\frac{1}{1{,}000}$ is the same as multiplying by 1,000.

Let's try another example. To convert 5 g to milligrams, divide 5 g by $\frac{1}{1{,}000}$ (or multiply it by 1,000).

$$X = \frac{5\text{ g}}{\frac{1}{1{,}000}}$$

$$X = 5\text{ g} \times 1{,}000$$

$$X = 5{,}000\text{ mg}$$

Therefore, 5 g = 5,000 mg.

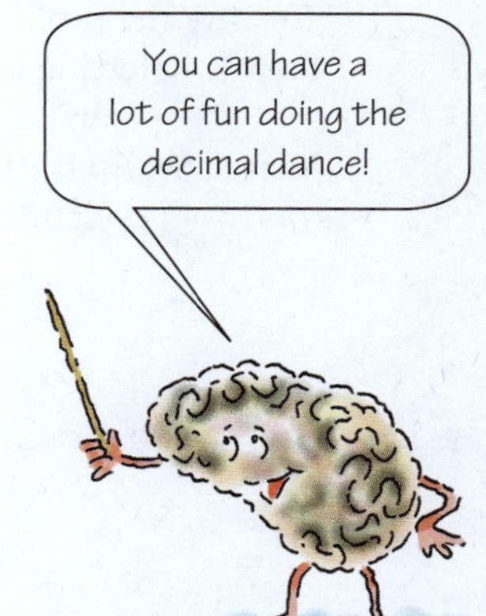

You can have a lot of fun doing the decimal dance!

Converting centiliters to liters

How is 350 cL converted to liters? Here's how, using both charts.

Dancing decimal never rests

Using the *Amazing metric decimal place finder*, p. 86, follow these incredibly easy steps:

Step 1: Count the number of places to the right or left of *centi* it takes to reach *liters*. Note that *liters* is two places to the left, indicating that a liter is 100 times larger than a centiliter.

Step 2: To show this, move the decimal point in 350.0 two places to the left, creating the number 3.5.

Therefore, 350 cL = 3.5 L.

Another vision of subdivision

Now refer to the chart in *What a little prefix can do*, p. 84.

Step 1: First, find *centi*. Notice that its subdivision is 0.01 or $\frac{1}{100}$. When using this chart to go from a smaller unit to a larger one (centiliters to liters), simply multiply by the subdivision.

Here's why: 1 L equals 100 cL. Therefore, 1 centiliter is $\frac{1}{100}$ L (or 1 liter divided by 100). To convert 350 cL to liters, multiply 350 cL by $\frac{1}{100}$ (which is the same as dividing by 100) to attain 3.5 L.

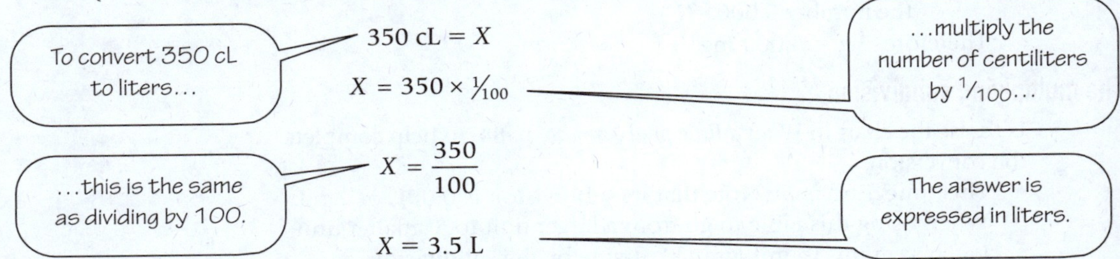

To convert 350 cL to liters...
350 cL = X
X = 350 × 1/100
...multiply the number of centiliters by 1/100...
...this is the same as dividing by 100.
X = 350/100
X = 3.5 L
The answer is expressed in liters.

Solving for *X*

Another way to convert between metric units is by solving for *X*. The following examples show how to solve for *X* in three clinical situations. Not comfortable working with fractions, see *Overcoming fear of fractions* on p. 89.

How much does that baby weigh?

An infant weighs 6.5 kg. How much does this infant weigh in grams? To solve the problem, follow these incredibly easy steps:

Step 1: Referring to the *Insta-metric conversion table*, p. 85, 1,000 g equals 1 kg.

Step 2: Set up the following equation, substituting *X* for the unknown weight in grams:

$$\frac{1{,}000\text{ g}}{1\text{ kg}} = \frac{X}{6.5\text{ kg}}$$

Step 3: Cross-multiply the fractions:

$$\frac{1{,}000\text{ g}}{1\text{ kg}} \times \frac{X}{6.5\text{ kg}}$$

$$X \times 1\text{ kg} = 6.5\text{ kg} \times 1{,}000\text{ g}$$

For math phobics only

Overcoming fear of fractions

Don't like working with fractions? Here's an alternative to solving for *X* in problems. In the example about determining an infant's weight in grams (below), the equation that's expressed in fractions can also be set up as a ratio and proportion.

Step 1: Set up the equation:

$$1{,}000\text{ g}:1\text{ kg}::X:6.5\text{ kg}$$

This is read as 1,000 grams is to 1 kilogram AS *X* is to 6.5 kilograms.

Step 2: Multiply the means and extremes:

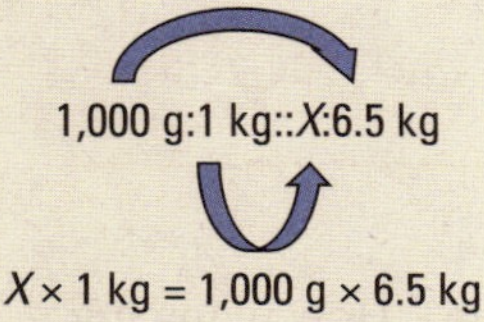

$$X \times 1\text{ kg} = 1{,}000\text{ g} \times 6.5\text{ kg}$$

Step 3: Divide both sides of the equation by 1 kg to isolate *X*.

Step 4: Cancel units that appear in both the numerator and the denominator:

$$X = 6{,}500\text{ g}$$

The infant weighs 6,500 g.

Memory jogger

To remember the difference between ***means*** and ***extremes*** in a ratio, think of:

Means = ***m***iddle numbers

Extremes = ***e***nd numbers

Step 4: Divide both sides of the equation by 1 kg to isolate *X*. Cancel units that appear in both the numerator and denominator:

$$\frac{X \times 1\text{ kg}}{1\text{ kg}} = \frac{6.5\text{ kg} \times 1{,}000\text{ g}}{1\text{ kg}}$$

$$X = 6{,}500\text{ g}$$

The infant weighs 6,500 g.

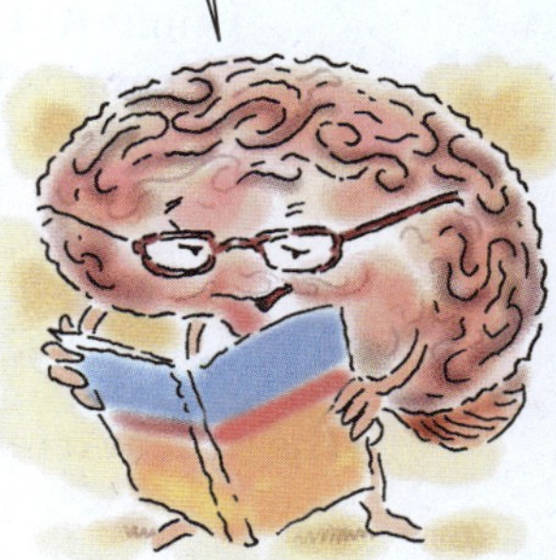

Remember that X stands for the unknown quantity in the equation.

How much IV fluid?

If a patient received 0.375 L of lactated Ringer solution, how many mL did the patient receive?

Referring to the *Insta-metric conversion table*, p. 85, 1 L is equal to 1,000 mL.

Step 1: Set up the following equation, substituting *X* for the unknown amount of IV solution in mL:

$$\frac{1\text{ L}}{1{,}000\text{ mL}} = \frac{0.375\text{ L}}{X}$$

Step 2: Cross-multiply the fractions:

$$\frac{1\text{ L}}{1{,}000\text{ mL}} \times \frac{0.375\text{ L}}{X}$$

$$X \times 1\text{ L} = 0.375\text{ L} \times 1{,}000\text{ mL}$$

Step 3: Divide both sides of the equation by 1 L to isolate *X*. Cancel units that appear in both the numerator and the denominator:

$$\frac{X \times 1\cancel{\text{L}}}{1\cancel{\text{L}}} = \frac{0.375\cancel{\text{L}} \times 1{,}000\text{ mL}}{1\cancel{\text{L}}}$$

$$X = 375\text{ mL}$$

The patient received 375 mL of IV fluid.

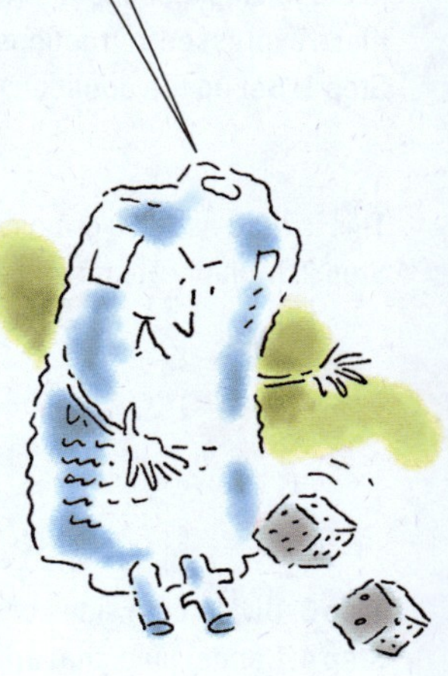

No need to gamble on this dosage. Just convert, cross-multiply, divide, and cancel!

How much medication?

A nurse administered 2 g of ceftriaxone (Rocephin). How many mg of this medication did the patient receive?

Referring to the *Insta-metric conversion table*, p. 85, 1 g is equal to 1,000 mg.

Step 1: Set up the following equation, substituting *X* for the unknown amount of medication in milligrams:

$$\frac{1\text{ g}}{1{,}000\text{ mg}} = \frac{2\text{ g}}{X}$$

Step 2: Cross-multiply the fractions:

$$\frac{1\text{ g}}{1{,}000\text{ mg}} \times \frac{2\text{ g}}{X}$$

$$X \times 1\text{ g} = 2\text{ g} \times 1{,}000\text{ mg}$$

Step 3: Divide each side of the equation by 1 g, to isolate *X*. Cancel units that appear in both the numerator and the denominator:

$$\frac{X \times 1\cancel{\text{g}}}{1\cancel{\text{g}}} = \frac{2\cancel{\text{g}} \times 1{,}000\text{ mg}}{1\cancel{\text{g}}}$$

$$X = 2{,}000\text{ mg}$$

The patient received 2,000 mg of Rocephin.

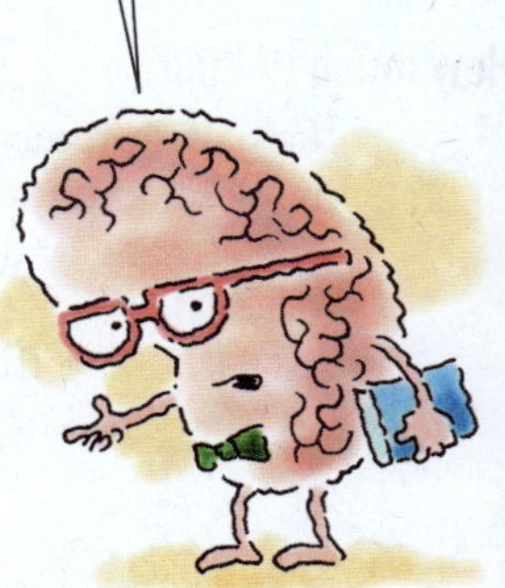

Don't forget to use commas when expressing whole numbers greater than 999 (e.g., 1,000 units; 1,000 mg)!

Dosage drill

Test your math skills with this drill

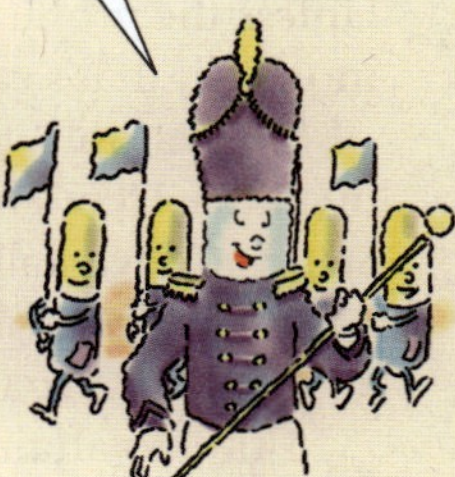
Be sure to show how you arrive at your answer.

The licensed practitioner prescribes lidocaine hydrochloride 4 g in 500 mL of dextrose 5% in water (D_5W) for a patient. How many mg of the medication is contained in the solution? (Hint: The medication is lidocaine hydrochloride and the fluid is D_5W.)

Your answer: ____________

Referring to the *Insta-metric conversion table*, p. 85, 1 g is equal to 1,000 mg.

Step 1: Set up an equation, substituting X for the unknown amount of medication in milligrams.

$$\frac{1\text{ g}}{1{,}000\text{ mg}} = \frac{4\text{ g}}{X}$$

Step 2: Cross-multiply the fractions.

$$X \times 1\text{ g} = 4\text{ g} \times 1{,}000\text{ mg}$$

Step 3: Divide each side of the equation by 1 g to isolate X. Cancel units that appear in both the numerator and the denominator.

$$\frac{X \times 1\cancel{\text{g}}}{1\cancel{\text{g}}} = \frac{4\cancel{\text{g}} \times 1{,}000\text{ mg}}{1\cancel{\text{g}}}$$

$$X = 4{,}000\text{ mg}$$

The solution contains 4,000 mg of lidocaine hydrochloride.

Metric mathematics

Before adding, subtracting, multiplying, or dividing different metric units, all the quantities must be first converted to the same unit. Unless the problem calls for an answer in a specific unit, use the common unit that's easiest to work with and then perform the math.

For example, let's add 2 kg, 202 mg, and 222 g, expressing the sum in grams. Here's how to do this:

Step 1: Convert all the measurements to grams. (Refer to the *Insta-metric conversion table*, p. 85.)

- Convert 2 kg to grams: 1 kg equals 1,000 g. Multiply 2 kg by 1,000 to attain 2,000 g. Thus 2 kg = 2,000 g.
- Convert 202 mg to grams: 1,000 mg equals 1 g and 1 mg equals $\frac{1}{1,000}$ g. Therefore, divide 202 mg by 1,000 to attain 0.202 g.
- 222 is already expressed in grams. No conversion is needed.

Step 2: Add of the numbers together. Remember to pay attention to the decimal places!

$$2,000 + 0.202 + 222 = 2,222.202 \text{ g}$$

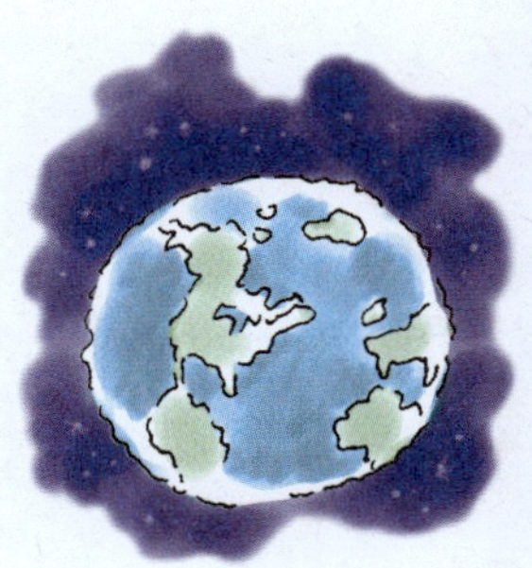

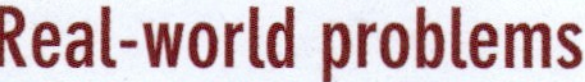

Real-world problems

A patient with a 1 L bag of IV fluid received 500 mL of fluid over the first shift, 225 mL over the second shift, and 150 mL over the third shift. How many mL of fluid remain in the IV bag?

Step 1: Determine how much fluid the patient has already received. To do this, add each of the amounts together (since the amounts are all the same units of measure, no conversion is needed):

$$500 + 225 + 150 = 875 \text{ mL}$$

Step 2: The question is asking how many mL are remaining in the IV bag; therefore, convert 1 L to mL. Referring to the *Insta-metric conversion table*, p. 85, 1 L = 1,000 mL.

Step 3: Calculate the amount of fluid remaining in the IV bag by subtracting 875 mL from 1,000 mL.

There is 125 mL of fluid remaining in the 1 L IV bag.

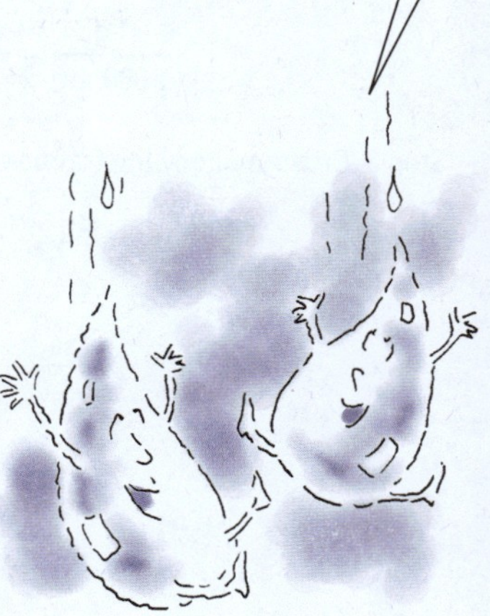

How many of us are left? Just add, convert, and subtract. Wheeee!

A tantalizing tablet tabulation!

A patient is ordered to receive 4 g of erythromycin (Erythrocin) in a 24-hour period. If erythromycin is available in 500-mg tablets, how many tablets should the nurse administer?

Step 1: Convert all the units of measures to the same units. It may be easier to convert 4 g to mg since the nurse needs to determine the number of 500-mg tablets to administer.

Referring to the *Insta-metric conversion table*, p. 85, 1 g is equal to 1,000 mg.

Step 2: To find how many milligrams are in 4 g, set up this proportion using fractions:

$$\frac{1{,}000 \text{ mg}}{1 \text{ g}} = \frac{X}{4 \text{ g}}$$

Step 3: Cross-multiply the fractions then solve for *X* by dividing each side of the resulting equation by 1 g:

$$\frac{1{,}000 \text{ mg}}{1 \text{ g}} \times \frac{X}{4 \text{ g}}$$

$$X \times 1 \text{ g} = 1{,}000 \text{ mg} \times 4 \text{ g}$$

$$\frac{X \times 1 \cancel{\text{g}}}{1 \cancel{\text{g}}} = \frac{1{,}000 \text{ mg} \times 4 \cancel{\text{g}}}{1 \cancel{\text{g}}}$$

$$X = 4{,}000 \text{ mg}$$

Therefore, $X = 4{,}000$ mg.

Step 4: Determine the number of 500-mg tablets that need to be administered to provide 4,000 mg. Set up another proportion using fractions:

$$\frac{500 \text{ mg}}{1 \text{ tablet}} = \frac{4{,}000 \text{ mg}}{X}$$

Step 5: Cross-multiply the fractions then solve for *X* by dividing each side of the resulting equation by 500 mg.

$$\frac{500 \text{ mg}}{1 \text{ tablet}} \times \frac{4{,}000 \text{ mg}}{X}$$

$$X \times 500 \text{ mg} = 4{,}000 \text{ mg} \times 1 \text{ tablet}$$

$$\frac{X \times \cancel{500 \text{ mg}}}{\cancel{500 \text{ mg}}} = \frac{1 \text{ tablet} \times 4{,}000 \cancel{\text{mg}}}{500 \cancel{\text{mg}}}$$

$$X = 8 \text{ tablets}$$

Therefore, $X = 8$ tablets.

The nurse should administer 8 tablets of erythromycin. (See *Did I get it right?*)

Did I get it right?

There may be times when you work with a dosage calculation problem and the answer doesn't seem right. If this happens, try verifying the answer by substituting it for *X* in the equation and doing the math. Both sides of the equation should be equal. As an example, let's use the previous problem about erythromycin tablets.

In this problem, $X = 8$ tablets; let's substitute that in the equation for *X*:

$$\frac{500 \text{ mg}}{1 \text{ tablet}} = \frac{4{,}000 \text{ mg}}{8 \text{ tablets}}$$

$$\frac{500 \text{ mg}}{1 \text{ tablet}} \times \frac{4{,}000 \text{ mg}}{8 \text{ tablets}}$$

$$8 \text{ tablets} \times 500 \text{ mg} = 4{,}000 \text{ mg} \times 1 \text{ tablet}$$

$$\frac{8 \text{ tablets} \times \cancel{500 \text{ mg}}}{\cancel{500 \text{ mg}}} = \frac{1 \text{ tablet} \times 4{,}000 \cancel{\text{mg}}}{500 \cancel{\text{mg}}}$$

$$8 \text{ tablets} = \frac{4{,}000 \text{ tablet}}{500}$$

$$8 \text{ tablets} = 8 \text{ tablets}$$

Observe that both sides of the equation are equal. Congratulations! The answer is right!

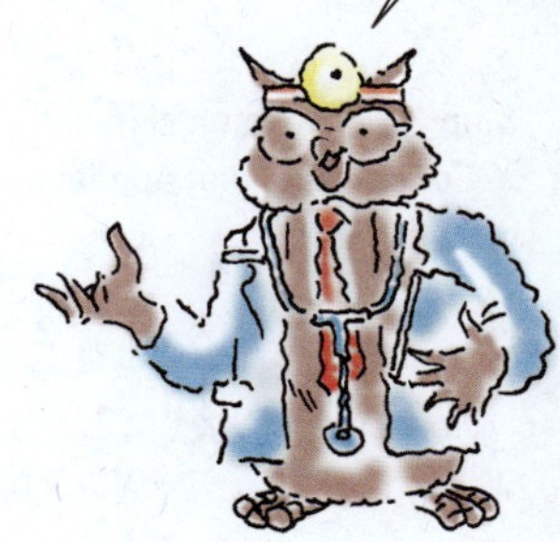

Nice Job! You have mastered metric math and measurements!

Dosage drill

Test your math skills with this drill

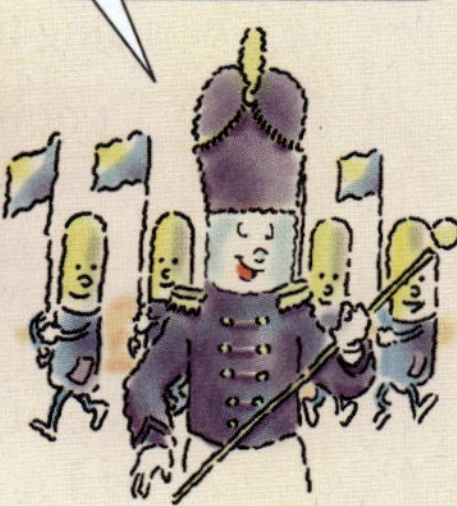
Be sure to show how you arrive at your answer.

A patient is prescribed a single dose of tinidazole (Tindamax) 2 g PO (by mouth) for treatment of trichomoniasis. If tinidazole is available in 500-mg tablets, how many tablets should the patient receive?

Your answer: ______________

Step 1: Convert all the units of measures to the same units. Convert grams to mg. Referring to the *Insta-metric conversion table*, p. 85, 1 g is equal to 1,000 mg.

Step 2: Set up an equation substituting *X* for the unknown amount of mg:

$$\frac{1\text{ g}}{1{,}000\text{ mg}} = \frac{2\text{ g}}{X}$$

Step 3: Cross-multiply the fractions:

$$X \times 1\text{ g} = 2\text{ g} \times 1{,}000\text{ mg}$$

Step 4: Divide each side of the equation by 1 g to isolate *X*. Cancel units that appear in both the numerator and the denominator:

$$\frac{X \times 1\cancel{\text{g}}}{1\cancel{\text{g}}} = \frac{2\cancel{\text{g}} \times 1{,}000\text{ mg}}{1\cancel{\text{g}}}$$

$$X = 2{,}000\text{ mg}$$

Step 5: To determine how many 500-mg tablets the patient should receive to provide the 2,000-mg dose, set up the following equation:

$$\frac{500\text{ mg}}{1\text{ tablet}} = \frac{2{,}000\text{ mg}}{X}$$

Step 6: Cross-multiply the fractions:

$$X \times 500\text{ mg} = 2{,}000\text{ mg} \times 1\text{ tablet}$$

$$\frac{X \times \cancel{500\text{ mg}}}{\cancel{500\text{ mg}}} = \frac{1\text{ tablet} \times 2{,}000\cancel{\text{mg}}}{500\cancel{\text{mg}}}$$

$$X = 4\text{ tablets}$$

The patient should receive a total of 4 tablets.

Pulling it together

Dimensional analysis can also be used to solve the same types of problems presented in this chapter! What is the given information? What is the desired amount? Set it up! Refer to Chapter 4 if help is needed!

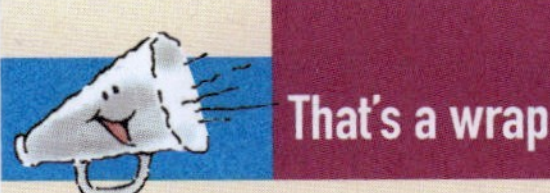

That's a wrap!

Metric system review

Knowing these important facts about the metric system will make calculations incredibly easy!

Metric basics

- It's the most widely used system for measuring amounts of medications.
- It's a decimal system (based on the number 10 and its multiples and subdivisions).
- Three basic units of measurement are used in the metric system:
  - *meter*, basic unit of length.
  - *liter*, basic unit of volume.
  - *gram*, basic unit of weight.
- Multiples and subdivisions of meters, liters, and grams are indicated by using a prefix before the basic unit, such as *kilo, centi*, or *milli*.

Metric conversions

- To convert a smaller unit to a larger unit:
  - move the decimal point to the left.
  - OR divide by the appropriate multiple.
  - OR multiply by the appropriate subdivision.
- To convert a larger unit to a smaller unit:
  - move the decimal point to the right.
  - OR multiply by the appropriate multiple.
  - OR divide by the appropriate subdivision.

Solving for *X*

- Set up an equation, substituting *X* for the unknown quantity.
- Cross-multiply the fractions.
- Divide both sides to isolate *X* on one side.
- Cancel units that appear in both the numerator and the denominator.
- Do the math!

Metric math

- All quantities in the problem must be the same unit, convert if necessary.
- When converting, choose the most common unit unless the problem calls to find a specific unit.
- Do the math!

Quick quiz

1. Which one is the correct symbol representing a gram according to the International System of Units?
   A. gm
   B. g
   C. Gm
   D. GM

Answer: B. The standard abbreviation for gram is g.

2. How many milligrams (mg) are in 3,120 mcg?
   A. 3,120,000 mg
   B. 0.312 mg
   C. 31.2 mg
   D. 3.12 mg

Answer: D. Locate milli and micro on the *Amazing metric decimal place finder*, p. 86. Count the number of places milli is to the left of micro; then move the decimal three places to the left.

3. What is the total volume of fluid in milliliters when adding 312 mL, 3.12 L, and 312 L together?
   A. 327.12 mL
   B. 315,432 mL
   C. 31,543.2 L
   D. 3,154 mL

Answer: B. Convert all the measurements to milliliters and then add all three numbers.

4. Which measurement is equivalent to a milliliter?
   A. cubic centimeter
   B. kiloliter
   C. hectoliter
   D. hentiliter

Answer: A. A milliliter of fluid occupies a cubic centimeter of space.

5. What is the weight in grams for an infant who weighs 5.2 kg?
   A. 5.2 g
   B. 5.02 g
   C. 50.2 g
   D. 5,200 g

Answer: D. Knowing that 1 kg is equal to 1,000 g, set up an equation with X grams as the unknown quantity and multiply 5.2 kg by 1,000 g/kg.

6. A patient has a fluid restriction order for a total of 2 L over 24 hours. The patient consumed a total of 50 mL, 1 L, 240 mL, and

80 mL over the past 12 hours. How many mL does the patient have left for the remaining 24-hour period?

A. 1,370 mL
B. 720 mL
C. 50 mL
D. 40 mL

Answer: B. Convert all the measurements to milliliters then add all the volumes together. Next, subtract the total volume consumed from the original 24-hour restriction amount.

Scoring

☆☆☆ If you answered all six items correctly, dig those decimals! You are a metric master.

☆☆ If you answered five items correctly, give yourself five points! If each point equaled a gram, you would have 60 dg or 600 cg.

☆ If you answered fewer than five items correctly, then leaping milliliters! Review the chapter and soon you will be doing a hector of a good job.

Suggested References

Institute for Safe Medication Practices (ISMP). (2010). ISMP Guidelines for Standard Order Sets. ISMP. https://www.ismp.org/guidelines/standard-order-sets

Institute for Safe Medication Practices (ISMP). (2024). ISMP List of Error-Prone Abbreviations, Symbols, and Dose Designations. ISMP.

Learn. US Metric Association. (2023). https://usma.org/basics

Chapter 6

Alternative measurement systems

Just the facts

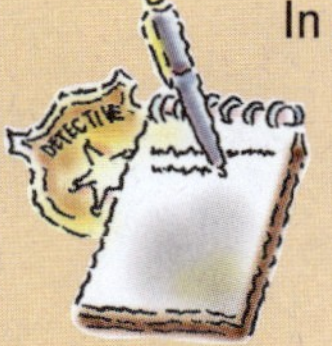

In this chapter, you'll learn how to:

- define the apothecaries' system and how it works
- define the household system and how it works
- define the avoirdupois system and how it works
- define the unit system and how it works
- define the milliequivalent system and how it works
- perform common conversions

A look at alternative systems

Although the metric system is most commonly used in clinical settings, nurses also work with other systems from time to time. These systems include the apothecaries', household, avoirdupois, unit, and milliequivalent systems.

When the alternative is the answer...

When might these other systems be used? A nurse might use these other systems when:

- medication orders are written using the apothecaries' system.
- teaching a patient to use a measuring device calibrated in the household system.
- using the avoirdupois system to calculate a dose that's based on a patient's weight.

Prepare for these occasions by becoming familiar with these alternative measurement systems.

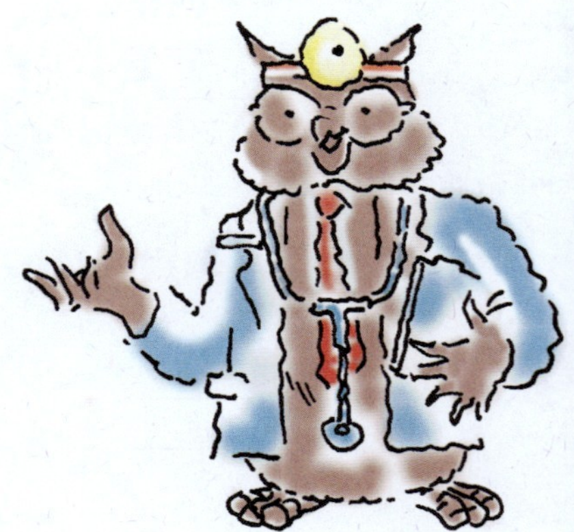

Choosing an alternative measurement system could make all the difference!

Apothecaries' system

Before the metric system was introduced, health care providers and pharmacists used the apothecaries' system. Since the widespread adoption of the metric system, use of this older system has sharply declined. Even though the apothecaries' system is rarely seen anymore, nurses should familiarize themselves with it.

Basic minims and grains

Unlike the metric system, which is used to measure length, volume, and weight, the apothecaries' system is only used to measure liquid volume and solid weight. The basic unit for measuring liquid volume is the minim, and the basic unit for measuring solid weight is the grain.

Think water and wheat

One way to remember these units is to visualize the minim as about the size of a drop of water, which weighs about the same as a grain of wheat. The following mathematical statement sums up this relationship:

1 drop = 1 minim = 1 grain

Other units of measure in the apothecaries' system build on these two basic units. Many of these units are also common household measurements. (See *Ye olde apothecaries' system*.)

Ye olde apothecaries' system

The apothecaries' system uses the following units to measure liquid volume and solid weight.

Liquid volume
60 minims (m) = 1 fluidram
8 fluidrams = 1 fluid ounce (fl oz)
16 fl oz = 1 pint (pt)
2 pt = 1 quart (qt)
4 qt = 1 gallon (gal)
Solid weight
60 grains (gr) = 1 dram
8 drams = 1 ounce (oz)
12 oz = 1 pound (lb)

The dram-a of conversions

Measurements of liquids and solids that are expressed in the apothecaries' system can easily be converted from one unit of measure to another. Here are a few examples:

- How many fluidrams are in 60 minims? Refer to the table shown in *Ye olde apothecaries' system*, p. 99, 60 minims equal 1 fluidram.
- How many quarts are in 1 gallon? One gallon equals 4 quarts of fluid.
- How many drams are in 30 grains? Because 60 grains equal 1 dram, 30 grains equal ½ dram.

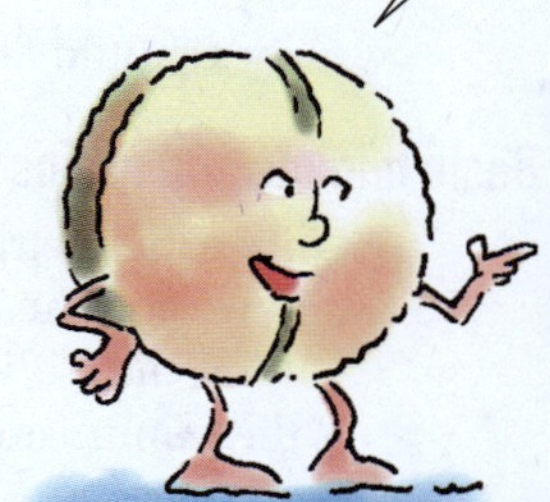

Some nurses may prefer to use a calculator to solve problems!

Roman numerals

When using the apothecaries' system, some licensed practitioners may express dosages in Arabic numerals followed by units of measure. However, the apothecaries' system traditionally uses Roman numerals. (See *The road to Roman numerals*.)

The road to Roman numerals

Here's a handy review of Roman numerals.

½ = ss	11 = XI	40 = XL
1 = I	12 = XII	50 = L
2 = II	13 = XIII	60 = LX
3 = III	14 = XIV	70 = LXX
4 = IV	15 = XV	80 = LXXX
5 = V	16 = XVI	90 = XC
6 = VI	17 = XVII	100 = C
7 = VII	18 = XVIII	500 = D
8 = VIII	19 = XIX	1,000 = M
9 = IX	20 = XX	
10 = X	30 = XXX	

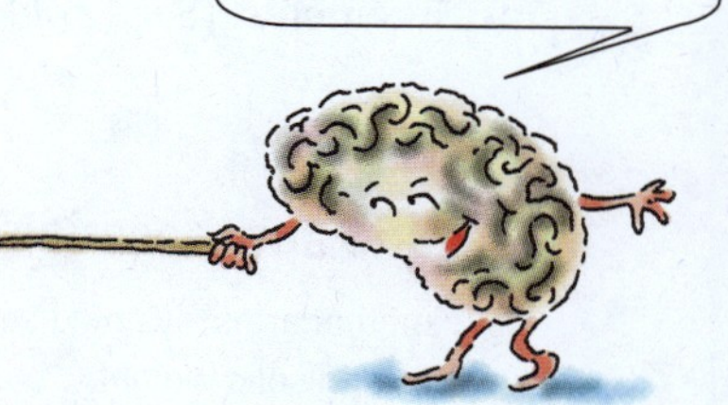

When in Rome...

When used in pharmacologic applications, Roman numerals ss (½) through × (10) are usually written in lower case. When Roman numerals are used, the unit of measure goes before the numeral. For example, 5 grains is written *grains v.* Fractions of less than ½ are written as common fractions using Arabic numerals. Other quantities are expressed by combining letters according to two general rules.

- When a smaller numeral precedes a larger numeral, subtract the smaller numeral from the larger numeral. For example:

$$IX = 10 - 1 = 9$$

- When a smaller numeral follows a larger numeral, add the numerals. For example:

$$XI = 10 + 1 = 11$$

Breaking up is easy to do

To convert an Arabic numeral to a Roman numeral, first break the Arabic numeral into its component parts; then translate each part into Roman numerals. For example:

$$36 = 30 + 6 = XXX + VI = XXXVI$$

Roman numeral conversions

Let's practice on converting the numbers below:

- Write 53 using Roman numerals:

$$53 = 50 + 3 = L + III = LIII$$

- Write CXXVI using Arabic numerals:

$$CXXVI = C + X + X + VI = 100 + 10 + 10 + 6 = 126$$

- Write 1,558 using Roman numerals:

$$1{,}558 = 1{,}000 + 500 + 50 + 8 = M + D + L + VIII = MDLVIII$$

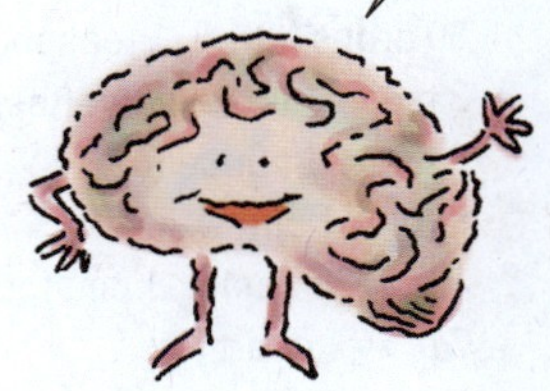

You are now numerically bilingual—fluent in Roman and Arabic—numbers, that is!

Household system

The household system of measurement uses droppers, teaspoons, tablespoons, and cups to measure liquid medication doses. However, because these measuring devices aren't all alike, the household system is useful only for approximate measurements, and it is not used in health care settings. For exact and accurate measurements, use the metric system. (See *Making sure the cup doesn't runneth over*, p. 102.)

Making sure the cup doesn't runneth over

Will your patient be taking medication at home? If so, teach them to use the devices below to help ensure accurate measurements.

Medication cup
A medication cup is calibrated in household, metric, and apothecaries' systems. Tell the patient to set the cup on a counter or flat surface and to check the fluid measurement at eye level.

Dropper
A dropper is calibrated in household or metric systems or in terms of medication strength or concentration. Advise the patient to hold the dropper at eye level to check the fluid measurement.

Hollow-handle spoon
A hollow-handle spoon is calibrated in teaspoons and tablespoons. Teach the patient to check the dose after filling by holding the spoon upright at eye level. Instruct them to administer the medication by tilting the spoon until the medicine fills the bowl of the spoon and then placing the spoon in their mouth.

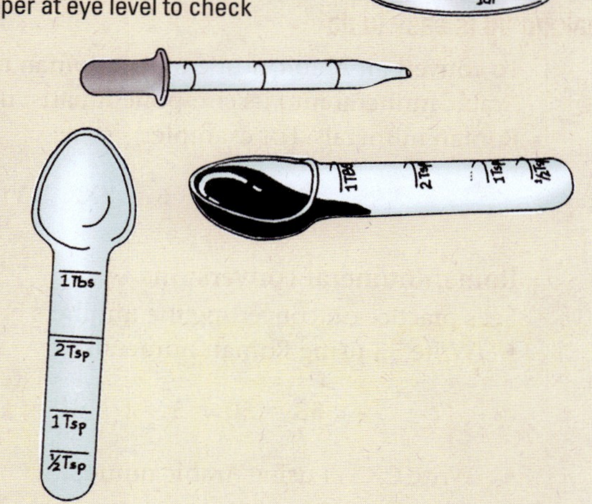

To measure prescribed medication doses at home, teach the patient the household system. (See *Common household units of measure.*)

Common household units of measure

Here's a rundown of the most commonly used household units of measure and their equivalent liquid volumes. Note: Don't use the abbreviations or symbol "t" for teaspoon and "T" for tablespoon because it's easy to make errors when writing them quickly.

60 drops (gtt) = 1 teaspoon (tsp)
3 tsp = 1 tablespoon (tbs)
2 tbs = 1 ounce (oz)
8 oz = 1 cup
16 oz (2 cups) = 1 pint (pt)
2 pt = 1 quart (qt)
4 qt = 1 gallon (gal)

Household system conversions

The examples that follow show how to convert measurements using the household system.

Cough syrup conundrum

The licensed practitioner has ordered 120 drops (gtt) of an expectorant cough syrup every 6 hours for a patient. The medication label gives instructions in teaspoons. How many teaspoons should be administered?

- There are 60 gtt of liquid in 1 teaspoon (tsp). To find out how many teaspoons are in 120 gtt, set up the following equation, using *X* as the unknown quantity:

$$\frac{60 \text{ gtt}}{1 \text{ tsp}} = \frac{120 \text{ gtt}}{X}$$

- Cross-multiply the fractions:

$$X \times 60 \text{ gtt} = 1 \text{ tsp} \times 120 \text{ gtt}$$

- Solve for *X* by dividing both sides of the equation by 60 gtt and canceling units that appear in both the numerator and the denominator:

$$\frac{X \times 60 \cancel{\text{gtt}}}{60 \cancel{\text{gtt}}} = \frac{1 \text{ tsp} \times 120 \cancel{\text{gtt}}}{60 \cancel{\text{gtt}}}$$

$$X = \frac{1 \text{ tsp} \times 120}{60}$$

$$X = 2 \text{ tsp}$$

The patient should receive 2 tsp of cough syrup.

Wait

Dimensional Analysis can also be used to solve this problem. Do you remember how? Check back with Chapter 4 if you get stuck!

Broth brain buster

A patient is on a clear liquid diet. For lunch, they drank 6 tablespoons (tbs) of chicken broth. How many ounces of broth did the patient drink?

- There are 2 tbs of liquid in 1 ounce (oz). To find out how many oz are in 6 tbs, set up the following equation, using *X* as the unknown quantity:

$$\frac{2 \text{ tbs}}{1 \text{ oz}} = \frac{6 \text{ tbs}}{X}$$

- Cross-multiply the fractions:

$$X \times 2 \text{ tbs} = 1 \text{ oz} \times 6 \text{ tbs}$$

- Find X by dividing each side of the equation by 2 tbs and canceling units that appear in both the numerator and the denominator:

$$\frac{X \times \cancel{2\ \text{tbs}}}{\cancel{2\ \text{tbs}}} = \frac{1\ \text{oz} \times 6\ \cancel{\text{tbs}}}{2\ \cancel{\text{tbs}}}$$

$$X = 3\ \text{oz}$$

The patient consumed 3 oz of chicken broth.

Dosage drill

Test your math skills with this drill

The licensed practitioner has ordered acetaminophen (Tylenol) 2 tablespoons (tbs) by mouth every 4 hours, as needed, for temperature greater than 101.5°F (38.6°C). The medication label gives instructions in teaspoons (tsp). How many tsp should be administered?

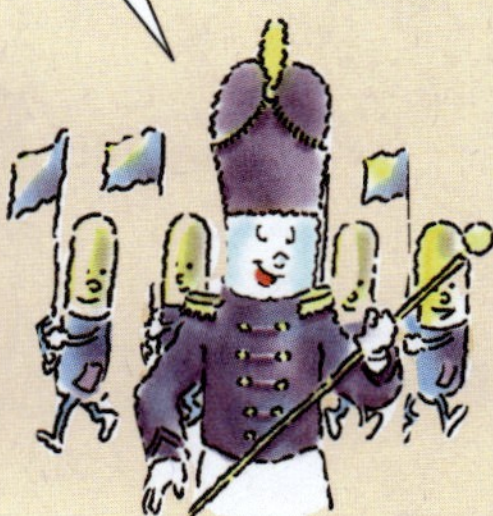
Use this drill to work out the problems!

Your answer: ______________

To find the answer, remember there are 3 tsp of liquid in 1 tbs. Set up the following equation to find out how many tsp are in 2 tbs:

$$\frac{3\ \text{tsp}}{1\ \text{tbs}} = \frac{X}{2\ \text{tbs}}$$

Cross-multiply the fractions.

$$1\ \text{tbs} \times X = 3\ \text{tsp} \times 2\ \text{tbs}$$

Divide each side of the equation by 1 tbs to isolate X. Cancel units that appear in both the numerator and the denominator:

$$\frac{X \times \cancel{1\ \text{tbs}}}{\cancel{1\ \text{tbs}}} = \frac{3\ \text{tsp} \times 2\ \cancel{\text{tbs}}}{1\ \cancel{\text{tbs}}}$$

$$X = 6\ \text{tsp}$$

The patient will receive 6 tsp of acetaminophen.
Prefer Dimensional Analysis? Refer to Chapter 4 for help!

Milk of magnesia mystery

A patient has an order for 4 tbs of milk of magnesia. How many tsp would this equal?

- There are 3 tsp of liquid in 1 tbs. To find out how many teaspoons are in 4 tbs, set up the following equation using *X* as the unknown quantity:

$$\frac{3 \text{ tsp}}{1 \text{ tbs}} = \frac{X}{4 \text{ tbs}}$$

- Solve for *X* by cross-multiplying the fractions, dividing each side of the equation by 1 tbs, and canceling units that appear in both the numerator and the denominator:

$$\frac{X \times \cancel{1 \text{ tbs}}}{\cancel{1 \text{ tbs}}} = \frac{3 \text{ tsp} \times 4 \ \cancel{\text{tbs}}}{1 \ \cancel{\text{tbs}}}$$

$$X = 12 \text{ tsp}$$

The patient will receive 12 tsp of milk of magnesia.

Avoirdupois system

This difficult-to-pronounce system of measurement (av-wah-doo-PWAH) is used for ordering and purchasing some pharmaceutical products and for weighing patients.

In this system, which means *goods sold by weight*, the solid measures or units of weight include grains (gr), ounces (oz), and pounds (lb). One ounce equals 480 gr, and 1 lb equals 16 oz or 7,680 gr. Note that the apothecaries' pound equals 12 oz, but the avoirdupois pound equals 16 oz.

Avoirdupois system conversions

The following examples show how to perform conversions in the avoirdupois system:

- How many pounds equal 32 oz? One pound equals 16 oz; therefore, 2 lb equal 32 oz.
- How many ounces equal 7,680 gr? One ounce equals 480 gr; therefore, 16 oz equal 7,680 gr.
- How many grains are in 2 lb? There are 7,680 gr in 1 lb; therefore, 15,360 gr are in 2 lb. (See *Measure for measure*, p. 106.)

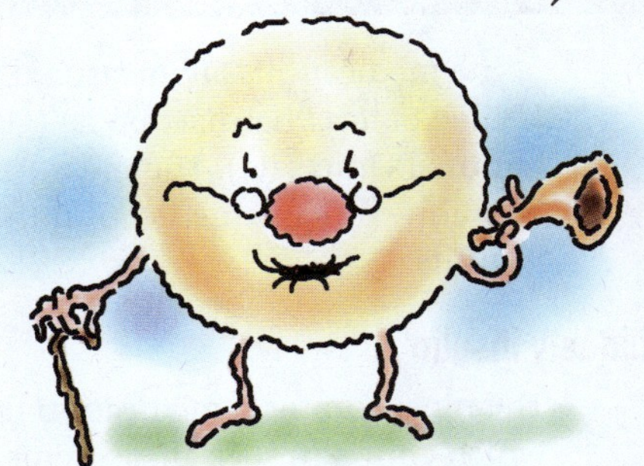

The avoirdupois system has been around since at least the 14th century… a very, very long time, indeed!

Measure for measure

Here are some approximate liquid and solid equivalents among the household, apothecaries', avoirdupois, and metric systems. Use your facility's protocol for converting measurements from one system to another.

Liquids		
Household	*Apothecaries'*	*Metric*
1 drop (gtt)	1 minim (m)	0.06 milliliter (mL)
15–16 gtt	15–16 m	1 mL
1 teaspoon (tsp)	1 fluidram	5 mL
1 tablespoon (tbs)	½ fluid ounce (fl oz)	15 mL
2 tbs	1 fl oz	30 mL
1 cup	8 fl oz	240 mL
1 pint (pt)	16 fl oz	480 mL
1 quart (qt)	32 fl oz	960 mL
1 gallon (gal)	128 fl oz	3,840 mL
Solids		
Avoirdupois	*Apothecaries'*	*Metric*
1 grain (gr)	gr i	0.06 gram (g)
1 gr	gr i	60 milligrams (mg)
15.4 gr	15 gr	1 g
1 oz	480 grains	28.35 g
1 pound (lb)	1.33 lb	454 g
2.2 lb	2.7 lb	1 kilogram (kg)

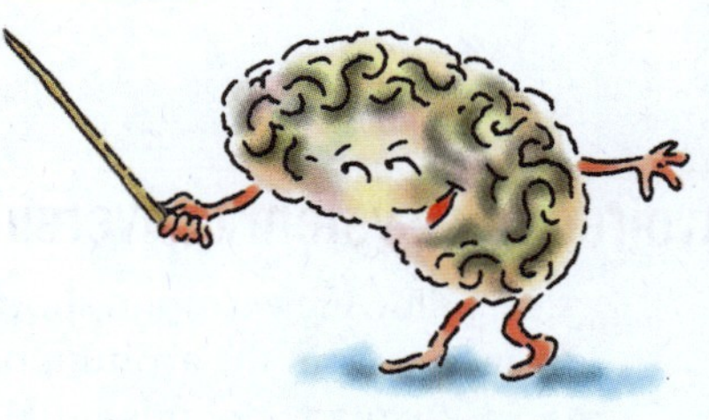

This chart will help make measurement math incredibly easy!

Unit system

Some medications are measured in units, such as United States Pharmacopoeia (USP) units or International Units (IU). The measurement of the unit is unique to each medication that's expressed in units.

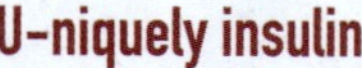

U-niquely insulin

The most common medication that's measured in units is insulin, which comes in such measurements as U-100 strength.

With insulin, the U refers to the number of units per milliliter. For example, 1 mL of U-100 insulin contains 100 units.

More units singled out

Some other medications are also measured in units, for example, the anticoagulant heparin, the topical antibiotic bacitracin, and penicillin G. The hormone calcitonin and the fat-soluble vitamins A, D, and E are measured in IU. Some forms of vitamin A and D are measured in USP units.

All out of proportion

To calculate the dose to be administered when the medication is available in units, use this proportion:

$$\frac{\text{amount of drug in mL or other measure}}{\text{dose required in units}} = \frac{\text{1 mL or other measure}}{\text{drug available in units}}$$

Unit system conversions

The unit calculation examples covered in this chapter are basic examples. Detailed information regarding insulin and heparin calculations is discussed in Chapter 17. The examples in this section show how to perform conversions in the unit system.

Penicillin problem

A patient has been prescribed 500,000 units of penicillin by IM injection. The available vial of penicillin contains 1,000,000 units/mL. How many mL of medication should the nurse administer? Here is how to solve this problem:

- Set up a proportion using X as the unknown quantity:

$$\frac{X}{\text{500,000 units}} = \frac{\text{1 mL}}{\text{1,000,000 units}}$$

- Cross-multiply the fractions:

$$X \times \text{1,000,000 units} = \text{1 mL} \times \text{500,000 units}$$

- Find X by dividing each side of the equation by 1,000,000 units and canceling units that appear in both the numerator and the denominator:

$$\frac{X \times \cancel{\text{1,000,000 units}}}{\cancel{\text{1,000,000 units}}} = \frac{\text{1 mL} \times \text{500,000 } \cancel{\text{units}}}{\text{1,000,000 } \cancel{\text{units}}}$$

$$X = 0.5 \text{ mL}$$

The patient should receive 0.5 mL of penicillin.

Milliliter mystery

The licensed practitioner orders heparin 3,000 units subcutaneous every 8 hours for a patient, with the first dose to be given now. The heparin vial available contains 1,000 units/mL. How many milliliters should be administered now by the nurse?

- Set up a proportion using *X* as the unknown quantity of heparin:

$$\frac{X}{3{,}000 \text{ units}} = \frac{1 \text{ mL}}{1{,}000 \text{ units}}$$

- Cross-multiply the fractions:

$$X \times 1{,}000 \text{ units} = 1 \text{ mL} \times 3{,}000 \text{ units}$$

- Find *X* by dividing both sides of the equation by 1,000 units and canceling units that appear in both the numerator and the denominator:

$$\frac{X \times \cancel{1{,}000 \text{ units}}}{\cancel{1{,}000 \text{ units}}} = \frac{1 \text{ mL} \times 3{,}000 \ \cancel{\text{units}}}{1{,}000 \ \cancel{\text{units}}}$$

$$X = 3 \text{ mL}$$

The nurse should administer 3 mL of heparin subcutaneously.

Milliequivalent system

Some electrolytes, such as potassium and sodium, are measured in milliequivalents (mEq). Drug manufacturers dispense information about the number of metric units required to provide the prescribed number of milliequivalents. For example, the manufacturer's instructions may indicate that 1 mL equals 4 mEq.

Electrolyte example

Licensed practitioners usually order the electrolyte potassium chloride in milliequivalents. Potassium preparations are available for use in IV fluids, as oral suspensions or elixirs, and in solid tablet or powder form. Potassium is also available in the combination medication called potassium phosphate. The phosphate in this medication is measured in millimoles.

A promising proportion

To calculate the dose to be administered when the medication is available in milliequivalents, use this proportion:

$$\frac{\text{amount of medication in mL or other measure}}{\text{dose required in mEq}} = \frac{1 \text{ mL or other measure}}{\text{medication available in mEq}}$$

Dosage drill

Test your math skills with this drill

A loading dose of streptokinase (Streptase) 250,000 international units (IU) has been ordered for a patient. The vial of streptokinase contains 750,000 IU/mL. How many mL of the medication should be administered?

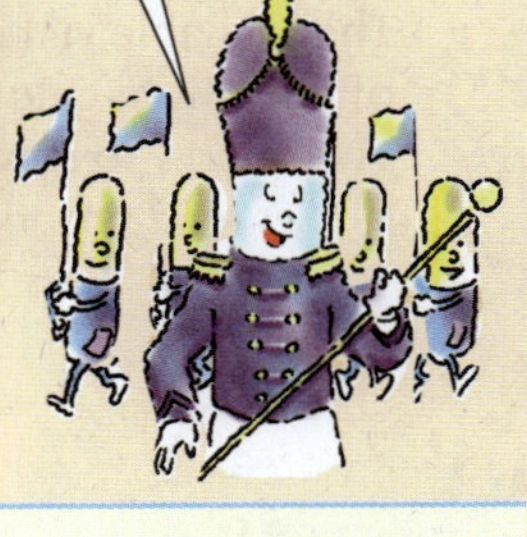

Use this drill to work out the problems! Be sure to show how you arrive at your answer.

Your answer: ______________

To find the answer, first set up a proportion using *X* as the unknown quantity:

$$\frac{X}{250{,}000 \text{ international units}} = \frac{1 \text{ mL}}{750{,}000 \text{ international units}}$$

Cross-multiply the fractions:

$$X \times 750{,}000 \text{ international units} = 1 \text{ mL} \times 250{,}000 \text{ international units}$$

Find *X* by dividing each side of the equation by 750,000 IU and canceling units that appears in the numerator and the denominator:

$$\frac{X \times \cancel{750{,}000 \text{ international units}}}{\cancel{750{,}000 \text{ international units}}} = \frac{1 \text{ mL} \times 250{,}000 \cancel{\text{ international units}}}{750{,}000 \cancel{\text{ international units}}}$$

$$X = 0.3 \text{ mL}$$

The patient should receive 0.3 mL of the medication.

Milliequivalent system conversions

The problems below show how to perform conversions using the milliequivalent system.

Finding the solution

The licensed practitioner has ordered an IV infusion of 40 mEq of potassium chloride in 100 mL of normal saline solution for a patient. The available vial of potassium contains 10 mEq/mL. How many mL of potassium chloride should be added to the normal saline solution? This is how to solve this problem.

- Set up a proportion using *X* as the unknown quantity:

$$\frac{X}{40\text{ mEq}} = \frac{1\text{ mL}}{10\text{ mEq}}$$

- Cross-multiply the fractions:

$$X \times 10\text{ mEq} = 1\text{ mL} \times 40\text{ mEq}$$

- Find *X* by dividing each side of the equation by 10 mEq and canceling units that appear in both the numerator and the denominator:

$$\frac{X \times \cancel{10\text{ mEq}}}{\cancel{10\text{ mEq}}} = \frac{1\text{ mL} \times 40\ \cancel{\text{mEq}}}{10\ \cancel{\text{mEq}}}$$

$$X = 4\text{ mL}$$

The nurse should add 4 mL of potassium chloride to the 100 mL of normal saline solution.

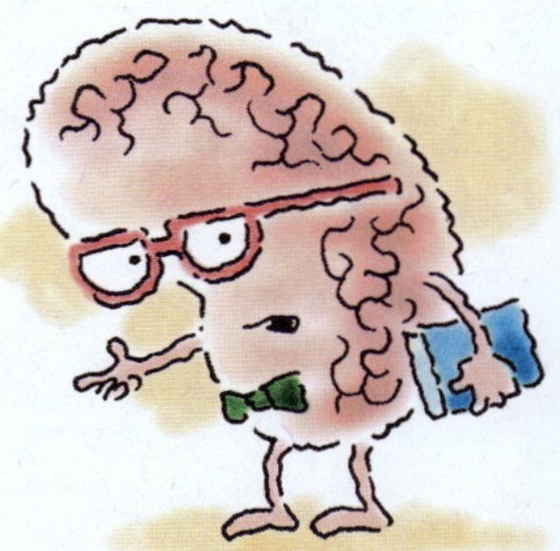

Milliequivalents sound small but they can be a big dosage problem without the right calculation tools!

Calculate that sodium bicarbonate!

A patient has an order for 25 mEq of sodium bicarbonate. The vial from the pharmacy contains 50 mEq of sodium bicarbonate in 50 mL of solution. How many mL of the solution should the nurse administer? Here's how to solve this problem:

- Set up a proportion using *X* as the unknown quantity:

$$\frac{X}{25\text{ mEq}} = \frac{50\text{ mL}}{50\text{ mEq}}$$

- Cross-multiply the fractions:

$$X \times 50\text{ mEq} = 50\text{ mL} \times 25\text{ mEq}$$

- Find X by dividing both sides of the equation by 50 mEq and canceling units that appear in both the numerator and the denominator:

$$\frac{X \times \cancel{50\ \text{mEq}}}{\cancel{50\ \text{mEq}}} = \frac{\cancel{50}\ \text{mL} \times 25\ \cancel{\text{mEq}}}{\cancel{50}\ \cancel{\text{mEq}}}$$

$$X = 25\ \text{mL}$$

The nurse should administer 25 mL of sodium bicarbonate solution.

Potassium puzzle

The licensed practitioner prescribes 30 mEq of potassium chloride oral solution for a patient. The solution contains 60 mEq of potassium chloride in every 15 mL. How many mL of solution should the nurse administer to the patient? Here's how to solve this problem:

- Set up a proportion using X as the unknown quantity:

$$\frac{X}{30\ \text{mEq}} = \frac{15\ \text{mL}}{60\ \text{mEq}}$$

- Cross-multiply the fractions:

$$X \times 60\ \text{mEq} = 15\ \text{mL} \times 30\ \text{mEq}$$

- Find X by dividing both sides of the equation by 60 mEq and canceling units that appear in both the numerator and denominator:

$$\frac{X \times \cancel{60\ \text{mEq}}}{\cancel{60\ \text{mEq}}} = \frac{15\ \text{mL} \times 30\ \cancel{\text{mEq}}}{60\ \cancel{\text{mEq}}}$$

$$X = 7.5\ \text{mL}$$

The nurse should administer 7.5 mL of oral potassium chloride solution to the patient.

Frequently used conversions

In clinical practice, a licensed practitioner may write a medication order in one measurement system, but the medication may be available in a different system. For example, they might order gr x of a medication that's available only in milligrams.

To convert medication orders from one system to another, the nurse must know the equivalent measures. Having difficulty remembering the most commonly used equivalents? Try jotting down the equivalents on an index card, laminate the card, and place it in an easily accessible place, such as a pocket, for easy reference.

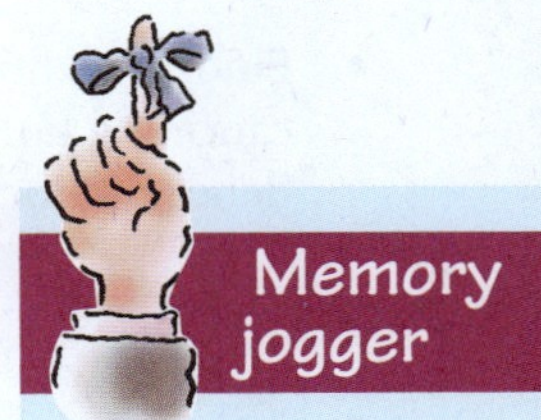

Memory jogger

Remember this jingle when converting inches to centimeters and vice versa: "2.5, that's 1 inch and no more."

A conversion excursion

Two conversions that are commonly used, especially in adult and pediatric intensive care units, are pounds (lb) to kilograms (kg) and inches (") to centimeters (cm). These conversions are used to determine body weight and body surface.

Remembering the general rules makes these conversions easy!

- Remember that 1 kg equals 2.2 lb. To convert pounds into kilograms, just divide the number of pounds by 2.2. To convert kilograms to pounds, multiply the number of kilograms by 2.2.
- Remember that 1″ equals 2.5 cm. To convert inches to centimeters, just multiply the number of inches by 2.5. To convert centimeters to inches, divide the number of centimeters by 2.5.

Equivalent measure conversions

The following examples show how to perform equivalent measure conversions.

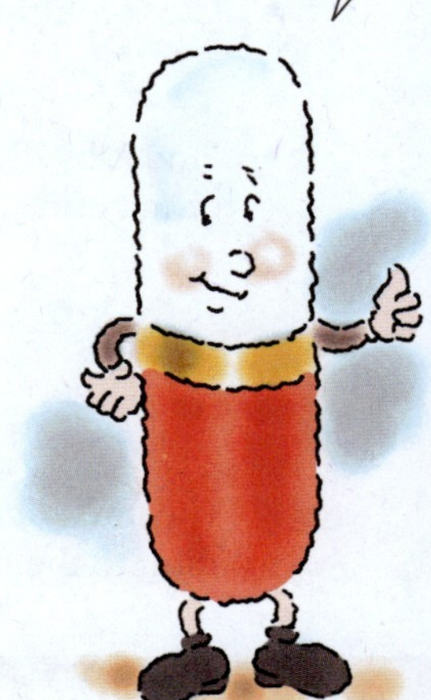

Remember that 2.2 lb = 1 kg! When converting from lb to kg, kg will always be a smaller number!

You say pounds, I say kilograms

To prepare medications for a hypotensive patient, the nurse must determine the patient's weight in kilograms. The patient weighs 125 lb. What would be the weight in kg? Here's how to perform the conversion:

- Since 1 kg equals 2.2 lb, set up a proportion using *X* as the unknown weight:

$$\frac{X}{125\text{ lb}} = \frac{1\text{ kg}}{2.2\text{ lb}}$$

- Cross-multiply the fractions:

$$X \times 2.2\text{ lb} = 1\text{ kg} \times 125\text{ lb}$$

- Find *X* by dividing both sides of the equation by 2.2 lb and canceling units that appear in both the numerator and the denominator:

$$\frac{X \times \cancel{2.2\text{ lb}}}{\cancel{2.2\text{ lb}}} = \frac{1\text{ kg} \times 125\ \cancel{\text{lb}}}{2.2\ \cancel{\text{lb}}}$$

$$X = 56.8\text{ kg}$$

The patient weighs 56.8 kg.

You say milliliters, I say cups

A patient who's on a clear liquid diet must drink 480 mL of water for lunch. The patient wants to know many cups this would equal. What would the nurse tell them? Here's how to calculate the answer:

- Since 1 cup equals 240 mL, set up a proportion using X as the unknown number:

$$\frac{X}{480\ \text{mL}} = \frac{1\ \text{cup}}{240\ \text{mL}}$$

- Cross-multiply the fractions:

$$X \times 240\ \text{mL} = 1\ \text{cup} \times 480\ \text{mL}$$

- Find X by dividing both sides of the equation by 240 mL and canceling units that appear in both the numerator and the denominator:

$$\frac{X \times \cancel{240\ \text{mL}}}{\cancel{240\ \text{mL}}} = \frac{1\ \text{cup} \times 480\ \cancel{\text{mL}}}{240\ \cancel{\text{mL}}}$$
$$X = 2\ \text{cups}$$

The nurse informs the patient that they must drink 2 cups of water.

You say tablespoons, I say milliliters

The licensed practitioner orders 30 mL of milk of magnesia for a patient's heartburn. The patient asks how many tablespoons would that be? What would the nurse tell them? Here's how to find out.

- Since 1 tbs contains 15 mL, set up a proportion using X as the unknown number:

$$\frac{X}{30\ \text{mL}} = \frac{1\ \text{tbs}}{15\ \text{mL}}$$

- Cross-multiply the fractions:

$$X \times 15\ \text{mL} = 1\ \text{tbs} \times 30\ \text{mL}$$

- Find X by dividing both sides of the equation by 15 mL and canceling units that appear in both the numerator and the denominator:

$$\frac{X \times \cancel{15\ \text{mL}}}{\cancel{15\ \text{mL}}} = \frac{1\ \text{tbs} \times 30\ \cancel{\text{mL}}}{15\ \cancel{\text{mL}}}$$
$$X = 2\ \text{tbs}$$

The patient would take 2 tbs of milk of magnesia.

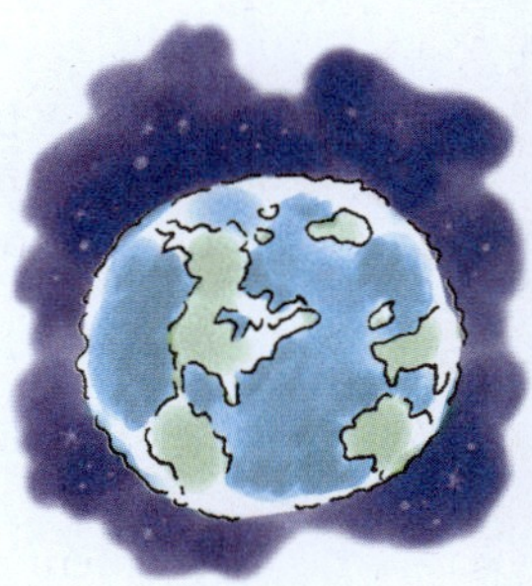

Real-world problems

Here are real-world examples using alternative measurement systems.

Calcium question

The licensed practitioner orders the following IV fluid for a patient: 2,000 mg calcium gluconate in 500 mL of dextrose 5% in water (D_5W). The calcium gluconate is available in a vial containing 100 mg calcium gluconate per 1 mL. How many milliliters of calcium gluconate should be added to the D_5W?

- Set up a proportion using *X* as the unknown quantity.

$$\frac{X}{2{,}000 \text{ mg}} = \frac{1 \text{ mL}}{100 \text{ mg}}$$

- Cross-multiply the fractions:

$$X \times 100 \text{ mg} = 1 \text{ mL} \times 2{,}000 \text{ mg}$$

- Find *X* by dividing both sides of the equation by 100 mg and canceling units that appear in both the numerator and the denominator:

$$\frac{X \times \cancel{100 \text{ mg}}}{\cancel{100 \text{ mg}}} = \frac{1 \text{ mL} \times 2{,}000 \cancel{\text{ mg}}}{100 \cancel{\text{ mg}}}$$

$$X = 20 \text{ mL}$$

The nurse should add 20 mL of calcium gluconate to the 500 mL of D_5W.

A tall order

A patient's height measures 68″. How many centimeters would this equal?

- Remember that 1″ = 2.5 cm. Set up a proportion using *X* for the unknown quantity.

$$\frac{X}{68''} = \frac{2.54 \text{ cm}}{1''}$$

- Cross-multiply the fractions:

$$X \times 1'' = 2.54 \text{ cm} \times 68''$$

- Solve for *X* by dividing both sides of the equation by 1″ and canceling units that appear in both the numerator and the denominator:

$$\frac{X \times \cancel{1''}}{\cancel{1''}} = \frac{2.54 \text{ cm} \times 68\cancel{''}}{1\cancel{''}}$$

$$X = 172.72 \text{ cm}$$

The patient measures 172.72 cm.

That's a wrap!

Alternative measurement systems review

Keep these important facts in mind when performing calculations with alternative measurement systems.

Apothecaries' system

- Measures liquid volume and solid weight
- Minim—basic unit of liquid volume
- Grain—basic unit of solid weight
- 1 drop = 1 minim = 1 grain
- Traditionally uses Roman numerals

Roman numerals

To convert a Roman numeral to an Arabic numeral, remember:

- if a smaller Roman numeral precedes a larger Roman numeral, subtract the smaller numeral from the larger numeral.
- if a smaller Roman numeral follows a larger Roman numeral, add the numerals.

To convert an Arabic numeral to a Roman numeral:

- break the Arabic numeral into its component parts.
- translate each part into Roman numerals.

Household system

- Uses droppers, teaspoons, tablespoons, and cups to measure liquid medication doses.
- Common household conversions:
  3 tsp = 1 tbs
  8 oz = 1 cup
  4 qt = 1 gal

Avoirdupois system

- Pronounced "av-wah-doo-PWAH."
- Solid measures or units of weight, including grains, ounces, and pounds.
- Common avoirdupois conversions:
  1 oz = 480 gr
  1 lb = 16 oz = 7,680 gr

Unit conversions

- Insulin is the most common medication measured in units.
- Divide the units required by the amount of medication available in units.

Milliequivalent conversions

- Measures some electrolytes.
- Divide the amount of milliequivalents required by the amount of medication available in milliequivalents.

Commonly used conversions

- Pounds to kilograms: Divide the number of pounds by 2.2.
- Kilograms to pounds: Multiply the number of kilograms by 2.2.
- Inches to centimeters: Multiply the number of inches by 2.5.
- Centimeters to inches: Divide the number of centimeters by 2.5.

Quick quiz

1. What is the Arabic numeral 575 in Roman numerals?
   A. DXXXXXXXV
   B. DLXXV
   C. CCCCCLXXV
   D. DXC

Answer: B. To convert 575, break it into its component parts (500, 70, and 5); then translate the parts into Roman numerals.

2. What does the symbol ss represent?
   A. one-half
   B. the abbreviation for "without"
   C. the dram symbol
   D. the grain symbol

Answer: A. The symbol ss represents one-half in Roman numerals.

3. Which medications are measured in units?
   A. penicillin G, insulin, and heparin
   B. cotrimoxazole, Lasix, and digoxin
   C. cough medicine, antihistamines, and decongestants
   D. erythromycin, atropine, and calcium

Answer: A. Penicillin G, insulin, and heparin are all measured in units.

4. How are electrolytes measured?
   A. in grains
   B. in milligrams
   C. in milliequivalents
   D. in fluidrams

Answer: C. Most electrolytes, such as potassium chloride, are measured in milliequivalents.

5. How would a nurse convert pounds to kilograms?
   A. multiply pounds by 2.54
   B. divide pounds by 2.2
   C. divide pounds by 2.54
   D. multiply pounds by 2.2

Answer: B. One kilogram equals 2.2 lb. By dividing pounds by 2.2, the nurse obtains kilograms.

6. Before the metric system was established, which system did health care practitioners and pharmacists use?
   A. apothecaries' system
   B. avoirdupois system
   C. household system
   D. unit system

Answer: A. Used before the metric system, the apothecaries' system is being phased out today.

7. The licensed practitioner prescribes 5,000 units of heparin IV for a patient. The heparin vial that's available contains 1,000 units/mL. How many milliliters should the nurse administer?
   A. 0.5 mL
   B. 0.05 mL
   C. 5 mL
   D. 50 mL

Answer: C. To solve this problem, set up the proportion.

$$\frac{X}{5{,}000\text{ units}} = \frac{1\text{ mL}}{1{,}000\text{ units}}$$

Cross-multiply the fractions; then divide both sides of the equation by 1,000 units and cancel units that appear in both the numerator and the denominator.

$$\frac{X \times \cancel{1{,}000\text{ units}}}{\cancel{1{,}000\text{ units}}} = \frac{1\text{ mL} \times 5{,}000\ \cancel{\text{units}}}{1{,}000\ \cancel{\text{units}}}$$

$$X = 5\text{ mL}$$

8. What is the equivalent of 1 tsp of medication in mL?

A. 15 mL
B. 5 mL
C. 30 mL
D. 10 mL

Answer: B. 1 tsp equals 5 mL.

Scoring

☆☆☆ If you answered all eight items correctly, fantastic! Reward yourself with a minim of ice cream. (Okay, you can have a pint!)

☆☆ If you answered five to seven items correctly, good job! Have a fluidram of champagne. (Enjoy every minim!)

☆ If you answered fewer than five items correctly, keep at it. In the meantime, have a dram of chocolate. (Savor every grain!)

Part III

Medication administration consideration

Chapter 7

Medication orders

Just the facts

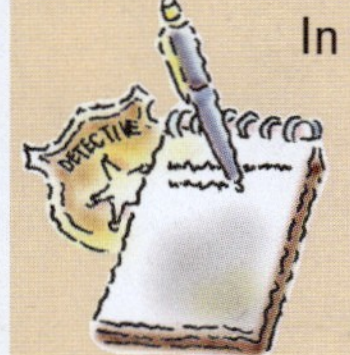

In this chapter, you'll learn how to:

- decipher what a medication order consists of
- interpret medication orders using standard abbreviations
- use military time
- handle unclear medication orders

A look at medication orders

Administering medications is one of the most critical nursing responsibilities. It's also the area with the smallest margin for error. How can nurses prevent medication errors? The best way is by knowing how to read and correctly interpret medication orders. To do this, nurses need to understand what a medication order is and how it's used. A licensed practitioner is a health care professional who is licensed to prescribe medications. Nurses can take medication orders from licensed practitioners which may include doctors (MD or DO), Nurse Practitioners (APN, NP), or Physician's Assistants (PA). Medication orders are required before a nurse may administer medications. In order for nurses to carry out the orders, nurses must know the terminology, abbreviations, and symbols used in generating the orders. Orders may be communicated in writing, electronically, or verbally in person or over the telephone. Here are some examples:

- Handwritten: an order written on a prescription form and given directly to the patient or by writing an order on an order sheet in a patient's chart.
- Electronic: orders that are electronically entered directly into a secure computer system in inpatient and ambulatory settings. Referred to as CPOE (Computerized Provider Order Entry), medication orders then become a part of a patient's electronic medication administration record (eMAR) and can be digitally transmitted to the patient's preferred pharmacy.
- Verbal/Telephone: communication of a medication order by a licensed practitioner either in person or over the phone where the

order is then recorded by a nurse. These forms of orders are typically discouraged but may still be required in some circumstances.

Verbal or Telephone orders

Verbal communication of medication orders should be limited to urgent situations where immediate written or electronic communication is not feasible. If it is not feasible for a licensed practitioner to write or electronically enter an order, the nurse may obtain the order verbally or over the phone. Although discouraged, the Joint Commission has established guidelines for receiving verbal orders including the following:

- Talk directly to the licensed practitioner. Make sure not to accept a third-party communication of a verbal order.
- Record the order and read it back to the licensed practitioner for verification. Make any corrections or additions needed, and then read back the final version to the licensed practitioner for confirmation. The Joint Commission emphasizes this confirmation process.
- Remember to notify the licensed practitioner of any urgent matters such as allergies or changes in vital signs.
- Orders must include the same required information as written orders: date and time order is received, name and dosage of the medication, route and frequency of administration, and any special conditions or instructions.
- Verbal/telephone orders should be documented in the patient's medical record, reviewed, and countersigned by the prescriber as soon as possible following the institution's policy.

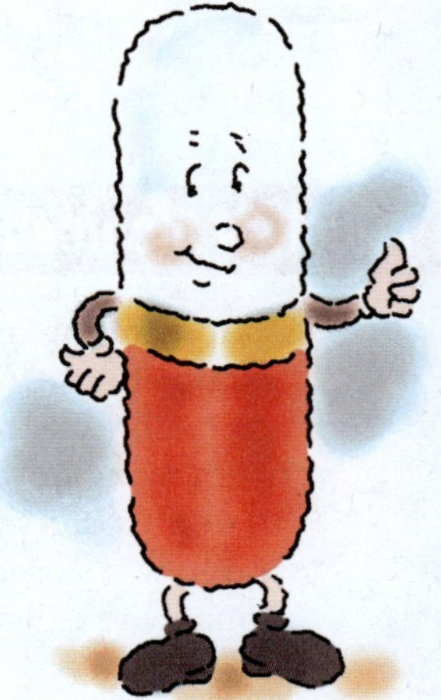

Regardless of how it's transmitted, a medication order is serious business and requires the nurse's utmost attention.

What's in a medication order?

Written orders by a licensed practitioner should be written on a physician's order sheet located in a patient's hospital chart or record. This order sheet must include the patient's full name and date of birth, which is usually provided with a printed admission label. If the facility is using a computerized documentation system, the licensed practitioner will sign in with a computerized signature and place the medication order on a specific patient chart, which then needs pharmacy verification. After the pharmacy reviews and verifies the medication order, it then becomes available on the patient's MAR. All orders, no matter the form they are received in, must include the following information:

- date and time of the order
- name of the medication (either generic or trade name)
- dosage of the medication
- route of administration
- frequency of medication administration

- restrictions, specific conditions, or instructions related to the order
- licensed practitioner's signature, or name, and code number in a computerized system
- For controlled medications: the licensed practitioner must provide their Drug Enforcement Agency (DEA) number—a number registered and assigned by the DEA
- Orders must contain standard abbreviations only. (See *A brief look at abbreviating*.)

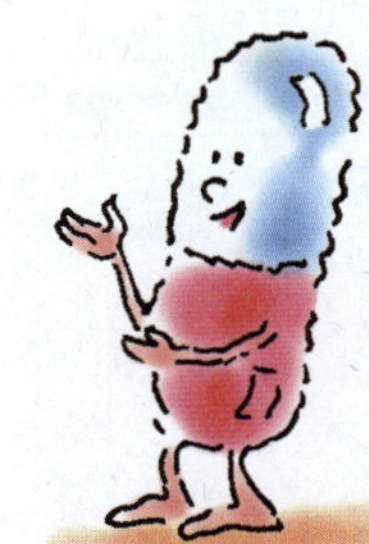
Being aware of
standard guidelines
will help interpret
medication orders.

Following orders

Standard guidelines exist for writing medication orders. Being aware of these guidelines help nurses interpret medication orders and prevent serious errors:

- The generic name of a medication is written entirely in lowercase letters (unless it starts the beginning of a sentence).
- The trade or brand name of a medication begins with a capital letter.
- Medication names should NOT be abbreviated to avoid errors.
- Information is written down following a standard sequence: date and time of medication order first, then medication name, dose, route and frequency of administration, and any special instructions.

A brief look at abbreviating

Standard abbreviations are used to describe medication measurements, dosages, routes, and frequency of administration, and other related terms. The Joint Commission recommends facilities to have a standard approach to standardized abbreviations for all staff to follow. (See *Standard abbreviations*.)

Standard abbreviations

Standard abbreviations are handy for quick and accurate transcription of medication orders and documentation of medication administration. However, some abbreviations used commonly in the past have been identified as possible patient safety risks; these are labeled below as "Do not use!"

Abbreviation	Meaning	Use or do not use
Medication and solution measurements		
cc	cubic centimeter	Do not use! Use "mL".
fl oz or oz	fluid ounce	✓
g	gram	✓
mg	milligram	✓
gtt	drop	✓

(*continued*)

Standard abbreviations (*continued*)

Abbreviation	Meaning	Use or do not use
kg	kilogram	✓
L	liter	✓
mcg	microgram	✓
mL	millilitre	✓
Medication dosage forms		
cap	capsule	✓
XL	extra-long release	✓
elix	elixir	✓
LA	long acting	✓
liq	liquid	✓
SA	sustained action	✓
SR	sustained release	✓
Sol	solution	✓
Susp tab	suspension tablet	✓
U or u	unit	Do not use! Use "unit."
Routes of medication administration		
A.D.	right ear	Do not use! Use "right ear."
A.S.	left ear	Do not use! Use "left ear."
A.U.	each ear	Do not use! Use "each ear."
I.M.	intramuscular	✓
I.V.	intravenous	✓
NG tube	nasogastric tube	✓
O.D.	right eye	Do not use! Use "right eye."
O.S.	left eye	Do not use! Use "left eye."
O.U.	each eye	Do not use! Use "each eye."
NGT	nasogastric tube	✓
P.O. or p.o.	by mouth	✓
P.R.	rectally	✓
P.V.	vaginally	✓
S.C.	subcutaneously	Do not use! Use "subcut" or "subcutaneously."
S.L.	sublingually	✓

Standard abbreviations (*continued*)

Abbreviation	Meaning	Use or do not use
Frequency of medication administration		
a.c.	before meals	✓
b.i.d.	twice a day	✓
t.i.d	three times a day	✓
h.s.	at bedtime	Do not use! Use "at bedtime."
MN	at midnight	✓
p.c.	after meals	✓
p.r.n. or PRN	as needed	✓
q.a.m.	every morning	✓
q.d. Q.D., QD, or qd	every day	Do not use! Use out "daily."
q.o.d. Q.O.D., QOD, or qod	every other day	Do not use! Use "every other day."
q4h	every 4 hours	✓
stat	immediately	✓
Miscellaneous abbreviations		
ASAP	as soon as possible	✓
BPM	breaths (or beats) per minute	✓
$\bar{c}$	with	✓
D/C or dc	discontinue	Do not use! Use "discontinue" or "discharge."
KVO	keep vein open	✓
NKA	no known allergies	✓
NKDA	no known drug allergies	✓
NPO	nothing by mouth	✓

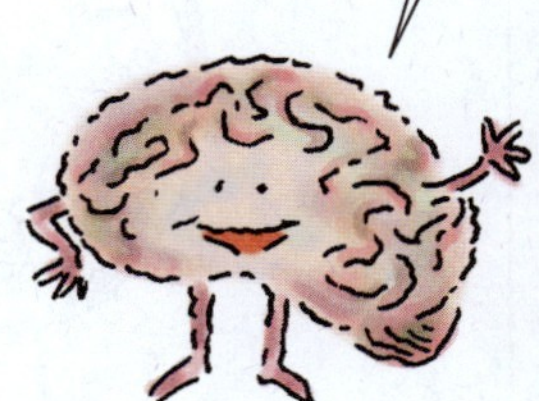

To use or not to use ... that is the question.

However, The Joint Commission has also developed a "Do not use" list of abbreviations known for causing medication errors. Refer to Chapter 9, for more information on this list.

Remember that abbreviations can be easily misinterpreted, especially if they're written or entered into a computer carelessly or quickly. If an abbreviation seems unusual or doesn't make sense, contact the licensed practitioner for clarification. Then, clearly write the correct term in the revision and transcription or have the licensed practitioner correct the abbreviation in the computer.

Marching in time (military time, that is)

Some health care facilities require pharmacologic orders to be written and transcribed in military time. For example, an order might read furosemide *40 mg I.V. b.i.d. at 0900 and 2100 hours*. (See *Military time*.)

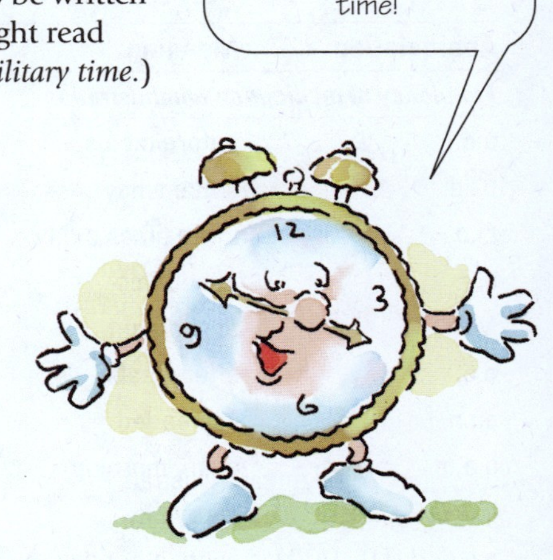

Simply confusing or confusingly simple?

Military time might seem confusing at first, but it's actually simple to use. This method of time is based on a 24-hour system. Here's how it works:

- To write single-digit times from 1:00 AM to 9:59 AM, put a zero before the times and remove the colon. For example, 1:00 AM is written 0100 hours.
- To write double-digit times from 10:00 AM to 12:59 PM, just remove the colon. For example, 11:00 AM becomes 1100 hours.
- The minutes after the hour remain the same. For example, 4:45 AM becomes 0445 hours.
- To write times from 1:00 PM to 12 midnight, simply add 1200 to the hour and remove the colon. For example, 1:00 PM becomes 1300 hours (1:00 + 12:00); 3:30 PM becomes 1530 hours (3:30 + 12:00); and 12:00 AM (midnight) becomes 2400 hours (12:00 + 12:00).

Military time

Study the two clocks below to better understand military time. The clock on the left represents the hours from 1 AM (0100 hours) to noon (1200 hours). The clock on the right represents the hours from 1 PM (1300 hours) to midnight (2400 hours).

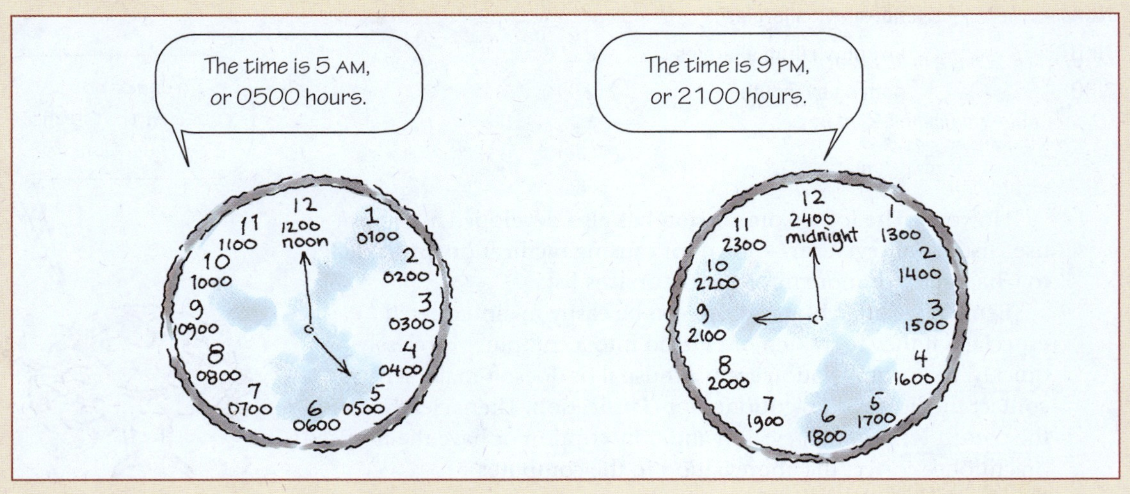

- To write the minutes between 12:01 AM and 12:59 AM, start over with zero. For example, 12:33 AM becomes 0033 hours.

Dealing with medication orders

After determining that a medication order contains all the necessary information, the nurse can begin to interpret it. Read on to find guidelines for dealing with illegible handwriting, timing medication administration, renewing medication orders, and discontinued medication orders. (See *Say it in English*.)

Say it in English

The following examples illustrate how to read and interpret a wide range of medication orders.

Medication order	Interpretation
Colace 100 mg P.O. b.i.d. p.c.	Give 100 mg of Colace by mouth twice per day after meals.
Vistaril 25 mg I.M. q3h p.r.n. anxiety	Give 25 mg of Vistaril intramuscularly every 3 hours as needed for anxiety.
Increase morphine to 2 mg I.V. q8h	Increase morphine to 2 mg intravenously every 8 hours.
Folic acid 1 mg P.O. daily	Give 1 mg of folic acid by mouth daily.
Lisinopril 10 mg P.O. daily, hold for SBP less than 100	Give 10 mg of Lisinopril by mouth daily, withhold the medication if the systolic blood pressure falls below 100 mm Hg.
Nitroglycerin 0.4 mg tablet S.L. every 5 minutes × 3 doses p.r.n. chest pain	Give 0.4 mg of nitroglycerin tablet sublingually every 5 minutes for a maximum dose of three tablets as needed for chest pain.
Aspirin 325 mg P.O. daily starting tomorrow AM	Give 325 mg of aspirin by mouth daily starting tomorrow in the AM
Vasotec 2.5 mg P.O. daily	Give 2.5 mg of Vasotec by mouth daily.
$D_5W\bar{c}$ KCl 20 mEq in 1L I.V. at 100 mL/hr	Give 1 L of dextrose 5% in water with 20 mEq of potassium chloride intravenously at a rate of 100 mL/hr.
Discontinue penicillin I.V., start penicillin G 800,000 units P.O. q6h	Discontinue intravenous penicillin; start 800,000 units of penicillin G by mouth every 6 hours.
Diphenhydramine 25 mg P.O. at bedtime p.r.n. insomnia	Give 25 mg of diphenhydramine by mouth at bedtime as needed for insomnia.

Hospital hieroglyphics

If any of the required information is missing or if the licensed practitioner's handwriting is illegible, follow up with the licensed practitioner to clarify the information before acknowledging the order. The nurse should also follow up to seek clarification if nonstandard abbreviations are used.

Once the nurse verifies that the order is clear and is appropriate, then the order can be acknowledged.

Computerized provider order entry

CPOE is the computer system that allows direct entry of medication orders by the licensed practitioner. These medication orders are communicated over a secure computer network directly to other departments, such as the pharmacy. The pharmacist can review and then verify the medication order. The nurse must still check the accuracy of the medication on the MAR before administration. The CPOE system is designed to prevent and reduce medication errors. The CPOE is usually integrated with the electronic health record (EHR). The EHR is a digital version of the patient's paper chart.

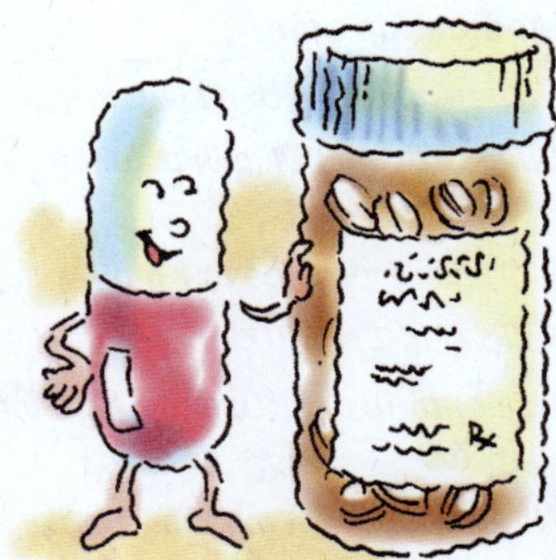
Medication administration time depends on a facility's policy and the nature of the medication, as well as its onset and duration.
Rx

Calibrating the clinical clock

Timing of medication administration is dependent on three conditions:

1. The facility's policy (for medications given a specific number of times per day)
2. The nature of the medication itself (i.e., in the morning or at bedtime)
3. The medication's onset and duration of action

Be sure to administer medications within the institution's policy. Most facilities require administration within a half-hour or an hour of the times specified on the MAR. After giving a medication, record the actual time that the medication was administered.

Reevaluate, renew, reorder

Health care facilities also have policies for how often medication orders must be renewed. For example, opioids may need to be reordered every 24, 48, or 72 hours. This requirement allows health care professionals to reevaluate the patient's need for the medication and to adjust the dosage or frequency of administration, if necessary.

Remember that I.V. fluids—such as normal saline solution, dextrose and water, and total parenteral nutrition (TPN) solutions—are considered medications. Check all I.V. fluid orders carefully. Most health care facilities provide guidelines for the renewal of I.V. fluids, as well as for other medications.

Stop! That's an order

If the licensed practitioner decides to discontinue a medication before the original order runs out, they must discontinue that particular medication through a written order. These orders must also be precise.

For example, if an order reads *discontinue K* and the patient is receiving vitamin K and potassium chloride, the nurse will need to contact the licensed practitioner to clarify which exact medication needs to be discontinued.

Handling ambiguous medication orders

All too often, written medication orders are unclear because of the use of nonstandard abbreviations, illegible handwriting, incorrect dosages, or missing information. It helps if handwritten orders are neat, with medications spelled correctly. (See *Don't struggle with difficult orders*, p. 130.) Remember that CPOE systems help prevent and reduce medication errors.

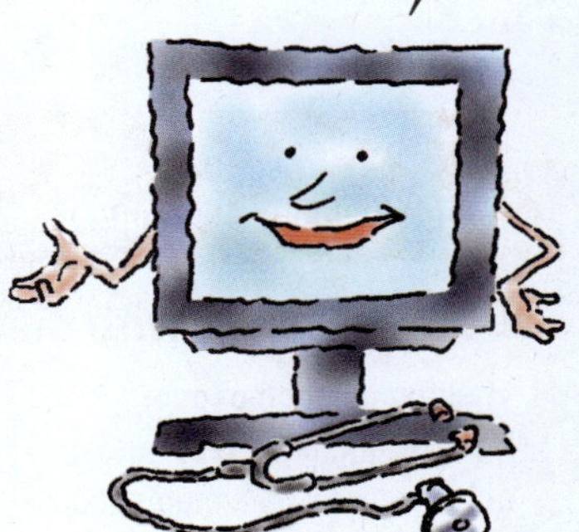

Although CPOE has reduced medication errors, they still can happen. Nurses need to be vigilant in verifying orders!

Rule #1: Bad input equals bad output

Even if the licensed practitioner enters medication orders into the computer system, nurses' interpretation skills are still extremely important. Although computers solve the problem of illegible handwriting, they can't correct human error. A computer will accept the wrong medication, the wrong dose, the wrong route, and the wrong frequency. Some newer computer software systems can actually check the medication order against the patient's allergies, weight, and interactions with their other medications. Remember, some safeguards are programmed into computer systems to minimize errors, but it's still up to the nurse to verify the orders.

Rule #2: Advocate appropriate administration

Not only do nurses need to interpret medication orders, but they also need to assess if the orders are appropriate. Nurses, as patient advocates, need to verify that any ordered medication is appropriate to give specific to a patient's needs and current situation. For example, nurses should do the following:

- Think critically; do not be timid about asking for clarification and justification.
- Know the action of each ordered medication, the purpose for which it's given, and its possible adverse and side effects.
- Know the patient. Medications should be used with caution in very young or very old patients, as well as those who are pregnant, have known kidney or liver disease, have a compromised immune system, or suffer from diabetes.
- Use all available resources if a medication order seems questionable. Ask a licensed practitioner, a pharmacist, a nurse leader, or refer to a drug library reference/book.

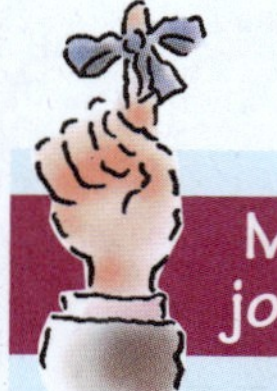

Memory jogger

Repetition is key!

Use repetition to remember responsibilities when it comes to medication administration. When preparing to administer each medication, think of each of the following actions. To remember the steps in sequence, think of the phrase "*Until Clear, Ask Many Times*":

Understand the medication and how it works.

Clarify the medication order as needed.

Administer the medication.

Monitor the patient for therapeutic response to the medication and for adverse effects.

Teach the patient about the medication as needed.

Before you give that medication!

Don't struggle with difficult orders

The combination of poor handwriting and inappropriate abbreviations on a medication order can lead to confusion and medication errors. Ask the licensed practitioner to clarify an order that's difficult to understand or one that seems wrong.

FREEDOM HOSPITAL

UNIT NO. 4 SOUTH, 432A
NAME JOE JACKSON
ADDRESS 33 SHORT STREET
CITY HOPE, NJ BIRTH 2·21·24

DOCTOR'S ORDERS

INSTRUCTIONS
1. Each time a physicians writes a medication order, detach top copy and send to pharmacy.
2. Rule off unused lines after last copy (Pink) has been sent to pharmacy.

DO NOT USE THIS SHEET UNLESS A NUMBER SHOWS. 1

DATE	TIME	ORDERS	DOCTOR'S SIGNATURE	NURSE'S SIGNATURE
2/14/09	12³⁰ p	[illegible]		
		[illegible]		
		[illegible]		
		[illegible]		
		[illegible]		
		[illegible]		[illegible]
4/29/09		[illegible]		
4/30/09		[illegible]		

Discharge diagnoses in order of decreasing priority must be supplied at time of patient's discharge.

If something is not legible on a medication order, ask the licensed practitioner for clarification. All this goes for I.V. fluids too!

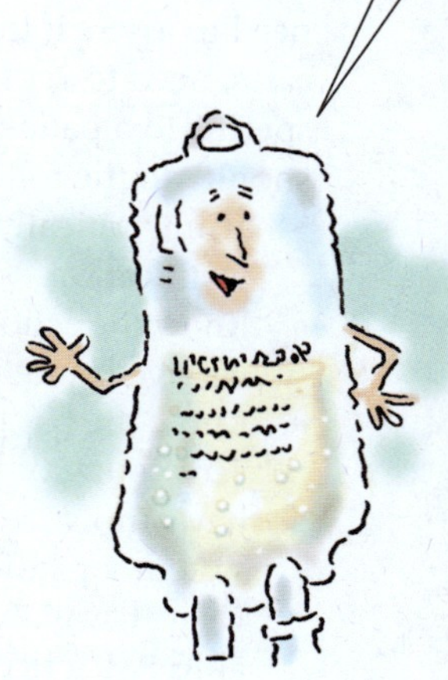

Advice from the experts

Right on target

No matter how careful nurses are when administering medications, occasional errors can still occur. The pharmacy may even send the wrong medication. To avoid errors and keep patients safe, never administer a medication without first checking off the "six rights" of medications!

1. Right patient
2. Right medication
3. Right dose
4. Right route
5. Right time
6. Right documentation

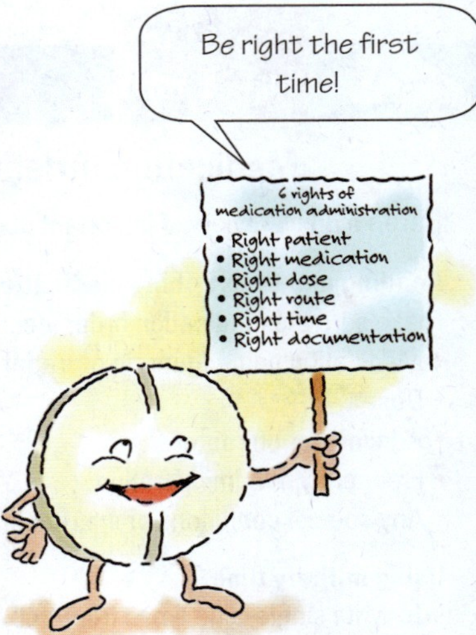
Be right the first time!
6 rights of medication administration
• Right patient
• Right medication
• Right dose
• Right route
• Right time
• Right documentation

- Always check the six "rights" before giving a medication. (See *Right on target*.)
- Check and recheck all medication calculations.
- Never administer a medication that's improperly labeled, missing a label, or drawn up in a syringe prepared by another person.
- Never use opened, leaking, or unmarked I.V. solution bags.

Real-world problems

The following are examples of poorly written medication orders that need to be clarified by the licensed practitioner who wrote them.

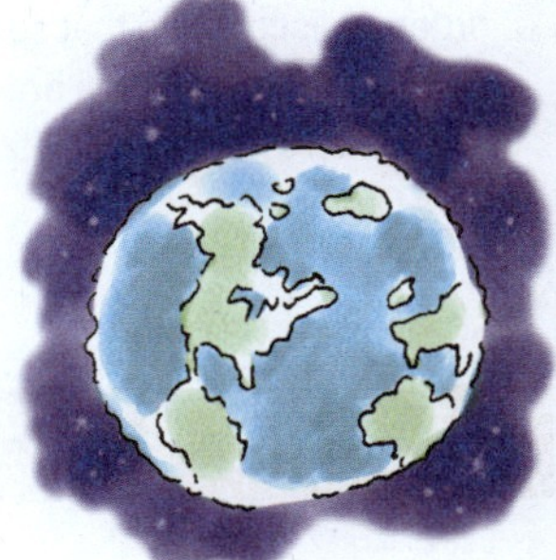

What?

K 40 mEq I.V. daily—It's unclear what medication is being ordered. Is it vitamin K or potassium chloride (KCl)? If it's KCl, remember that this electrolyte must be diluted in a large volume of I.V. fluid before administration.

How?

Digoxin 0.25 mg daily—The administration route is missing. Digoxin may be given orally as a pill or elixir or may be given I.V.

When?

Lisinopril 10 mg P.O.—The frequency of administration is missing. This order is incomplete as the nurse needs to know how often a medication needs to be given.

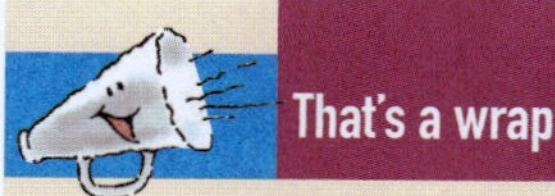

That's a wrap!

Medication orders review

Here's a quick review of important points about medication orders.

Reading and transcribing medication orders

Make sure the medication order includes all of the following information:

- Medication name (generic or trade)
- Dose
- Administration route
- Frequency of administration
- Any special conditions or instructions

Using military time

- To write single-digit times from 1:00 AM to 12:59 PM, put a zero before the time and remove the colon. (Example: 4:00 AM is 0400 hours)
- To write double-digit times from 1:00 AM to 12:59 PM, just remove the colon. (Example: 12:00 PM [noon] is 1200 hours)
- To write times from 1:00 PM to 12 AM (midnight), add 1200 to the hour and remove the colon. (Example: 9:00 PM is 2100 hours)
- Minutes after the hour remain the same. (Example: 10:36 PM is 2236 hours)

Administering medications

- Give within 30–60 minutes of the specified time according to a facility's protocol.
- Record the actual administration time.
- If a medication is to be discontinued, make sure the licensed practitioner writes an order to discontinue that specific medication.
- With each medication order, ensure that the order is appropriate for the patient and the patient's current condition.

Quick quiz

1. Which statement about medication abbreviations is true?
   A. They are written in lowercase letters.
   B. They are written in capital letters.
   C. They are written with the first letter in capitals.
   D. They are to be avoided.

Answer: D. Medication abbreviations should generally be avoided to prevent errors.

2. Which is the correct abbreviation for "after meals?"
   A. P.O.
   B. P.R.
   C. p.c.
   D. a.c.

Answer: C. P.O. stands for "by mouth," P.R. stands for "by rectum," and a.c. stands for "before meals."

3. Which abbreviation is unacceptable according to The Joint Commission's "Do not use" list?
   A. p.r.n.
   B. p.o.
   C. mcg
   D. S.C.

Answer: D. The abbreviation S.C. should be avoided. Instead, write out *subcut* or *subcutaneously.*

4. What is the correct meaning of this order: morphine 4 mg I.M. q4h p.r.n. pain scale of 7–10, hold for respiratory rate less than 10 BPM?
   A. Administer morphine 4 mg intramuscularly four times per day for pain on a pain scale of 7–10; hold for respiratory rate less than 10 breaths per minute.
   B. Administer morphine 4 mg intramuscularly every 4 hours for pain on a pain scale of 7–10; hold for respiratory rate greater than 10 breaths/min.
   C. Administer morphine 4 mg intramuscularly every 4 hours as needed for pain on a pain scale of 7–10; hold for respiratory rate less than 10 breaths/min.
   D. Administer morphine 4 mg intramuscularly every 6 hours for pain on a pain scale of 7–10; hold for respiratory rate greater than 10 breaths/min.

Answer: C. "Every 4 hours" is abbreviated q4h and the abbreviation p.r.n. means "as needed."

5. Using military time, how should this medication order be properly written: "Administer phenytoin sodium (Dilantin) 150 mg by mouth twice per day at 9:00 AM and 9:00 PM; draw Dilantin levels every other day"?
   A. Phenytoin sodium (Dilantin) 150 mg P.O. b.i.d. at 0900 and 2100, draw Dilantin levels every other day.
   B. Phenytoin sodium (Dilantin) 150 mp P.O. t.i.d. at 9:00 AM and 9:00 PM, draw Dilantin levels q.d.
   C. Phenytoin sodium (Dilantin) 150 mg I.V. b.i.d. at 9:00 AM and 9:00 PM, draw Dilantin levels q.o.d.
   D. Phenytoin sodium (Dilantin) 150 mg P.R. b.i.d. at 0900 and 2100, draw Dilantin levels q.o.d.

Answer: A. In option B, t.i.d. means "three times per day," and q.d., meaning daily, shouldn't be used. In option C, I.V. means "intravenously," and "q.o.d" shouldn't be used. In option D, "P.R." means "per rectum" and "q.o.d." shouldn't be used.

Scoring

☆☆☆ If you answered all five items correctly, wow! You're error-free!

☆☆ If you answered four items correctly, you're almost there! You can spot an incorrect order and read hospital hieroglyphics.

☆ If you answered fewer than four items correctly, keep going! You're acquiring the art of the medication order.

Suggested References

The Joint Commission. (2022). Managing health information: use of abbreviations, acronyms, symbols and dose designations—understanding the requirements. Retrieved October 31, 2023, from https://www.jointcommission.org/standards/standard-faqs/hospital-and-hospital-clinics/information-management-im/000001457

The Joint Commission. (2023). *Joint Commission eliminates licensed independent practitioner term*. https://www.jointcommission.org/resources/news-and-multimedia/newsletters/newsletters/joint-commission-online/dec-14-2022/joint-commission-eliminates-licensed-independent-practitioner-term

Chapter 8

Administration records

Just the facts

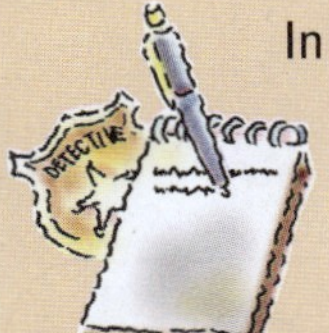
DETECTIVE

In this chapter, you'll learn how to:

- distinguish between different types of medication administration record systems that are used
- document patient information on the administration record
- record medication information on the administration record
- document administration of controlled substances

A look at administration records

Maintaining accurate medication administration records (MARs) is a vital nursing responsibility, both for legal reasons and for patient safety. The liability risk of the health care provider may increase if medication administration isn't properly documented. Missing or inaccurate documentation can lead to medication errors that may jeopardize patients' health.

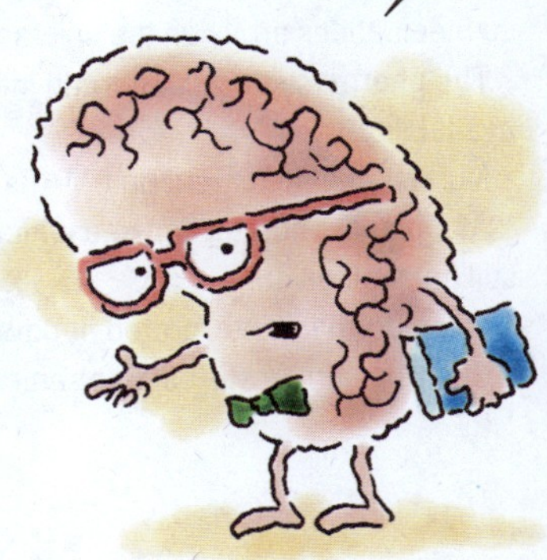
Missing or inaccurate documentation may jeopardize a patient's health.

Record-keeping systems

Two main types of MAR systems are used today: the MAR and eMAR through computer charting.

The MAR

The MAR is an 8 ½″ × 11″ form that goes into the patient's chart. It tracks what medications are currently ordered, when medications are given, as well as important information such as allergies. A MAR also may be kept in the medication room on the medication cart in a three-ring binder or may be attached to the patient's chart or clipboard while the patient is hospitalized. On discharge, the MAR is placed in the patient's chart with the other MARs already used for that patient.

Computer charting

Another system, computer charting or electronic medication administration record (eMAR), is being used increasingly by more health care facilities. Information is entered into a computer that automatically generates a list of administration times for all scheduled medications. Computer systems cut the risk of medication errors caused by illegible handwriting, therefore improving patient safety. (See *Record keeping in the computer age.*)

Record keeping in the computer age

As health care facilities purchase or develop computer systems, manufacturers offer an increased number of choices among medication monitoring programs.

From simple...

Computerized record systems range from simple to sophisticated. In the simplest systems, the computer is used as a word processor.

...to sophisticated

In more sophisticated systems, licensed practitioners can order medications from the pharmacy by typing the medication's name, or they can select specific medications by searching through various listings, such as pharmacologic categories, pharmacokinetic categories, and disease-related uses.

The computer indicates whether the pharmacy has the medication. The order then goes into the pharmacy's computer for filling. The order also generates a copy of the patient's record, on which the nurse can document medication administration. In some cases, the nurse can document medication administration right on the computer with a date-and-time stamp.

Benefits bit by bit

Computer systems offer the following advantages:

- When medication orders are changed, the pharmacy receives immediate notification, so medications arrive on the unit faster.
- The pharmacy's computer can immediately confirm or deny a medication's availability.
- Nurses can document on eMARs quickly and easily.
- At a glance, nurses can see which medications have been administered and which still must be given.
- Errors from misinterpreted handwriting are eliminated.
- Records can be stored electronically in addition to, or instead of, paper copies.

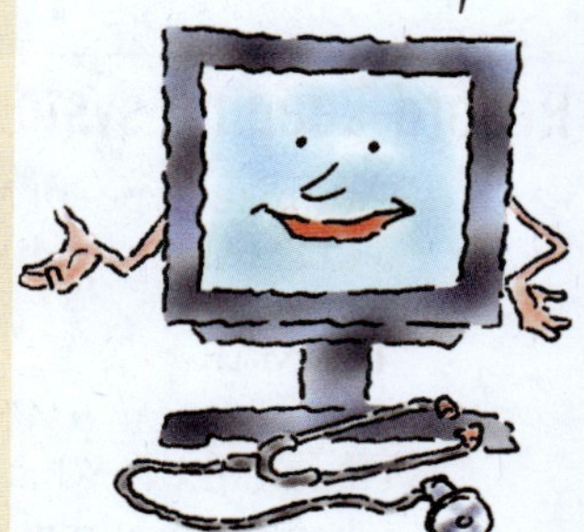
Using computerized physician order entry (CPOE) for medication orders not only eliminates errors from illegible handwriting, but it also provides instant notification—and less delay.

Different forms, same info

The MAR below illustrates the kind of information that is required on all different types of administration forms. Although different facilities may use different forms, virtually all require the patient's information, date and time the order was written, medication information, time of administration, and the nurse's initials (or electronic signature) after administering the medication.

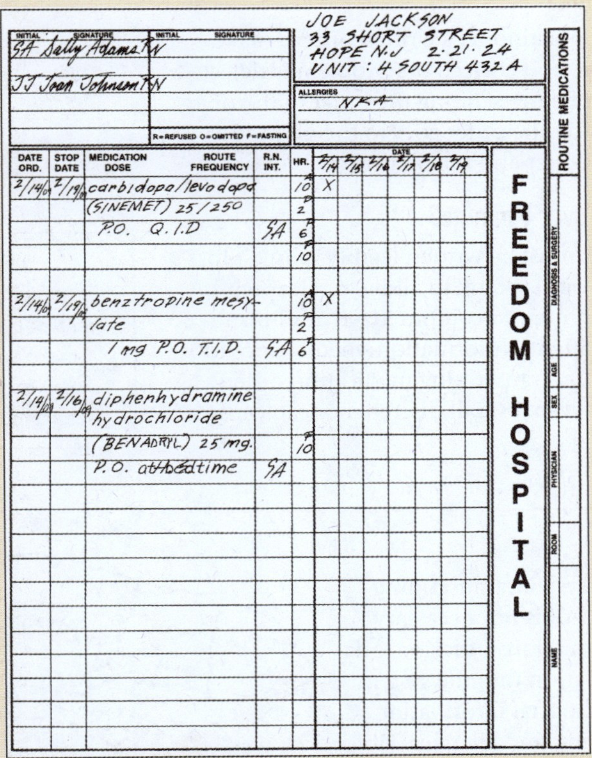

INITIAL	SIGNATURE	INITIAL	SIGNATURE
SA	Sally Adams RN		
JJ	Joan Johnson RN		

R=REFUSED O=OMITTED F=FASTING

JOE JACKSON
33 SHORT STREET
HOPE N.J 2·21·24
UNIT: 4 SOUTH 432A

ALLERGIES: NKA

DATE ORD.	STOP DATE	MEDICATION DOSE ROUTE FREQUENCY	R.N. INT.	HR.	2/14	2/15	2/16	2/17	2/18	2/19
2/14/―	2/19/―	carbidopa/levodopa (SINEMET) 25/250 P.O. Q.I.D	SA	10 A	X					
				2 P						
				6 P						
				10 P						
2/14/―	2/19/―	benztropine mesylate 1 mg P.O. T.I.D.	SA	10 A	X					
				2 P						
				6 P						
2/14/―	2/16/―	diphenhydramine hydrochloride (BENADRYL) 25 mg. P.O. at bedtime	SA	10 P						

FREEDOM HOSPITAL

ROUTINE MEDICATIONS

DIAGNOSIS & SURGERY | AGE | SEX | PHYSICIAN | ROOM | NAME

See you in court

No matter what type of medication charting system a facility uses, certain standard information must still be recorded. Standardization allows MARs to be used as legal documents if it ever becomes necessary to prove that a medication dose was or was not given. (See *Different forms, same info*.) As a rule of thumb, chart it to prove it. In other words, if a nurse is questioned under oath about a situation that occurred 5 years ago, will that nurse be able to remember every medication given to a patient? Probably not very clearly. This is yet another example of the importance of proper documentation!

Documentation

In general, documentation reflects the tasks, assessments, and procedures nurses perform. Documenting on the administration record indicates that the order placed by a licensed practitioner was carried out by the nurse.

Does that say subcutaneous or subcuticular?

Before transcribing the licensed practitioner's written orders, make sure that they are complete, clear, and correct. If a problem is detected, contact the licensed practitioner before sending the order to the pharmacy. If a problem is detected after the order goes to the pharmacy, contact both the licensed practitioner and the pharmacy.

Is that 1 mg IV over 10 minutes or 10 mg over 1 minute?

Information recorded on a MAR must be written legibly in ink. Most facilities require the use of blue or black ink to allow for clear reproduction of the record. All handwritten or computerized administration records must contain the patient's information, medication information, and signatures. *Remember:* Transcribing medication orders requires close attention because even a small discrepancy can cause a major medication error.

Before transcribing medication orders, make sure that they're complete, clear, and correct!

Recording patient information

If a facility uses a computerized system, transcribing patient information onto the eMAR is not necessary. It's already there because the admissions office or registration enters the patient information into the system. The pharmacy may also add additional information such as the patient's height, weight, and allergies. However, the nurse may enter this information as well.

If using a MAR, affix a preprinted patient label onto the form. If this isn't available, copy the information from the patient's identification bracelet.

Identification, please

Record the patient's full name, date of birth, hospital identification number, unit number, bed assignment, and allergies, even those that aren't medication related. If the patient doesn't have any known allergies, write "NKA" or "NKDA." Make sure, of course, to confirm all this information with the patient or their durable power of attorney (DPOA).

Recording medication information

Next, transcribe from the licensed practitioner's order complete information about every medication the patient is taking. If admitting the patient or upon transfer of care, the process of compiling the most accurate list of medications a patient is taking is called medication reconciliation. Obtaining this information on admission or transfer of care is critical to avoiding potential adverse reactions. According to the Joint Commission, to avoid dosing or other errors, the necessary medication information a nurse needs to obtain includes all the medication names, dosages, strengths, dosage forms, administration routes and frequency, and any special instructions. The date and time of when the patient last took the medication is also very important in the medication reconciliation process.

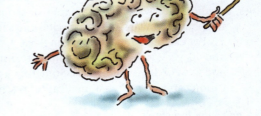

A lot of important information needs to be transcribed... the ordering licensed practitioner's name, medication name, dosage and form, administration route and frequency, and any special conditions or instructions.

It's a date!

Always record the dates on the administration record: the date and time the order was written; the date the medication should begin, if this is different from the original order date; and the date the medication should be discontinued. If a discontinuation time is not provided, many facilities have a standard length of time a medication may be given before it's automatically discontinued.

Full name, please

Record the medication's full generic name. If the licensed practitioner ordered the medication using a proprietary (trade or brand) name, record this name as well. Don't use abbreviations, chemical symbols, research names, or special facility names. Doing so can cause medication errors or delay therapy.

Be sure to record the dosage form and strength, too.

Working on your strength

When recording medication strength, be sure to write the amount of the medication to be administered.

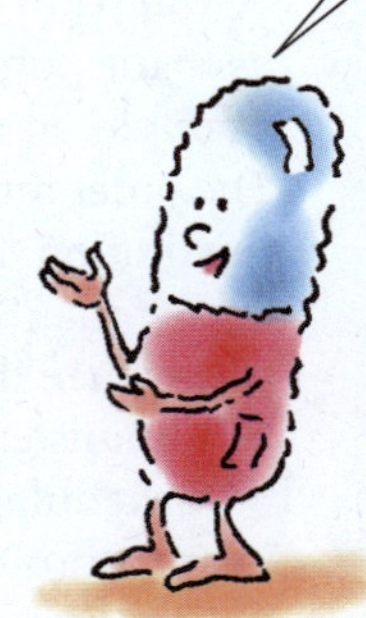

As a matter of form...

Also, record the medication dosage form that the licensed practitioner ordered. Then decide whether the form is appropriate, considering the patient's special needs.

For example, a patient who has difficulty swallowing may not be able to swallow large pills or tablets. The nurse may need to contact the licensed practitioner to discuss possible alternatives (i.e., liquid form).

Tracking the route

Recording the route of administration is especially critical for medications that may be given by many different routes. For example, acetaminophen can be given orally, intravenously, or rectally. However, some medications may only be given through one correct route; for example, NPH insulin may only be given subcutaneously. The nurse must also decide whether the route is appropriate taking into consideration the patient's special needs.

For example, if a patient has an order for a PO tablet but the patient is NPO and has a nasogastric tube in place, the patient won't be able to take the oral medication. The nurse would need to clarify this order with the licensed practitioner.

Schedule scheme

The licensed practitioner's order should include an administration schedule, such as *t.i.d.* or *q6h.* Transcribe the schedule or frequency of administration onto the MAR. Based on the facility's policy and the medication's availability, characteristics, onset, and duration of action, the pharmacy will schedule specific times for the medication to be given.

For example, t.i.d. may mean 9 AM, 1 PM, and 5 PM in one facility and 10 AM, 2 PM, and 6 PM in another. Similarly, b.i.d. may be 10 AM and 6 PM or 10 AM and 10 PM. Sometimes the *peak* or *onset* of the medication can affect when a medication is scheduled to be given.

Working round the clock

Remember that time notations are based on a 24-hour clock (see "Military time" in Chapter 7), unless otherwise specified.

Under special circumstances

Some facilities have separate administration records or specially designated areas of the regular administration record for transcribing single orders or special medication orders. Special orders may include medications ordered as p.r.n., large volume parenteral medications, and dermatologic and ophthalmic medications dispensed in bottles or tubes.

All p.r.n. orders must contain specific instructions (or parameters) as to the purpose or condition the medication should be given. For example, acetaminophen can be prescribed for both a fever and for pain. The order must contain instructions as to when the nurse can give the medication. If the p.r.n. acetaminophen is ordered for a temperature greater than 101°F, then the nurse would be able to give the acetaminophen when this condition is met. However, the nurse would not be able to administer the acetaminophen for a patient's treatment of pain.

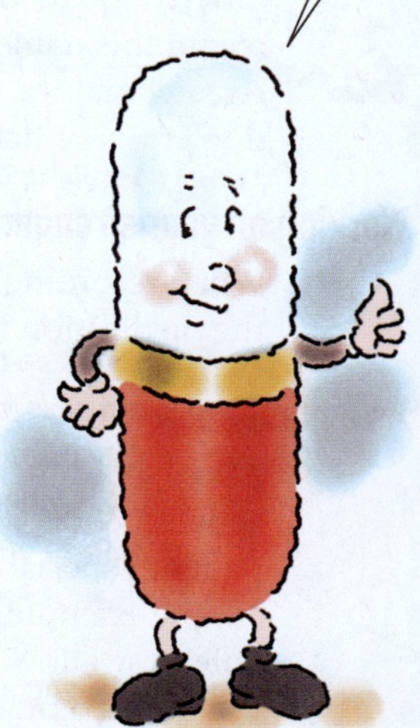
Recording the administration route is especially critical for medications that may be given by two or more different routes.

Scheduled medication orders do not have to contain any special instructions or parameters unless the licensed practitioner is requesting additional information to be considered for the administration of the medication. For example, a patient has an order for metoprolol XL

50 mg PO daily; hold for heart rate less than 100 bpm; SBP less than 100. The nurse would then need to obtain the patient's heart rate and blood pressure before administering the medication and based on the results would either give or hold the medication.

Some facilities put single orders or special medications on the regular administration record. Nurses need to be careful to distinguish these medications from those that are regularly scheduled. All facilities utilizing a MAR for medication documentation will have special forms for recording controlled substances. (See *Controlling controlled substances*.)

Controlling controlled substances

Federal and state laws regulate the dispensation, administration, and documentation of controlled substances. When these substances are issued to a unit, they're accompanied by a perpetual inventory record, commonly called a *controlled inventory record.*

A paper trail

If the licensed practitioner orders a controlled substance for a patient, document the administration on the MAR and the perpetual inventory record or *controlled inventory record.* When a dose is removed from the locked storage site, note this information on the perpetual inventory record:

- date and time the dose is removed
- amount of the medication remaining in the locked storage site
- patient's full name
- licensed practitioner's name
- medication dose
- nurse's signature

If any amount of the dose needs to be discarded, another nurse must verify (witness) the amount discarded and then sign the form, too.

Note that controlled substances should be kept under a *double lock.* In other words, medications are usually kept in some sort of locked cart or storage mechanism. Controlled substances could then be in a locked drawer of the locked cart. Get it? Yes, it's a big deal.

Paperless trail

Most facilities now utilize computerized medication dispensing systems such as a Pyxis Medstation on every unit. These systems may dispense controlled substances as well as other medications. A nurse's username and password serve as the signature to access and withdraw medications. Some dispensing systems may use a username and a fingerprint scan to serve as access to withdraw medications. However, another nurse is still needed to witness any part of a controlled substance that is discarded—the system will display a prompt screen for the witnessing nurse to enter their username and password to serve as their signature.

Computerized medication dispensing systems provide access to medications that are commonly needed in the patient care area. So, when a new medication is ordered, it is readily available from the computerized medication dispensing system instead of waiting for the pharmacy to deliver it. A safety feature allows the pharmacist to review and approve the medication before medications can be selected and administered from the system.

Computerized medication dispensing systems also have software that promotes patient safety by utilizing readable bar-codes for restocking and choosing medications, providing automated refilling systems, giving medication safety alerts, and linking to satellite pharmacies after hours so medications can be verified and distributed.

Don't forget to sign

Remember that every time an order is transcribed onto the MAR, the nurse must sign it. First, initial the record after transcribing from the licensed practitioner's order sheet. Many facilities also require nurses to perform a 24-hour (or daily) chart check. With paper charting, the nurse indicates that this has been completed by drawing a line under the very last order followed by their initials. This indicates that all orders have been transcribed correctly onto the MAR. If someone other than the nurse transcribes the order, a nurse must cosign the order sheet and the MAR. In CPOE, the nurse acknowledges and signs the order through their username and password access.

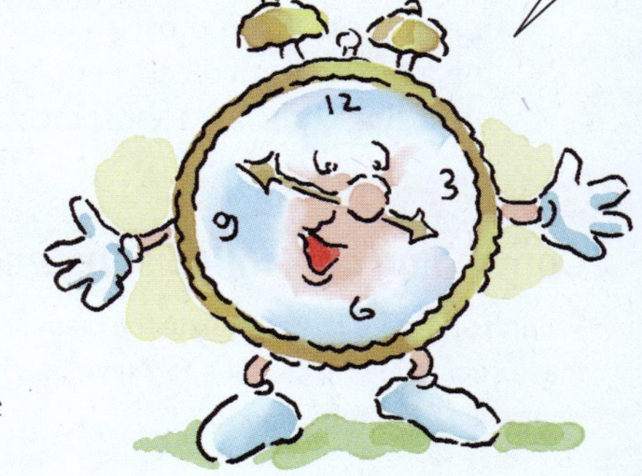

A nurse has to really keep track of the timing of medications!
12
3
9
6

After you give that medication, document!

Immediately after giving a medication, document the time of administration to prevent the medication from being inadvertently given again. For scheduled medications, nurses usually initial the appropriate time slot for the date that the medication was administered.

Scheduled medications are considered on time if they're given within a half-hour or an hour of the ordered time. This can depend on the geographical area where a facility is located. Regulations in the United States may change from state to state. For unscheduled medications, such as single doses and p.r.n. medications, record the exact time of administration in the appropriate slot on the MAR.

If the dose administered varies in any way from the strength or amount ordered, note this in a special area on the administration record or in the progress notes. For example, document whether a patient refused to take a medication, consumed only part of a medication, or vomited shortly after taking a medication. Additionally, if a medication is refused, document the patient's reasoning, any education provided, and when the licensed practitioner was notified.

Document detours

If a medication is administered by a different route from that which the licensed practitioner originally ordered, indicate that change, along with the reason and authorization for the change. Nurses must not change the route of any medication without consulting the licensed practitioner. Certain medications may not be interchangeable and/or a change in the dosage may be required. Don't forget to document if a special administration technique was used, such as a Z-track IM injection.

Citing the site

When administering a medication by a parenteral route, record the injection site to facilitate site rotation. Most administration forms include a numbered list of recognized sites, allowing the nurse to record the site by its number. However, if necessary, describe anatomical landmarks used to locate the specific site. The nurse should also document how the patient tolerated the injection.

When the timing's off

If a medication is not given on time or if the dose is missed entirely, document the reason on either the MAR or the patient's progress notes. Facility policy may require the nurse to circle and initial the time missed on the MAR to draw attention to it. The nurse must also notify the licensed practitioner as soon as possible and facilitate any orders consequently. Additionally, an incident form may need to be filed according to the facility's policy as well.

Initiate initialing

The nurse needs to sign the MAR after giving a medication by placing their initials in the appropriate space on the form. Make sure that the initials are legible and signed in the same way each time. Usually, most forms require the nurse's full name, title, and initials in the signature section of the MAR. If two or more nurses have the same initials, they should also include the initial of their middle name as part of their initials as well to avoid any potential confusion.

Real-world problems

Here are some examples of administration record problems that nurses may encounter in the real world.

The old NPO holdup

A patient has an order for oral potassium chloride supplements, but the patient was made NPO for a test, so the nurse withheld the dose. How would the nurse record this on the MAR?

In facilities still using written charts, the withheld dose is recorded by the nurse circling the time when the medication was held followed by placing their initials. The nurse can also record the reason the dose was withheld (in this case, the patient was made NPO) in the progress notes. Again, the nurse should notify the licensed practitioner to ensure it is safe to withhold the dose.

In control

A patient needs a dose of morphine sulfate, a controlled substance, but only needs 2 mg of the 4-mg prefilled syringe provided. On the MAR, how would the nurse indicate that the extra morphine was appropriately discarded?

First, the administering nurse would ask another nurse to witness the extra medication being discarded (by facility protocol). Then, the witnessing nurse needs to sign the controlled inventory record (or follow the facility's policy) to verify this process. If using a computerized medication dispensing system, discard as stated in *Controlling controlled substances*, p. 141.

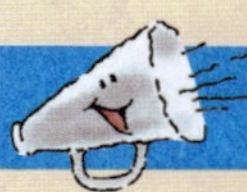

That's a wrap!

Administration records review

Keep these important points about medication administration records in mind.

Medication administration record systems

- MAR
  - Uses a form to record medication administration.
- Computer charting
  - Medication administration information entered into a computer (eMAR).
  - Automatic, computer-generated list of scheduled medications and their administration times.
  - Used increasingly over other systems.

Documenting medication administration

- Write legibly in blue or black ink.
- Record allergy information if it isn't already documented, using "NKA" or "NKDA" if no allergies are known.
- Transcribe from the licensed practitioner's order complete information about each medication (dates, times, medication names, dosages, strengths, dosage forms, administration routes, and administration times).
- If parenteral, record the injection site.
- Immediately document the times of all administrations.
- If unscheduled, record the exact time and reason that the medication was given
- If given late or not at all, document the reason and notify the licensed practitioner.
- Always sign any documentation on the MAR.

Recording controlled-substance administration

- Include date and time dose is removed from locked storage area.
- Include amount of medication remaining in locked storage area.
- Record the patient's full name.
- Document the licensed practitioner's full name.
- Enter the medication dose given.
- Include full signature (if a form is used; the nurse's password serves as a signature if a computer is used).
- If any part of the medication was discarded, obtain the signature of another nurse who verified the amount discarded (or have them enter their password as verification if using a computer).

Quick quiz

1. When is the nurse required to circle and initial the time slot of a medication?
   - A. when the dose was missed or administered late
   - B. when the administration time has changed
   - C. when another nurse forgot to administer a medication
   - D. when the medication has been discontinued

Answer: A. Circling and initialing the time slot signals to the next nurse that the dose was missed or late. The nurse then refers to the single-order or p.r.n. section of the MAR to find the actual administration time. This helps the nurse to avoid administering next dose too soon.

2. What does the abbreviation NKDA stand for?
   - A. no known adverse reactions
   - B. no known administration
   - C. no known alteration
   - D. no known drug allergies

Answer: D. Allergy information should always be recorded. If there are no known allergies, document NKDA.

3. To avoid confusion, how should nurses with the same initials sign the MAR?
   - A. with their identification numbers
   - B. with pens with different colors of ink
   - C. with their middle initials
   - D. with their birth dates

Answer: C. Middle initials should be used. In addition, be sure to write legibly and always sign the same way.

4. What should the nurse do immediately after administering a medication?
   - A. record the medication's effectiveness
   - B. document the time of administration
   - C. order the next dose of the medication from the pharmacy
   - D. take the patient's vital signs

Answer: B. Documenting the time of administration immediately after the medication is given prevents from it from being inadvertently given again.

Scoring

 If you answered all four items correctly, amazing! You've been voted best nurse at the Administration Academy Awards!

 If you answered three items correctly, fantastic! Here's your Oscar for best supporting nurse!

☆ If you answered fewer than three items correctly, keep your chin up! You're still a record setter!

Suggested References

Barnsteiner, J. H. (2008). Chapter 38: Medication reconciliation. In Hughes R. G. (ed.). *Patient safety and quality: An evidence-based handbook for nurses*. Agency for Healthcare Research and Quality (US). https://www.ncbi.nlm.nih.gov/books/NBK2648/

Ortiz, N. R., & Preuss, C. V. (2023). Controlled substance act. In: *StatPearls [Internet]*. StatPearls Publishing. [Updated 2023 March 24]. https://www.ncbi.nlm.nih.gov/books/NBK574544/

Patient Safety Network. (2019). Medication reconciliation. https://psnet.ahrq.gov/primer/medication-reconciliation

Chapter 9

Preventing medication errors

Just the facts

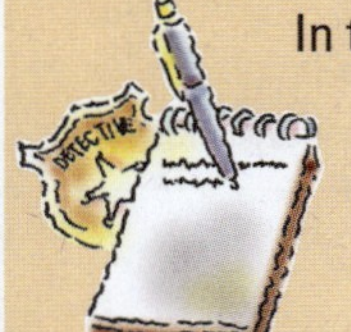

In this chapter, you'll learn how to:

- recognize types and causes of common medication errors
- prevent medication errors
- report medication errors

A look at medication errors

Medication errors cause thousands of injuries and deaths in health care settings every year. The U.S. Food and Drug Administration (FDA) alone receive more than 100,000 U.S. reports each year associated with a suspected medication error. In fact, between 7,000 and 9,000 people die in U.S. hospitals every year due to medication errors! Since approximately only 1 out of every 10 medication errors is reported, no one knows exactly how many errors actually occur. Despite such discouraging statistics, finding better ways to safeguard patients against these kinds of errors has become a national health care priority.

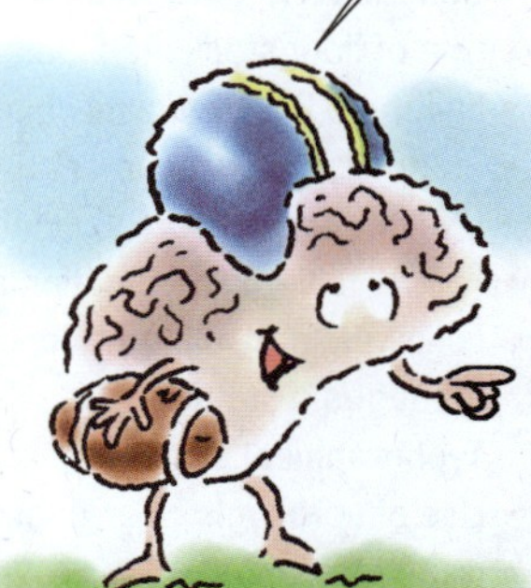

Time-out called to review that medication play!

Are you legal?

Depending on a facility's location, several different licensed practitioners—including doctors, advanced-practice registered nurses, physician assistants, dentists, podiatrists, and optometrists—may be legally permitted to prescribe, dispense, and/or administer medications. Usually, however, licensed practitioners prescribe medications, pharmacists prepare and dispense the medications, and nurses administer them to patients.

An integral team player

Nurses are almost always on the front line when it comes to medication administration. This means they also bear a major share of the responsibility in protecting patients from all types of medication errors. Be proactive! Nurses should get into good habits early in their careers, including double-checking themselves and not being afraid to ask for help or advice from colleagues.

Doing your part

Many kinds of medication errors can occur in everyday nursing practice. Consequently, each institution has its own set of guidelines for how and when to properly administer medications to patients, and each nurse is responsible for knowing what those guidelines are. Besides faithfully following a facility's administration policies, nurses can help prevent medication errors by studying and avoiding the common slip-ups that allow them to happen. (See *Common medication errors.*)

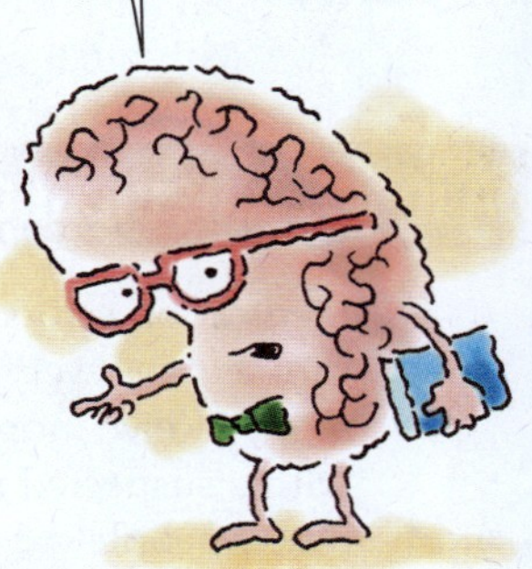

Medication errors are widely accepted as the most common and preventable cause of patient injury. It pays to be extra careful and to follow a facility's guidelines when administering medications.

Common medication errors

Certain situations or activities can place nurses at high risk for making a medication error. Some of the most common types and causes of errors are highlighted here.

Types of errors

- Giving the wrong medication
- Giving the wrong dose
- Using the wrong diluent
- Preparing the wrong concentration
- Missing a dose or failing to give an ordered medication
- Giving the medication at the wrong time
- Administering a medication to which the patient is allergic
- Infusing the medication too rapidly
- Giving the medication to the wrong patient
- Administering the medication by the wrong route

Causes

- Failing to identify the patient using two forms of identification
- Insufficient knowledge
- Chaotic work environment with distractions
- Use of floor stock medications
- Failure to follow facility policies and procedures
- Incorrect preparation or administration techniques
- Use of intravenous (IV) solutions that aren't premixed
- Failure to verify medication and dosage instructions
- Following oral, not written, orders
- Inadequate staffing
- Typographical errors
- Use of acronyms or erroneous abbreviations
- Math errors
- Poor handwriting
- Failure to check dosages for high-risk medications or pediatric medications
- Inadequate medication information
- Preparation of the medication in a clinical area instead of the pharmacy
- Unlabeled syringes

To prevent medication errors, avoid distractions and interruptions when preparing and administering medications. Nurses also need to adhere to the "six rights" of medication administration: identify the right patient using two patient identifiers, right medication, right dose, right time, right route, and right documentation. Some literature identifies up to nine rights of medication administration, which in addition to the six rights include the right action (or reason for the medication), the right form, and the right response.

Medication errors in practice

In addition to dosage calculation errors (which account for roughly 7% of all reported medication errors), common errors include mistakes with medication or patient names, missed allergy alerts, errors compounded by two or more practitioners, errors involving routes of administration, misinterpreted abbreviations, misinterpreted medication orders, preparation errors, reconciliation errors, and errors caused by stress.

If a medication order doesn't seem right for the patient's diagnosis, call the licensed practitioner to clarify the order.

Medication name errors

Medications with similar-sounding names are easy to confuse. Even different-sounding names can look similar when written out rapidly by hand on a medication order. Remember, if the patient's medication order doesn't seem right for the diagnosis; call the licensed practitioner to clarify the order. (See *Look-alike and sound-alike medication names*, p. 150.)

Tall Man Letters

One way that many pharmacies, health care institutions, and hospitals try to clarify these look-alike and sound-alike medications is to use Tall Man Letters. An example of this is with these look-alike and sound-alike medications: glyBURIDE and glipiZIDE. Both medications are antidiabetic agents that could be mistaken for one another. With emphasis on the difference in the spelling, it alerts the nurse to look closely at the names.

Morphing the name

For example, an order for morphine can be easily confused with one for hydromorphone. Both medications are available in 4-mg prefilled syringes, and both can cause respiratory depression. However, morphine has a greater effect on a patient's respiratory status. If morphine was administered when the licensed practitioner ordered hydromorphone, the patient could develop respiratory depression or even respiratory

Before you give that medication

Look-alike and sound-alike medication names

The medication names listed here resemble each other in terms of spelling or sound. This list contains some of the more common medications, but many more exist. Always double-check the medication order carefully before administering medication to patients. If there're any doubts about the appropriateness of the medication, consult the licensed practitioner, the pharmacist, or a medication reference:

- Adderall and Inderal
- Allegra and Viagra
- amantadine and rimantadine
- amiodarone and amiloride
- amoxicillin and amoxapine
- benztropine and bromocriptine
- Celebrex and Celexa
- Celebrex and Cerebyx
- cimetidine and simethicone
- codeine and Cardene
- dexamethasone and desoximetasone
- digoxin and doxepin
- diltiazem and diazepam
- epinephrine and ephedrine
- epinephrine and norepinephrine
- flunisolide and fluocinonide
- hydromorphone and morphine
- hydroxyzine and hydralazine
- imipramine and desipramine
- Imuran and Inderal
- insulin glargine and insulin glulisine
- levothyroxine and liothyronine
- metformin and metronidazole
- naloxone and naltrexone
- nifedipine and nicardipine
- nitroglycerin and nitroprusside
- oxycontin and oxycodone
- pentobarbital and phenobarbital
- propylthiouracil and Purinethol
- Ritalin and Rifadin
- sitagliptin and sumatriptan
- sulfisoxazole and sulfasalazine
- vinblastine and vincristine
- Xanax and Zantac
- Zyrtec and Zyprexa

arrest. Another example of a look-alike and sound-alike medication is Xanax and Zantac. Xanax, a benzodiazepine, is an antianxiety medication, while Zantac is a histamine 2 antagonist used to decrease gastric secretions. If a patient had no gastrointestinal symptoms or medical history, the nurse would need to clarify this order.

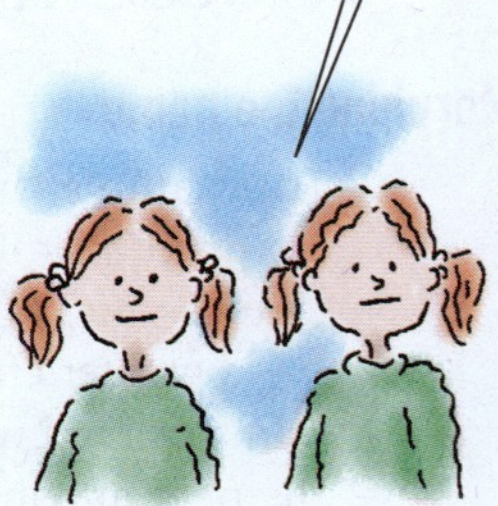

Caution with doubles! Be aware that even patients can have similar names which can cause problems if the nurse does not verify each patient's identity before giving a medication.

Posting prevention

The use of automated medication dispensing systems prevents and decreases medication errors. If a facility or unit does not have this system in place, consider posting a notice prominently on each unit where opioids are kept, to warn the staff about this common mix-up. Another prevention strategy includes attaching a fluorescent or brightly colored sticker with the words "NOT MORPHINE" to each hydromorphone syringe.

Patient name errors

Medication names aren't the only names subject to confusion. Sometimes, patient names can cause trouble as well, especially when nurses don't verify each patient's identity before administering medications. Caring for two patients with the same or similar first or last name can further complicate matters. Consider the following scenario.

A tale of two Bobs

Five-year-old Robert Brewer is hospitalized with abdominal pain. Robert Brinson, also age 5, is admitted to the same pediatric unit after a severe asthma attack. The boys are assigned to adjacent rooms and each of them have a nonproductive cough.

The nurse caring for Robert Brewer enters his room to give him an expectorant. As the nurse is about to administer the medication, the child's mother informs her that someone else came into the room a few minutes ago to give Robert a medication that he inhaled by mask. The nurse quickly determines that another nurse mistakenly gave Robert Brinson's medication (acetylcysteine—a mucolytic) to Robert Brewer.

Fortunately, no harmful adverse effects developed. However, if the other nurse had checked the patient's identity more carefully, this error would never have occurred.

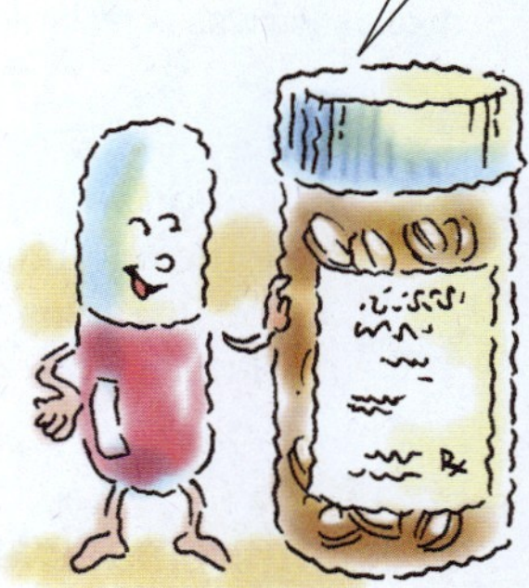

Providing patients and family with education about the patient's medications can help prevent errors at home.

Check and double-check

Always verify the patient's identity using two patient identifiers. The two identifiers may be included in the same location, such as the hospital identification bracelet. Acceptable identifiers include the patient's first and last names, assigned identification number (such as the medical record number), and birth date. Involve the patient and/or family in the identification process by asking for the full name and birthdate.

Teach the patient (or parents if the patient is a minor) to offer their identification bracelet for inspection when anyone enters the room to administer a medication. Patient identification bracelets should not be removed from a patient at any time during their stay. If an identification bracelet falls off, is removed, or becomes misplaced, the nurse should replace it immediately. (See *Raising the bar with bar coding*, p. 152.)

Patients should also be taught what medications have been ordered, the purpose or action of the medications, how often, and what times they will be receiving them. In addition, patients should be taught any potential side effects they may experience. Nurses should also provide education about any potential adverse effects of a medication such as the signs and symptoms of an allergic reaction with antibiotics. This

Raising the bar with bar coding

Barcode medication administration technology is one way to help prevent medication errors before they reach the patient. With this technology, a barcode is placed on each medication the patient is to receive. Each medication barcode contains the National Medication Code, which includes the medication's name, its dose, and packaging information. Another barcode is placed on the patient's hospital identification bracelet.

Before administering a medication, the nurse accesses a copy of the medication administration record (MAR) or electronic medication administration record (eMAR), properly identifies the patient using two patient identifiers, and then scans the patient's barcode located on their identification bracelet followed by scanning the medication barcode. Scanning both barcodes in this manner helps ensure that the nurse is administering the right medication to the right patient at the right time. If there are any discrepancies at this time, a notification will alert the nurse to the discrepancy. There are a variety of discrepancy alerts a nurse could receive, including but not limited to the following: look-alike/sound-alike medications, patient allergy, medication contraindications, dosage mistakes, and administration time mistakes. Some facilities have computer systems that put extra safeguards on high-risk medication administrations like insulin, blood products, and controlled substances. Even with all the safeguards in place, errors can still occur. Nurses must take this responsibility seriously and follow policy and nursing knowledge.

Barcodes in action

Here are two examples of how barcode medication technology prevented medication errors:

A nurse attempting to administer furosemide (Lasix) 40 mg IV to a patient scanned the medication label at the patient's bedside and received a warning message that read "No order in the system." The nurse didn't administer the medication and immediately reviewed the patient's chart. After reviewing the chart, the nurse realized that the medication wasn't intended for that patient.

In another incident, a nurse scanned the barcode on the patient's identification bracelet and then scanned the barcode on the levofloxacin (Levaquin) medication container. The nurse received a warning message that read "Dose early." This could be considered a "near miss" situation where the error was caught before being given to the patient. As a result of the warning message, the nurse administered the medication at the proper time—2 hours later when the medication was actually due to be administered.

education will also help prepare patients to take the medication safely at home upon discharge. Medication administration should be interactive, involving the patient and family in the process. (See *Preventing medication errors through teaching*.)

Preventing medication errors through teaching

Medication errors aren't limited to hospital settings. Patients sometimes make medication errors when taking their medications at home. To prevent such errors, nurses need to take the time to educate patients thoroughly about each medication they will be taking. Always print out a copy of the medication list to review with the patient and/or caregiver to ensure understanding. Whether on the discharge form in the hospital, in a clinic, nursing home discharge, or home health visit; be sure to cover these points:

Preventing medication errors through teaching (*continued*)

- medication's name (generic and trade name)
- medication's purpose
- correct dosage and how to calculate it (such as breaking scored tablets or mixing liquids when necessary)
- how to take the medication
- when to take the medication
- what to do if a dose is missed
- how to monitor the medication's effectiveness (e.g., checking blood glucose levels when taking an antidiabetic medication)
- potential medication interactions (including the need to avoid certain over-the-counter and herbal medications)
- required dietary changes (including the use of alcohol)
- possible adverse effects and what to do if they occur
- proper storage, handling, and disposal of the medication or supplies (such as syringes)
- required follow-up

Missed allergy alerts

After a nurse verifies a patient's identity, they need to check to see if the patient is wearing allergy identification, such as MedicAlert® jewelry. All allergy identification tags or jewelry should have the name of the specific allergen conspicuously written or embossed on them. This same allergy information should be recorded in the patient's chart. Patients admitted to the hospital must wear a band that identifies the patient has an allergy. Most facilities utilize a universal red band for the identification of an allergy. For safety, nurses must refer to the chart to review the allergy list and reaction to all allergies. Most electronic medical records (EMR) show the allergy across the top of the header. Regardless of whether the patient is wearing allergy identification, nurses still need to ask patients directly about their medication allergies and the reactions that occur with them. Sometimes patients forget to add an allergy to their list at the primary care provider's (PCP) office, and some patients don't regularly seek medical care. Therefore, asking the patient directly is sometimes a nurse's only safeguard against this type of error.

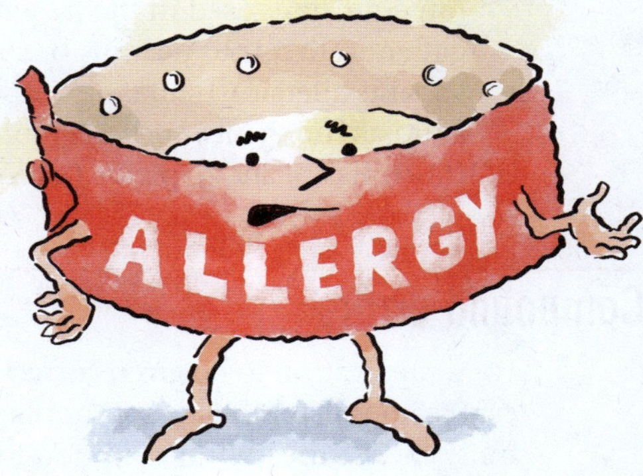

Placing an allergy bracelet on patients with identified allergies alert staff to be vigilant when administering medications.
ALLERGY

A distressing situation

Consider this example. The licensed practitioner issues a stat order for lorazepam (Ativan) for a distressed patient. By the time the nurse arrives with the medication, the patient has grown more visibly distressed. Unnerved by the patient's demeanor, the nurse quickly administers the medication—without verifying the patient's identity, checking the patient's allergy bracelet, or medication administration record first, and without verifying the order. The patient has an immediate allergic reaction.

This patient was wearing an allergy bracelet along with the allergy information clearly indicated on the chart and medication administration record; this error was fully preventable.

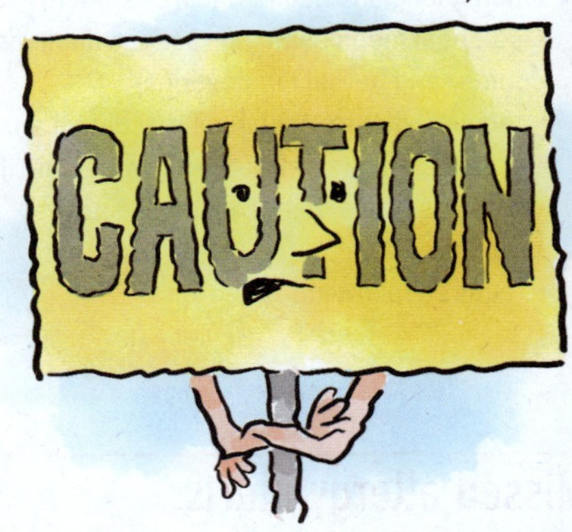
Be especially alert for the possibility of an anaphylactic reaction when a patient is allergic to peanuts, soy, or sulfa compounds.
CAUTION

Resisting temptation

Any time nurses find themselves in a tense situation with a patient who needs or wants medication fast, the nurse needs to resist the temptation to act first and document later. Skipping this crucial step can easily lead to a medication error.

Not just talking peanuts

Certain medications should never be given to patients allergic to peanuts, soy, or sulfa compounds. Keep these tips in mind to help prevent allergic reactions in these patients:

- A patient who's severely allergic to peanuts or soy may have an anaphylactic reaction (a severe, life-threatening reaction) to ipratropium (Atrovent) aerosol given by a metered-dose inhaler. Ask the patient (or parents) whether they are allergic to peanuts or soy before giving this medication. If this is the case, the nurse will need to use the nasal spray or inhalation solution (nebulizer) form of the medication. Since neither form contains soy lecithin (an emulsifier used in the metered-dose formula), it's safe for patients allergic to peanuts or soy.
- Patients allergic to sulfa medications shouldn't receive sulfonylurea antidiabetic agents, such as chlorpropamide (Diabinese), glyburide (Micronase), and glipizide (Glucotrol).

Compound errors

For a medication to be given correctly, each member of the health care team must fulfill an appropriate role. The licensed practitioner must choose the right medication for the patient, then write the order correctly and legibly or enter it into the computer correctly. Most electronic systems offer the correct and appropriate choices for the provider to choose from. The pharmacist must interpret the order, determine whether it's complete and safe, and prepare the medication using precise measurements. Finally, the nurse must evaluate whether the medication is appropriate for the patient, verify it's for the correct patient and time, and then administer the medication correctly according to facility guidelines.

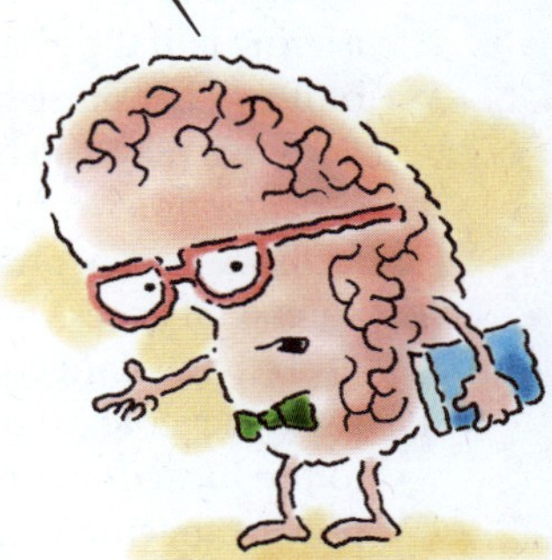

Nurses should not hesitate to seek out clarification of a medication order!

Never break the chain

A breakdown along this chain of events can easily lead to a medication error, an error that's further compounded because of the number of people who could have prevented it. That's why it's vital for all health care providers to work together as a team, supporting and helping each other to promote the best patient care. In some cases, working as a team may be as simple as asking for further clarification or as complicated as double-checking with another licensed practitioner.

Calling all pharmacists

For instance, the pharmacist can help clarify the number of times a medication must be given each day. Pharmacy can also help label medications or remind the nurse to always return unused or discontinued medications back to the pharmacy. Pharmacists also check into allergies, like not dispensing sulfa-containing antibiotics to patients allergic to sulfa.

I can see clearly now

Nurses are responsible for clarifying an order that doesn't seem clear or correct. Nurses must also correctly handle and store medications and administer only the medications that they have personally prepared. Never give a medication with an ambiguous label or no label at all. Here's an example of what could happen.

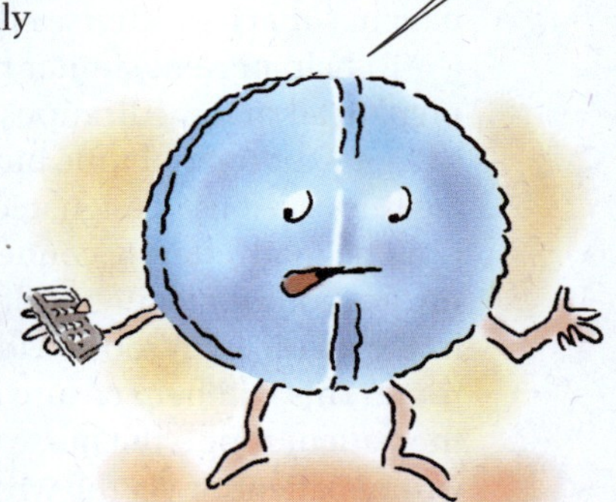

It's a good practice to double-check all math calculations. Ask a pharmacist or another nurse to check your math!

A shocking mistake

The nurse places an unlabeled syringe on a tray near a patient in the operating room. The nurse gets called away unexpectedly and the licensed practitioner administers the medication. The licensed practitioner thought the syringe contained bupivacaine (Marcaine), but instead it contained 30 mL of epinephrine 1:1,000, which the nurse had drawn up into the syringe. The patient developed ventricular fibrillation, was immediately defibrillated, and then needed to be transferred to the intensive care unit, where they later recovered.

Obviously, this was a compound medication error. The nurse should have labeled the syringe clearly, and the licensed practitioner should never have given an unlabeled medication to the patient.

Liters versus grams

In another example of a compound error, a nurse working in the neonatal intensive care unit prepares a dose of aminophylline to administer to an infant. No one checks the nurse's calculations. Shortly after receiving the medication, the infant develops tachycardia and other signs of theophylline toxicity and later dies. The nurse thought that the order read *7.4 mL of aminophylline.* Instead, it read *7.4 mg.*

This tragedy might have been avoided if the licensed practitioner had written a clearer order, if the nurse had clarified the order before administering it, if the pharmacist had prepared and dispensed the medication, or if another nurse had double-checked the dosage calculation. In addition, this may also have been avoided if the facility utilized computerized provider order entry (CPOE). To avoid these types of situations, many facilities require pharmacists to prepare and dispense all nonemergency parenteral doses whenever commercial unit doses aren't available.

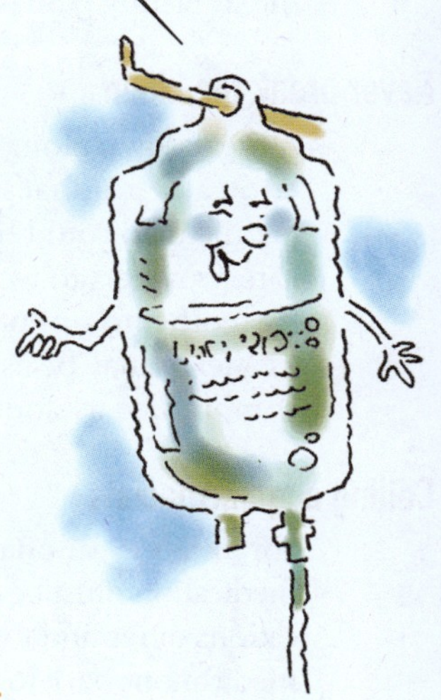

Never administer a medication or solution that isn't labeled or is labeled poorly.

Leaving dangerous chemicals near patient-care areas is extremely risky. Never leave medications at the patient's bedside. Return them to the locked medication room to be stored. All medications that are patient specific must be labeled with the patient information, medication name, and strength.

Route errors

Many medication errors stem, at least in part, from problems involving the route of administration. The risk of error increases when a patient has several different types of access devices as described in the following scenario.

Crossing the line

A nurse prepares a dose of digoxin elixir for a patient with a central IV line and a jejunostomy tube in place. The nurse mistakenly administers the oral medication into the central IV line. Fortunately, the patient suffers no adverse effects.

To help prevent similar mix-ups in the route of administration, prepare all oral medications in a syringe that has a tip small enough to fit an abdominal tube but too large to fit a central line. Some facilities even use designated tubing for enteral feedings, so that it can't be inadvertently connected to an IV line. When preparing all medications that will be administered by syringe, label the syringe in the medication room with the patient's name, medication, and route. This will help ensure that if a distraction occurs on the way to the patient room, the nurse will not administer the medication to the wrong patient or via the wrong route.

Clearing the air

Here's another error that could have been avoided: To clear air bubbles from a patient's insulin infusion, the nurse disconnects the tubing and increases the pump rate to 200 mL/hr, flushing the bubbles through quickly. The nurse then reconnects the tubing and restarts the infusion but forgets to reset the drip rate back to the original infusion rate of 2 units/hr. The patient receives a total of 50 units of insulin before the nurse detects the error.

To prevent this kind of mistake, never increase the drip rate to clear bubbles from a line. Instead, remove the tubing from the pump, disconnect it from the patient, and use the flow-control clamp to establish gravity flow of the IV fluid to purge the air from the line.

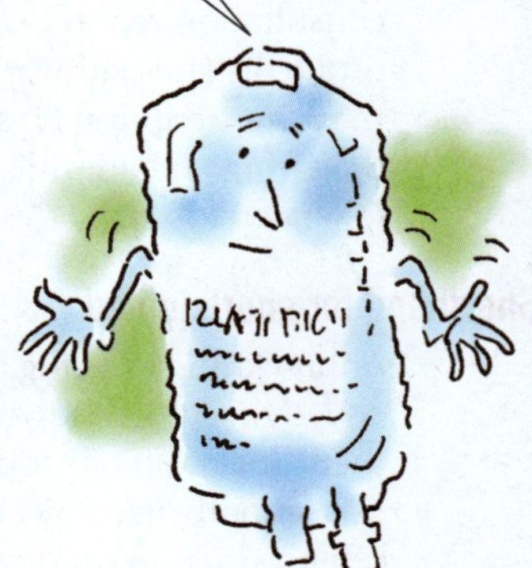
To safely clear air bubbles from an IV line, always remove the tubing from the pump and disconnect it from the patient.

High-alert medications and the independent double-check

The Joint Commission and each facility have identified certain medications that are considered high-alert and may require an independent double-check prior to administration to the patient. Examples of some of these medication types include antidiabetic agents, narcotics, anticoagulants, and chemotherapy medications. The independent double-check consists of two nurses reviewing the order and each nurse, independent of each other, calculating the amount and how the medication should be given. They both compare their findings to confirm accuracy prior to administrating it to the patient. This is mandatory. It ensures patient safety and is vital in preventing medication errors.

Smart IV pumps

Smart infusion pumps for the administration of IV medications help reduce the risk of infusion errors. These types of pumps combine computer technology and drug libraries to limit the potential for dosing errors. They also contain high and low alarm limits to control the flow rate ranges for which certain medications can be set, further helping to reduce errors.

Misinterpreted abbreviations

Some commonly used abbreviations are known to contribute significantly to medication errors. For example, in an order reading *levothyroxine (Synthroid) 50 µg PO daily*, the µg (meaning micrograms) may be easily misinterpreted to mean *milligrams*. The patient could mistakenly receive 50 mg of levothyroxine, or 1,000 times the ordered dose.

The Joint Commission guidelines

To prevent such devastating errors, every facility is encouraged to make a "Do not use" list readily available for all health care workers. This list identifies abbreviations that should *never* be used in any form, under any circumstances. In fact, The Joint Commission has compiled a list of dangerous abbreviations that should be avoided in all clinical documentation, including medication orders, patient charts, progress notes, consultation reports, operative reports, educational materials, and protocols and pathways. Although the use of EMR helps to correct these transcription errors, the nurse must still remain diligent when preparing and administering medications. (See *The Joint Commission's "Do not use" list*, p. 159.)

Shorthand for shortsighted

Abbreviating or using a shorthand version of a medication name is equally risky, as shown in this example: Epoetin alfa (Epogen), a synthetic form of erythropoietin that's commonly abbreviated as EPO, is occasionally used by anemic cancer patients to stimulate red blood cell production. In one case, a licensed practitioner wrote, "May take own supply of EPO" on the discharge orders of a patient whose cancer was in remission. However, the patient wasn't anemic.

Sensing that something was wrong with ordering epoetin alfa for a patient who isn't anemic, the pharmacist interviewed the patient, who confirmed that they were taking "EPO," or evening primrose oil, to lower their cholesterol level. Fortunately, the pharmacist became aware of his misinterpretation of the abbreviation before an error could occur in this situation.

To avoid this type of error, ask licensed practitioners to spell out all medication names.

Misinterpreted orders

As a rule of thumb, if a nurse is unfamiliar with a medication that is prescribed, always consult a medication reference before administering the medication to the patient. Also, ask the licensed practitioner to clarify vague or ambiguous terms. Nurses shouldn't assume that they will get it right on their own.

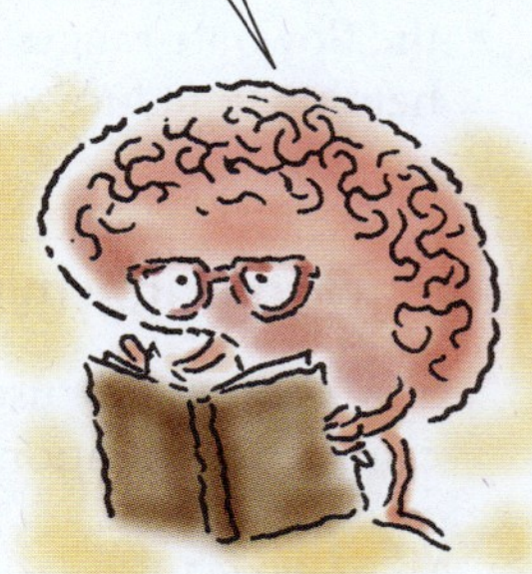

Nurses should always look up a medication or consult a pharmacist if they are unfamiliar with a medication.

Guessing is always wrong

Here's an example. A patient was supposed to receive one dose of the antineoplastic medication lomustine (Ceena) to treat brain cancer. Lomustine is typically given as a single oral dose once every 6 weeks. The order read, "Administer at night." Since the evening shift nurse misinterpreted the order to mean "every

The Joint Commission's "Do not use" list

All health care facilities accredited by The Joint Commission are encouraged to develop and maintain a "Do not use" list—a list of abbreviations that should never be used in any form (upper or lowercase, with or without periods) in clinical documentation because they're confusing and subject to misinterpretation.

Official "Do not use" list

These abbreviations must appear on a "Do not use" list and should be avoided in *all* orders and medication-related documentation that is handwritten (including free-text computer entry) or on preprinted forms.

Abbreviation	Potential problem	Preferred term
U, u (for unit)	Mistaken as 0 (zero), 4 (four), or cc	Write *unit.*
IU (for international unit)	Mistaken as IV (intravenous) or 10 (ten)	Write *international unit.*
Q.D., QD, q.d., qd (daily)	Mistaken for each other.	Write *daily.*
Q.O.D., QOD, q.o.d., qod (every other day)	The period after the *Q* may be mistaken for an *I*, and the *O* may be mistaken for an *I*.	Write *every other day.*
Trailing zero (as in *X.0 mg*), *absence of leading zero (as in *.X mg*)	Inaccuracies with numbers or values due to missed decimal point	Write *X mg* or *0.X mg.*
MS, MSO_4, $MgSO_4$	Confused for one another (can mean morphine sulfate or magnesium sulfate)	Write *morphine sulfate* or *magnesium sulfate.*

***Exception:** A "trailing zero" may be used only where required to demonstrate the level of precision of the value being reported, such as for laboratory results, imaging studies that report the size of lesions, or catheter/tube sizes. It may not be used in medication orders or other medication-related documentation.

Additional abbreviations

These abbreviations, acronyms, and symbols may represent a risk to patient safety. They are not part of the official "Do not use" list but are reviewed annually for possible inclusion.

Do not use	Potential problem	Use instead
> (greater than)	Misinterpreted as the number "7" (seven) or the letter "L"	Write *greater than.*
< (less than)	Confused for one another	Write *less than.*
Abbreviations for medication names	Misinterpreted due to similar abbreviations for multiple medications	Write medication names in full.
Apothecary units	Unfamiliar to many practitioners	Use metric units.
	Confused with metric units	
@	Mistaken for the number "2" (two)	Write *at.*
cc	Mistaken for U (units) when poorly written	Write *mL* or *milliliters.*
µg	Mistaken for mg (milligrams), resulting in one thousand fold overdose	Write *mcg* or *micrograms.*

night" when the licensed practitioner meant "once at bedtime," the patient received three daily doses of a medication when they should have only received it once. Consequently, the patient developed severe thrombocytopenia and leukopenia, and later died.

Remember to clarify confusing orders with the licensed practitioner and to read each order carefully. Always keep a medication reference book handy. Most facilities also provide computer access to digital medication references as well. Either way, it's important for nurses to look up any medications that they are unfamiliar with—doing so may prevent an error and save a life.

Did I hear you right?

In rare cases, nurses may have to follow a verbal order given from a licensed practitioner to administer a medication. These situations typically involve when a licensed practitioner does not have access to a computer or to a prescription form—perhaps in an emergency. If the nurse finds themselves in this type of situation, they must follow these incredibly easy but vital steps.

- Be sure to listen closely to the instruction.
- Repeat it back to the licensed practitioner to ensure the order was heard correctly.
- Listen for confirmation before administering the medication.
- If possible, promptly document the order and the details of the incident in the patient's chart. Make sure that the licensed practitioner reviews and signs all orders as necessary as soon as the patient has stabilized.

It's extremely important to know a facility's policy on accepting and documenting verbal orders. Be aware that many facilities have very specific protocols regarding verbal orders and telephone orders. With the increased prevalence of CPOE and availability of computers, this allows medical orders to be entered and retrieved quickly from virtually any location. CPOE allows providers to enter orders even while away from the health care setting.

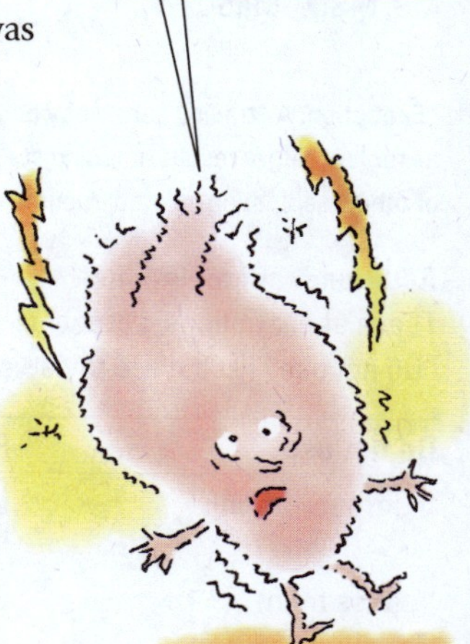

Even in an emergency, make sure all medication orders are complete, clear, and appropriate!

Preparation errors

Another type of error is when the nurse preparing a medication makes an incorrect selection of a medication compound or solution strength, which can be harmful or even fatal to the patient. With practice, nurses can develop a sharp eye for this type of error, as described in the following situations. In both cases, the alert nurses noticed that antineoplastics prepared in the pharmacy appeared suspiciously different and took the appropriate action.

The sleuthing Holmes...

The first case involves a 6-year-old child who was ordered to receive 12 mg of methotrexate intrathecally. The pharmacist handling the order mistakenly selected a 1-g vial of methotrexate instead of a 20-mg vial and reconstituted the medication with 10 mL of normal saline solution. The preparation containing 100 mg/mL was incorrectly labeled as containing 2 mg/mL, and 6 mL of the solution was drawn into a syringe. Although the syringe label indicated 12 mg of methotrexate, the syringe actually contained 600 mg of the medication.

The nurse who received the syringe observed that the medication's color didn't appear normal and returned it to the pharmacy for verification. The pharmacist retrieved the vial that was used to prepare the dose and withdrew the remaining solution into another syringe. Upon comparing the solutions in both syringes and, noting that they matched, concluded that the color change was due to a change in the manufacturer's formula. No one noticed the vial's 1-g label. The alert nurse prevented a potentially serious medication error.

... and Dr. Watson

In a similar case, a 20-year-old patient with leukemia was supposed to receive mitomycin (Mitozytrex) instead of mitoxantrone (Novantrone). These medications are both antineoplastic antibiotics; however, mitoxantrone is a dark blue liquid.

Upon receiving the medication from the pharmacy, the nurse noticed the unusual bluish tint of what was labeled mitomycin and immediately questioned the pharmacist. The pharmacist assured her that the color difference was due to a change in manufacturer, therefore the nurse administered the medication. Upon further investigation, however, it was discovered that the pharmacist had mislabeled a solution of mitoxantrone as mitomycin. Fortunately, the patient suffered no harmful effects.

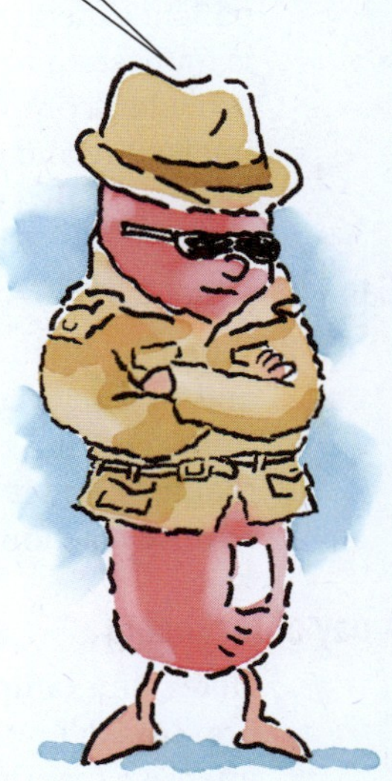

Astute observation is key for any good detective or nurse!

It's elementary!

If a familiar medication seems to have an unfamiliar appearance, investigate the cause. If the pharmacist cites a manufacturing change, ask them to double-check whether they have received verification from the manufacturer. Nurses should always document the appearance discrepancy, the action taken, and the pharmacist's response in the patient record.

Reconciliation errors

Medication errors can occur when communication about medications isn't clear as patients transfer from one health care setting to another.

To prevent this type of error, it's important to obtain, maintain, and communicate an accurate list of the patient's medications whenever new medications are ordered or medication dosages are changed. Some facilities require two registered nurses to reconcile new medication orders by having a chart check due every 12 hours or requiring two nurse signatures with new admissions.

List and compare

Whenever a patient is admitted to a facility, a list is created containing all the patient's current home medications. The nurse should involve the patient and/or their caregiver to make sure that the list is accurate and complete. The nurse can compare the patient's home medications to those ordered by the licensed practitioner and reconcile any discrepancies. Some facilities have strategically placed a pharmacist within the Emergency Department to help assist with medication reconciliation. However, it is ultimately the admitting nurse's responsibility to gather the home medication information and the reconciliation is the sole responsibility of the licensed practitioner.

Patients need education about the medications that they will be taking at home, including new and discontinued medications.

The big hand-off

If the patient is transferred to other areas within the same facility, nurses need to communicate the current list of medications to the next care team and document that communication took place in the patient's medical record. Likewise, if the patient is transferred to another health care facility, provide a complete reconciled list to the receiving facility and document in the patient's medical record that communication took place.

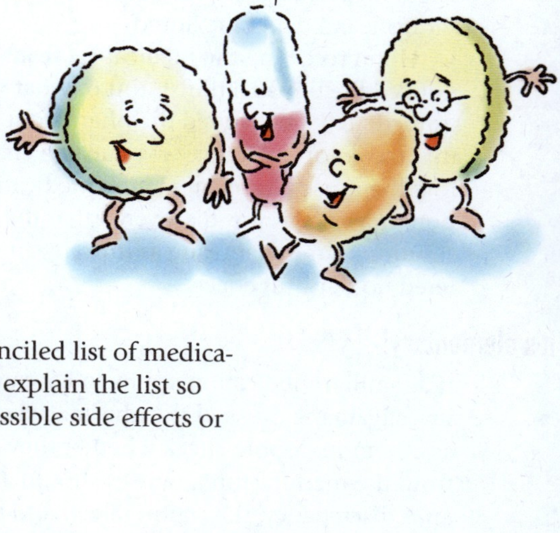

Can I have that to go?

When a patient is discharged home, the patient and/or caregiver needs to receive a complete reconciled list of medications. The nurse needs to take time to review and explain the list so that they understand the medications and any possible side effects or adverse reactions.

A day of reckoning

Here's an example of what can go wrong when a patient's medication list isn't reconciled. A 56-year-old man admitted to the cardiac intensive care unit, suffering from an acute myocardial infarction (heart attack), was prescribed nitroglycerin, morphine, metoprolol, aspirin, and betaxolol (a treatment for glaucoma). Within 2 days, the patient's condition improved, and then transferred to the cardiac step-down unit, where the medication regimen included nitroglycerin, morphine, metoprolol, and aspirin. The following morning, the patient asked the nurse why he hadn't received his eye drops. Had the medication list been reconciled on admission to the step-down unit, this error could have been prevented.

Stress can interfere with job performance and lead to medication errors. Nurses need to be aware of their stress level and seek assistance if it becomes overwhelming.

Stress-related errors

No one will argue that nursing is sometimes a difficult, stressful occupation, even under the best circumstances. Clearly, nurses carry a great deal of responsibility in medication administration, ensuring that the right patient gets the right medication, in the right concentration, at the right time, and by the right route. Interruptions can cause stress and errors when preparing medications. Take time in the medication room or a quiet area to review the medication order and review the rights for medications prior to interacting with a patient.

Recognizing stressors

Too much stress—whether personal, job-related, or environmental—can cause or contribute to medication errors. Nurses should attempt to avoid stress, or at least learn to recognize and minimize it. Doing this will help lower the risk of making errors and maximize the therapeutic effects of patients' medication regimen.

Added stress from error

Committing a serious medication error can cause enormous stress that might cloud a nurse's judgment. If a nurse realizes that a medication error has been made, the best practice is to speak up and seek help immediately instead of trying to remedy the situation themselves, as in the following situation.

A nurse anesthetist administered midazolam (Versed), a sedative, to the wrong patient. Discovering this error, the nurse anesthetist then reaches for a vial thought to be an antidote, flumazenil (Romazicon) and withdraws 2.5 mL of the medication and administers it to the patient. When the patient fails to respond, the nurse anesthetist realized that the vial that was grabbed was not an antidote, but instead a vial of ondansetron (Zofran), an antiemetic. Asking for assistance, another practitioner administered the proper IV administration of flumazenil. The patient recovers unharmed.

Assuring quality and preventing errors

Each facility has its own method of tracking errors in medication administration. Unfortunately, many errors aren't reported because the administering nurses are afraid or don't even recognize the event as an error. What nurses fail to realize, however, is that tracking and reporting errors allows the performance improvement (quality assurance) team to recommend ways to prevent future episodes, thereby benefiting both nurses and patients. Whether a nurse recognizes an error that they made themselves or by another nurse, errors must be reported–even if the nurse who committed the error is a good coworker. It's all about patient safety. Hiding errors benefits no one.

Stepping up to the challenge

On a more personal level, steps can be taken to help decrease the risk of making medication errors. Perhaps the easiest way is to strictly adhere to a facility's policies, suggested safety precautions, and performance improvement recommendations.

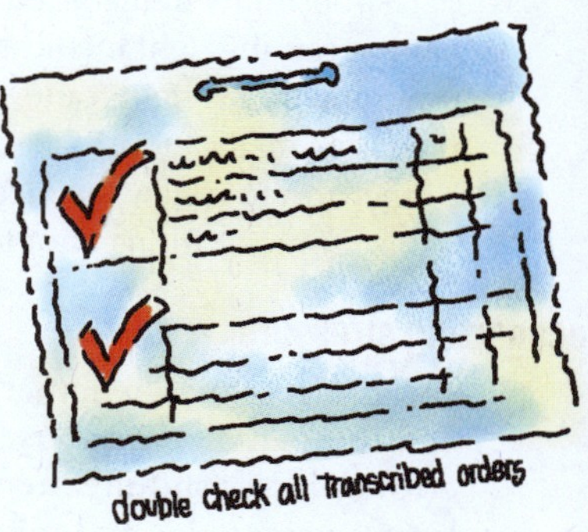
double check all transcribed orders

Other measures that can be taken to avoid errors include being especially careful when transcribing orders from the Physician's Order Sheet to the administration record, being aware of the right to refuse to administer potentially dangerous medications and maintaining a calm and professional demeanor.

Overcoming your fear

Keep in mind that despite the best intentions and circumstances, mistakes are bound to happen eventually. Nurses may very well find themselves in a situation where they have caused or contributed to a medication error. If this occurs, they need to swallow their own fears and take the proper measures and report the incident promptly. Many errors are the result of a system error. By reporting the error, future errors may be prevented.

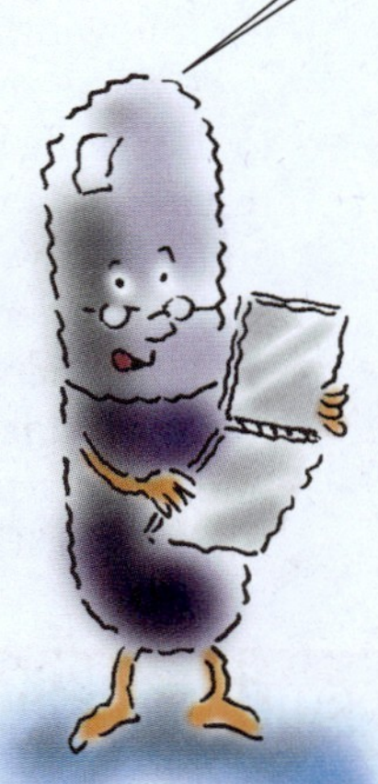
Completing 24-hour chart checks typically falls on the night shift nurses.

Transcribe carefully

Taking the time to carefully document medication orders is one of the easiest ways to prevent errors. To avoid transcription errors, follow these incredibly easy guidelines:

- Transcribe all orders from the Physician's Order Sheet to the administration record in a quiet area, where the nurse can concentrate without interruption.
- Before signing the order sheet and initialing the administration record, carefully check both forms to make sure that the orders have been copied accurately.
- Follow a facility's policy for reviewing orders. Some require nurses to check all patient charts for new orders several times each shift. Others require checking all orders written within the past 24 hours. In many cases, this responsibility falls on the night-shift nurses.

Know your rights

On rare occasions, nurses may be asked to administer a medication that they feel uncomfortable giving to a patient. Be aware that nurses can legally refuse to administer a medication under these circumstances:

- If the nurse thinks the dosage prescribed is too high.
- If the nurse thinks the medication might interact dangerously with other medications the patient is taking; this includes alcohol.
- If the nurse thinks the patient's physical condition contraindicates use of the medication.

The right way to just say "No"

When a nurse refuses to carry out a medication order, follow these steps:

1. Notify the nursing supervisor so alternative arrangements can be made (such as assigning a new nurse or clarifying the order).
2. Notify the licensed practitioner if the nursing supervisor hasn't already done so.
3. Document that the medication wasn't given and explain why (if the facility requires this to be completed).

Keep a cool head

Many medication errors occur because nurses are in a hurry, are under a great deal of stress, or are unfamiliar with a medication. Nurses should try and take their time to avoid distractions and stress. Remember that many medications are derivatives of other medications, and so they have similar names. If a nurse is unfamiliar with a medication, they should use available resources, such as medication references and online medical services, to find out all they can about it. (See *Conquering confusion*, p. 166.)

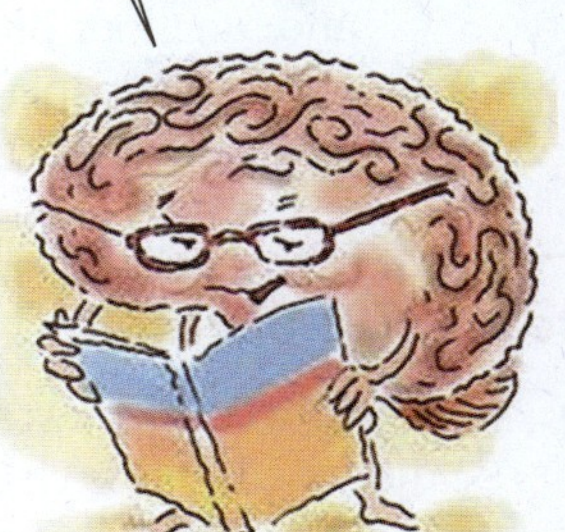

Let's see what the FDA says about this medication!

Report medication errors promptly

As mentioned before, whenever a nurse is involved in a medication error—regardless of who caused the mistake—it needs to be reported and documented immediately, meticulously, and factually.

The right response

If an error occurs, follow these steps:

1. Notify the licensed practitioner and nursing supervisor immediately.
2. Consult the pharmacist. The pharmacist can provide information about medication interactions, solutions to dose-related problems (such as what to do about an overdose or an omitted dose), and an antidote (if needed).

Before you give that medication

Conquering confusion

Before giving medications, nurses need to remind themselves these essential tactics:

Remember the six rights.
Before administering a medication, check that the right *medication*, at the right *dose*, by the right *route*, at the right *time*, to the right *patient*, and include the right *documentation*.

Double-check the math.
Nurses can never be too safe. Review the math at least twice to make sure all the calculations are correct. Have a pharmacist or coworker check the calculations as well.

Look at the label.
Examine medication labels closely—many of them look alike.

Notice the name.
Pay attention! Many medications have similar-sounding or similar-looking names.

3. Follow the facility's policy for documenting medication errors. An incident report may have to be completed for quality and legal purposes. If so, clearly document what happened, include only the facts, without defending any actions, or placing blame. Record the names and functions of everyone involved and what actions they took to protect the patient after the error was discovered. Do *not* document in the patient's chart that an "incident report was completed."

Real-world problem

Here's a complex scenario involving some of the medication errors discussed in this chapter. See if you can unravel what went wrong.

All the wrong moves

The nurse pages the licensed practitioner to ask for an order of an antiemetic for a patient who's complaining of nausea. The licensed practitioner calls the nurse back from the hospital cafeteria, giving a verbal order for the antiemetic prochlorperazine. The nurse documents the order on a patient's chart; however, it's the wrong chart. The nurse receives a call to float to the emergency department; therefore, asks another nurse to administer the medication before leaving the unit.

The second nurse reads the chart with the order for prochlorperazine and administers the medication to the wrong patient. Fortunately, the patient was not harmed after taking the prochlorperazine; however, the patient who should have received it continued to suffer from nausea until the error was corrected.

No hits, no runs... and how many errors?

This situation shows how carelessness and failure to follow proper procedures can lead to various errors. In this particular case, it involved two patients: one who received a medication that shouldn't have, and the other who should have received the medication to treat their complaints of nausea.

Starting from the beginning of the scenario, the verbal order should never have been accepted from the licensed practitioner as this clearly wasn't an emergency. Having the licensed practitioner write the order on the patient's chart or enter it into the computer system could have prevented the medication error.

This case also involved a transcription error; no matter how busy the nurse was, the nurse needed to take the time to make sure that they were documenting on the correct patient's chart. It also demonstrates a compound error because of the number of practitioners involved, each of whom could have taken an extra step to reduce the likelihood of error.

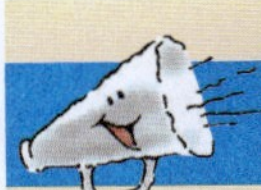

That's a wrap!

Preventing medication errors review

These bullets outline important points about preventing medication errors.

Common medication errors
- Dosage calculation errors
- Medication name errors
- Patient name errors
- Missed allergy alerts
- Compound errors
- Route errors
- Misinterpreted abbreviations
- Misinterpreted orders
- Preparation errors
- Reconciliation errors
- Stress-related errors

Avoiding transcription errors
- Transcribe orders in a quiet area
- Carefully check all work before signing
- Follow the facility's policy for reviewing orders

Refusing to carry out an order
- Notify the nursing supervisor
- Notify the licensed practitioner
- Document according to the facility's policy

The six "rights" of medication administration
- Right medication
- Right dose
- Right route
- Right time
- Right patient
- Right documentation

In case of error
- Notify the licensed practitioner and the nursing supervisor.
- Consult the pharmacist.
- Assess the patient throughout.
- Follow the facility's medication error documentation policy.

Quick quiz

1. Applying the six rights of medication administration will help nurses to do which one?
    A. Save time
    B. Increase medication awareness
    C. Ensure compliance with the medication regimen
    D. Prevent medication errors

Answer: D. The six rights (right medication, dose, patient, time, route, and documentation) help prevent medication errors, thereby promoting patient safety.

2. The nurse is preparing to administer a dose of piperacillin-tazobactam (Zosyn) to a patient with pneumonia. The nurse observes the patient is wearing an allergy alert bracelet and confirms with the patient that they have an allergy to penicillin. Which action should the nurse take?
    A. Administer the medication as ordered.
    B. Notify the nursing supervisor immediately.
    C. Withhold administering the medication and notify the licensed practitioner.
    D. Confirm that the dosage is correct, and then administer the medication.

Answer: C. Patients who are allergic to penicillin shouldn't receive this medication as it is a combination antibiotic containing penicillin. The nurse should withhold the medication and notify the licensed practitioner, who can order an alternative treatment.

3. The nurse prepares to administer ondansetron (Zofran) to a patient but was called to another patient's room. The nurse left the unmarked syringe at the patient's bedside and asked another nurse to administer it. What action should the second nurse take?
    A. Administer the medication in the unlabeled syringe.
    B. Confirm the contents of the syringe with the other nurse before administering it.
    C. Discard the unlabeled syringe in accordance with the facility's policy.
    D. Call the pharmacist to verify that the medication is safe to give.

Answer: C. By discarding this unlabeled syringe, the second nurse eliminates the risk of giving the wrong medication or solution to the patient. Never administer unlabeled syringes or solutions as there is no way to be certain that the right medication is being given. Even if the other nurse confirms the syringe's contents, it's possible that the syringe became mixed up with another one at the bedside. It's best to be safe—draw up and label a new syringe with the medication name and dosage to administer to the patient.

4. The nurse is to administer IV heparin (an anticoagulant), based on the weight of the patient. What would be the most appropriate way to ensure that the medication calculation is correct prior to administration?

A. Check the medication with the pharmacist.
B. Use two patient identifiers prior to administration.
C. Review the concentration of the medication.
D. Have two nurses perform an independent double-check of the calculations based on the patient's order, medication ordered, and patient's weight.

Answer: D. When administering high-alert medication such as an anticoagulant, an independent double-check would be appropriate to reduce the risk of error.

Scoring

☆☆☆ If you answered all four items correctly, fantastic! You haven't misinterpreted a thing.

☆☆ If you answered three items correctly, wonderful! You're avoiding mistakes and calculating your responses well.

☆ If you answered fewer than three items correctly, keep on trying! Dwelling on your errors will only compound the problem.

Suggested References

Condition of participation: Nursing services. The Federal Register: Code of Federal Regulations. (2023). https://www.ecfr.gov/current/title-42/section-482.23

The Federal Register. Federal Register: Code of Federal Regulations. (2023). https://www.ecfr.gov/current/title-42/section-482.24

Institute of Medicine of the National Academies Committee on Identifying and Preventing Medication Errors, Board on Health Care Services. (2007). *Preventing medication errors: Quality chasm series.* National Academies Press.

Institute for Safe Medication Practices (ISMP). (2011). ISMP acute care guidelines for timely administration of scheduled medications. ISMP. https://www.ismp.org/node/361

Institute for Safe Medication Practices (ISMP). (2018). ISMP list of high-alert medications in acute care settings. ISMP.

Institute for Safe Medication Practices. (2020). Error reporting. https://www.ismp.org/report-medication-error

Institute for Safe Medication Practices (ISMP). (2021). ISMP list of error-prone abbreviations, symbols, and dose designations. ISMP.

Institute for Safe Medication Practices (ISMP). (2022). ISMP targeted medication safety best practices for hospitals. ISMP. https://www.ismp.org/guidelines/best-practices-hospitals

Institute for Safe Medication Practices (ISMP). (2023). ISMP list of confused drug names. Plymouth Meeting. https://www.ismp.org/system/files/resources/2023-10/ISMP_ConfusedDrugNames_2023.pdf

Institute for Safe Medication Practices (ISMP). (2023) .Minimizing distractions and interruptions during medication safety tasks. ISMP Medication Safety Alert! Acute Care, *28*(20), 1–3.

ISMP develops guidelines for Standard Order sets. Institute for Safe Medication Practices. (2019). https://www.ismp.org/resources/ismp-develops-guidelines-standard-order-sets

The Joint Commission. (2004). Do not use list fact sheet. https://www.jointcommission.org/resources/news-and-multimedia/fact-sheets/facts-about-do-not-use-list/

The Joint Commission. (2021). Sentinel Event Policy (SE). https://www.jointcommission.org/-/media/tjc/documents/resources/patient-safety-topics/sentinel-event/sentinel-event-policy/camh_24_se_all_current.pdf

Requirements for hospital medication administration, particularly intravenous (iv) medications and post-operative care of patients receiving IV opioids. CMS.gov. (2014). https://www.cms.gov/Medicare/Provider-Enrollment-and-Certification/SurveyCertificationGenInfo/Policy-and-Memos-to-States-and-Regions-Items/Survey-and-Cert-Letter-14-15

Tariq, R. A., Vashisht, R., Sinha, A., Scherbak, Y. (2023). Medication dispensing errors and prevention. [Updated 2023 May 2]. In: *StatPearls [Internet]*. StatPearls Publishing. https://www.ncbi.nlm.nih.gov/books/NBK519065/

Westbrook JI, Woods A, Rob MI, Dunsmuir WTM, Day RO. (2010). Association of interruptions with an increased risk and severity of medication administration errors. *The Archives of Internal Medicine, 170*(8), 683–690. https://doi.org/10.1001/archinternmed.2010.65

Zhu, J., Weingart, S. N. (2022). Prevention of adverse drug events in hospitals. UpToDate. https://www.uptodate.com/contents/prevention-of-adverse-drug-events-in-hospitals?search=Prevention+of+adverse+medication+events+in+hospitals&source=search_result&selectedTitle=1~150&usage_type=default&display_rank=1#H31685292

Part IV

Oral, topical, and rectal medications

Chapter 10

Calculating oral medication dosages

Just the facts

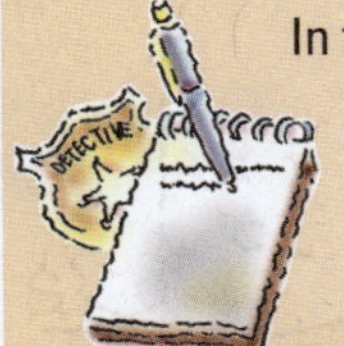

In this chapter, you'll learn how to:

- read medication labels to obtain accurate information for calculations
- administer medications safely
- correctly calculate oral dosages of tablets, capsules, and liquids
- calculate dosages using different measurement systems

A look at oral medications

Medications that are administered orally are usually in tablet, capsule, or liquid form. Most oral medications are available in a limited number of strengths or concentrations. A nurse's ability to calculate prescribed dosages for various medication forms and strengths is an important skill. Nurses don't have an unlimited supply of options.

Reading oral medication labels

To administer oral medication safely, nurses must verify the correct medication and the correct dosage. The first step is to read the label carefully, noting the medication's name, dose strength, and expiration date. Never give a medication from an unlabeled or poorly labeled package or container.

Medication names

All medication labels contain a generic name, the form (how it is supplied), the dose per unit, and the quantity included in the packaging. Some labels can also have the manufacturer's trade name (or name brand) in addition to the generic name.

Generic names

A medication may have several different brand names, but it has only one generic name. A medication is considered "Generic" and referred to the chemical name (aka active ingredient) found in both the generic and the name brands. The Food and Drug Administration (FDA) requires generic medication to contain the same active ingredient as name brands in dosage, route, safety, effectiveness, strength, stability, and quality (FDA, 2011). Generic medications are prescribed 9 out of 10 more times than name brands due to their lower cost to patients. When looking at a label, generic names typically appear in lowercase letters, sometimes in parentheses, and almost always under the manufacturer's trade name for name brands. (See *A look at the label,* p. 175.)

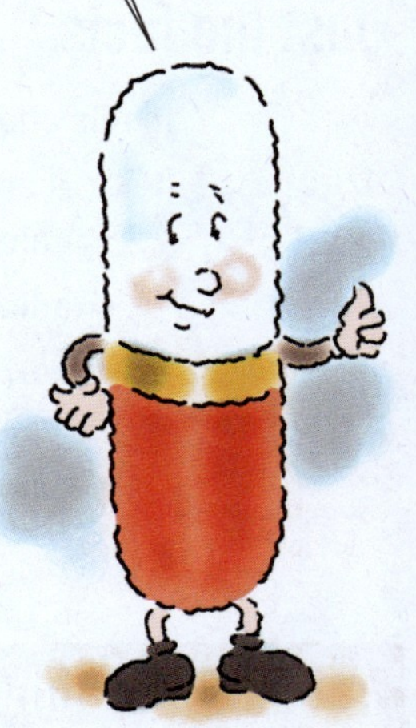

With all the different medications out there, make sure to read the labels carefully!

Trade names

Trade names, also called the *brand* or *proprietary* name, are the names, given by the manufacturer, which typically appear prominently on the label—usually above or before the generic name with the first letter capitalized, followed by the registration symbol. (See *A look at the label,* p. 175.) For example, the generic medication diltiazem goes by the brand names of Cardizem, Tiazac, Dilacor XR, and Cartia XT. Another example includes the generic medication ibuprofen which can be referred their brand names of Advil or Motrin. However, some medications are so widely used and so well known by their generic names that the manufacturer never gives them a trade name. One example is *atropine sulfate.*

Two in one

Some oral medications contain a mixture of two different medications. The labels for these combination medications list both generic names and their doses. These types of medications maybe ordered by their trade name and include the number of capsules, tablets, or the volume of elixir to be given—for example, the medication called Maxzide is a combination of triamterene and hydrochlorothiazide.

Worth a second glance

Whether a generic or trade name is used, be extra careful when reading the label to avoid errors.

Meeting the standard

The initials *U.S.P.* or *N.F.* may appear after the medication name. They stand for two legally recognized standards for medications: *United States Pharmacopeia* and *National Formulary.* These initials mean that a medication has met standards of purity, potency, and storage which are all enforced by the FDA. The FDA regulates and approves all new

Before you give that medication!

A look at the label

Before journeying into complex dosage computations, take a quick tour of this medication label. The brand name (trade name) is in all capitalized and very visible followed by the registered symbol. The generic name can be found directly below in lowercase letters. This medication comes as an oral suspension liquid and the dosage contains 200 mg/5 mL. Therefore, each 1 mL of the solution contains 40 mg of posaconazole. The entire bottle contains 105 mL of the liquid suspension medication.

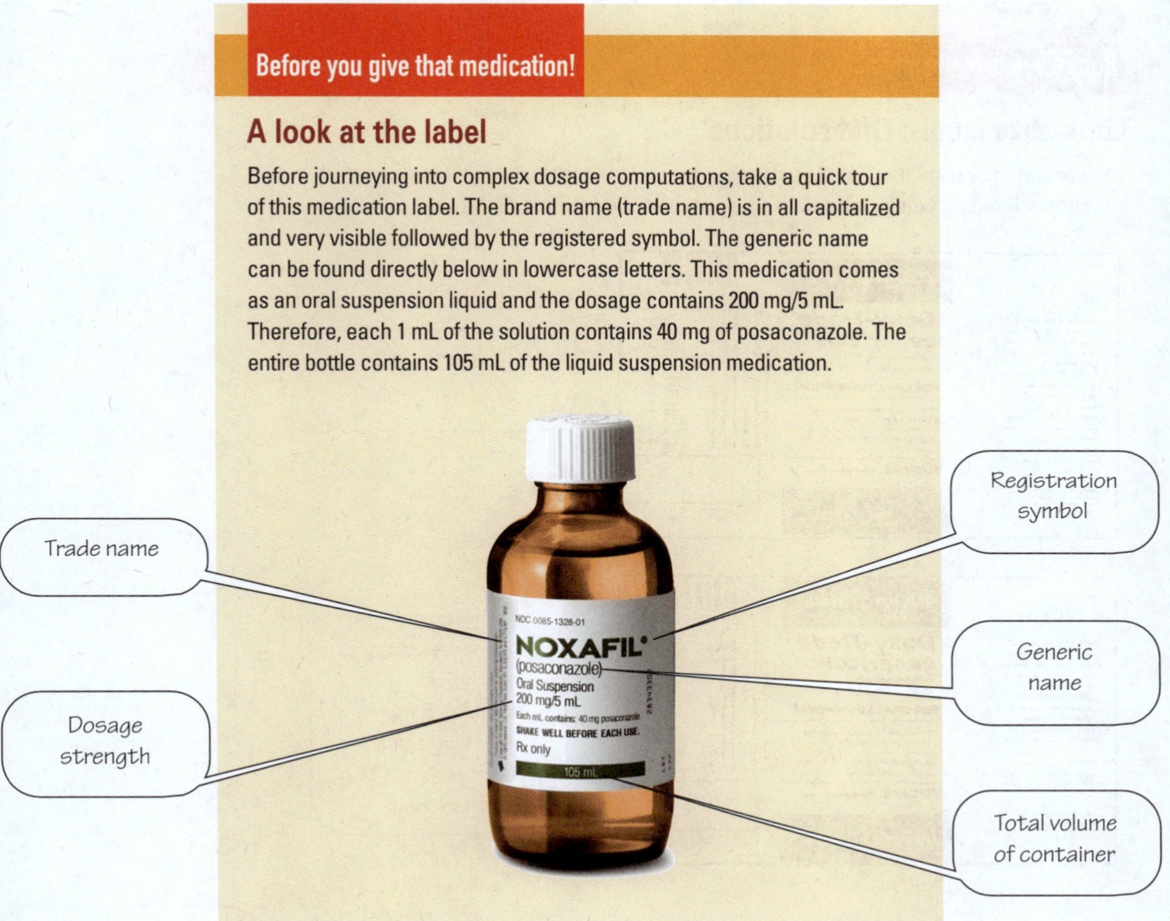

prescription drugs before they can be sold to the public. Over-the-counter drugs, dietary and herbal supplements are reviewed by the FDA for the active ingredient and labeling compliance.

Dose strength

After checking the medication name, look for the dose strength on the label. Pay close attention as some labels and containers may look very similar if not exactly alike but have different dosage concentrations. Other labels may have different medications but have similar packaging of the writing and color scheme. Nurses must be vigilant with verifying medications using the "rights" of medications in addition to three times safety checks. (See *Look-alike labels: Oral solutions*, p. 176.)

Before you give that medication!

Look-alike labels: Oral solutions

The simulated oral solution labels below are examples of look-alikes that you may encounter. Reading labels carefully can help you avoid medication errors.

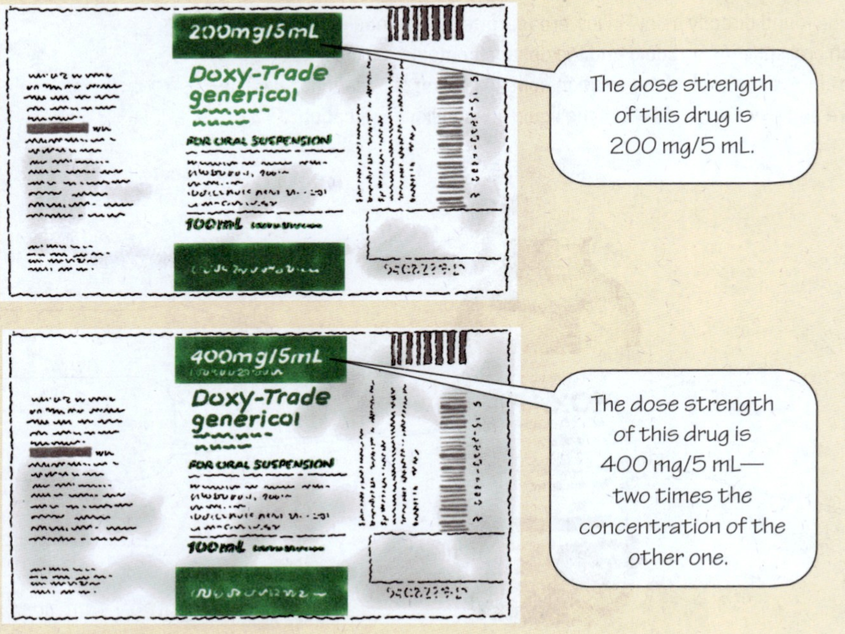

Expiration date

Last, nurses need to check the expiration date. This vital information is commonly overlooked. Expired medications may be chemically unstable or may no longer provide the correct dose. If a medication has expired, return it to the pharmacy so that it can be disposed of properly.

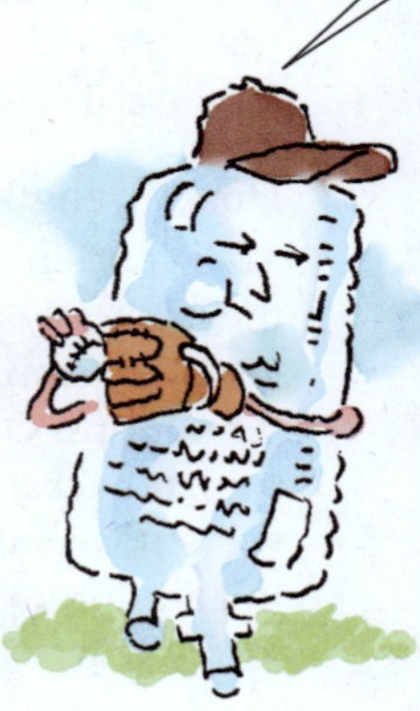

Caught another expired one! Way to go team!

Administering oral medications safely

As discussed earlier in Chapter 9, the most important rule in assuring the safest possible administration of medications is to check the "rights" of medication administration. Historically, nurses have been instructed on the "five rights" of medication administration to reduce medication errors. For this safety concept, one more right was added to total the six "rights" of medication administration:

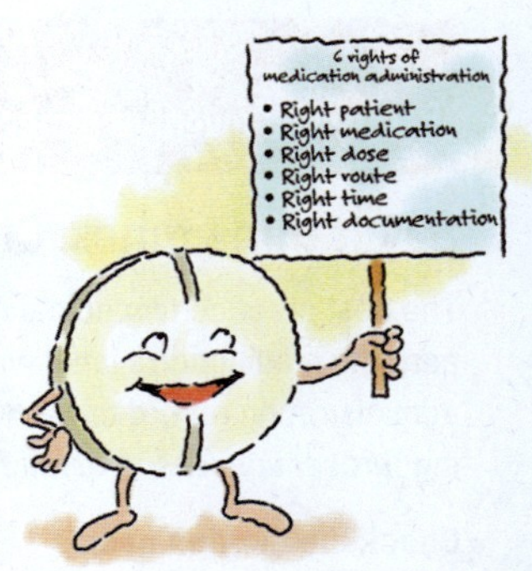

- The right patient
- The right medication
- The right dose
- The right route
- The right time
- and the sixth right of documentation.

Another important rule is to triple-check medication labels and medication orders. Safe medication administration requires nurses to compare the licensed practitioner's order as transcribed on the medication administration record (MAR) against the medication label three times.

(See *Say it three times: Check orders and labels*, p. 178.)

Safety Concerns

Never give medications prepared by someone else or one in an unlabeled container. If an unlabeled container is found, return it to the pharmacy or dispose of it as per the facility's policy. Controlled substances must be cosigned by another nurse prior to disposal. This is the law.

Proceed with safety in mind

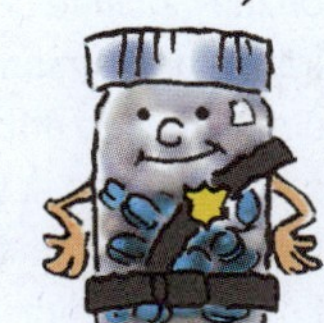

Here are some incredibly easy and essential steps for safe oral medication administration.

The licensed practitioner has ordered *nebivolol (Bystolic) 10 mg PO once daily* for a patient. Before giving this medication, the nurse follows these incredibly easy steps:

Step 1: Removes the medication, either from the patient's medication drawer or from the automated medication dispensing machine.

Step 2: Verifies the correct medication name, dose, and form which is labeled *nebivolol (Bystolic) 10 mg,* and notes that it's an oral tablet.

- If the medication is supplied in a bulk container, the nurse transfers one tablet from the supply to a medication cup, pouring from the supply to the lid and then into the cup without handling the tablet. However, if the medication will be scanned, the nurse leaves it in the unit dose package as the barcode needs to remain intact to scan.

Step 3: Checks the expiration date to ensure that it has not expired.

Step 4: Compares each part of the labeled medication carefully to the order on the MAR or eMar.

Step 5: Next, at the patient's bedside, the nurse verifies the patient's identity using two patient identifiers, and performs the

Before you give that medication!

Say it three times: Check orders and labels

The best practice to medication safety is to check, check, and check again. Before giving a medication, carefully compare the medication's label with each part of the medication administration record (MAR), holding the label next to the administration record to ensure accuracy. The example below walks through the incredibly easy steps for administering *furosemide (Lasix) 40 mg PO.*

Check medication names

- Read the medication's generic name on the MAR or eMAR and compare it to the generic name on the label. Both labels should list *furosemide* somewhere on the label.
- If available, the label may list the brand name of Lasix. Compare and verify this trade name.

Check the dosage, route, and record

- Read the dosage on the MAR or eMAR and compare it to the dose on the unit-dose package label. The nurse may have to remove more than a unit-dose package for the ordered dose. For example, the order is for 40 mg, but only individual 20 mg tablets are available. The nurse would have to remove two individual packages to equal the ordered *40 mg.*
- Read the route specified on the MAR or eMAR and note the dose form on the label. The MAR or eMAR should read *PO* or *by mouth*, and the label should have the word "oral" *in the available form provided (i.e., tablet, capsule, or liquid).*
- The nurse should note any special patient considerations which may include drug allergies or if the patient is on aspiration precautions.
- Nurses need to document not only the administration of all medications at the time they are given, but also any desired effects from the meds given. Examples of this include urine output following the administration of a diuretic, vital signs after administration of a blood pressure medication, or the effectiveness of an analgesic on a patient's complaints of pain.

Special considerations with certain medications

- Some medications can be affected by food or can cause GI upset. Nurses need to be aware of the importance of their timing and whether they should be given with food or on an empty stomach. For example, levothyroxine (Synthroid) a common thyroid medication should be taken daily at least 30 minutes before breakfast.
- Some medications have dietary considerations, such as warfarin (Coumadin), where foods containing vitamin K need to be monitored.
- Some medications should be given at certain times of the day to enhance the quality of life for the patient. One example of this is furosemide (Lasix), a diuretic. Administering a diuretic first thing in the morning allows the patient to void in the morning and sleep easier at night without getting up to use the restroom.

Check orders and labels three times

Follow this routine three times before giving the medication.

- The first time is when obtaining medications from the med cart or dosing machine.
- The second time is before placing the medication in the medication cup or other administration device.
- Last, removing the medication from the unit-dose package at the patient's bedside.

third medication check, comparing the label to the order and verifying the correct administration time. The nurse then administers the medication accordingly.

Remember, if a medication comes in a unit-dose packet, the nurse doesn't remove it from the packaging until at the patient's bedside and ready to administer it. (See *Unit-dose packaging,* p. 179.)

Unit-dose packaging

Tablets or capsules in unit doses may be dispensed on a card with the medications sealed in bubbles or in strips, with each medication separated by a tear line. Unit doses of liquids may be packaged in small, sealed cups with identifying information on the cover.

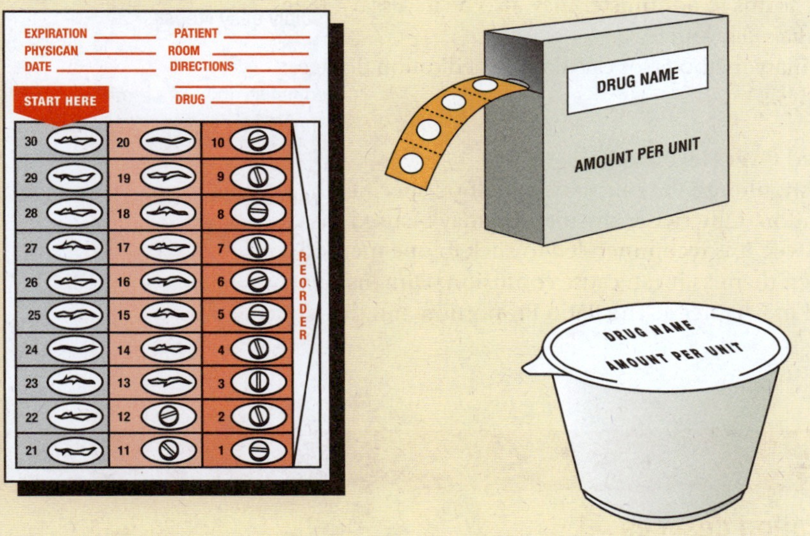

Save time with the unit-dose system

Using the unit-dose medication distribution system not only decreases medication errors, but helps nurses better manage their time with patients!

More exact (that's a fact)
This timesaving system provides the exact dose of medication needed for each patient. The pharmacist computes the number of tablets or the volume of liquid and prepares the proper dose for administration. Errors are decreased because the medication remains in its labeled container until ready to be administered.

Don't throw away your calculator yet
This does not mean nurses are exempt from performing dosage calculations. Some facilities don't use the unit-dose system, and others have systems that don't operate 24 hours per day. Therefore, dosage calculation skills are still vitally important.

Discovering discrepancies

If discrepancies are noted between the MAR or eMAR and the medication label, the nurse needs to clarify and verify the information. For example, suppose the eMAR lists acetaminophen to be given, but the medication available is labeled *cefaclor*. The nurse would need to contact the pharmacy regarding this discrepancy. Pharmacy workers can make mistakes as well as demonstrated in this example, hence the need for nurses to always perform the three safety checks.

Unit-dose systems

Many facilities use the unit-dose system, which provides prepackaged medications in single-dose containers and decreases the need for dosage calculations. (See *Save time with the unit-dose system*.)

Calculating dosages

Despite the prevalence of unit-dose systems, calculations are still necessary in many patient situations. For example, nurses may have to determine individualized dosages for special patients. Conversions between measurement systems to determine how many tablets, capsules, or other dosage forms to administer may also be necessary. (See *Special delivery medication dosages*.)

There are three primary methods for calculating medication dosages:

- Dimensional Analysis
- Ratio Proportion
- Formula or Desired Over Have Method

Nursing students should use the calculation method specified by their academic institution. Otherwise, any method may be used to arrive at the same answer. It is recommended to stick to one method and not to flip between them as it can cause confusion. Dimensional analysis was reviewed in Chapter 4. The Ratio Proportion and the

Advice from the experts

Special delivery medication dosages

Nurses may still need to calculate dosages for some patients even if a facility uses the unit-dose system. For example, patients requiring care in critical care, pediatric, or geriatric areas may need individualized medication dosages that may be unusually large or small.

Nurses may need to calculate specific medications needing to be carried out to the nearest hundredths or even thousands place. (See *Know your places,* p. 25.) The correct calculation of the exact dosage can mean the difference between an underdose or overdose and the correct dose. Many pediatric medications are calculated in this manner.

Changing the delivery route

Although the oral route is considered the safest and preferred route, some people can't tolerate oral medications due to problems with absorption, may be unconscious, or have difficulty swallowing. If this is the case, the nurse may need to contact the licensed practitioner to change PO meds to a different route, such as a parenteral form. The dosing between different routes is usually not interchangeable as noted with IV medications as smaller doses are needed related the "first pass" effect. In other words, IV medications go directly into the bloodstream and bypass the liver therefore having more medication available at the site of action.

Don't forget these special patients

Other patients who need individualized dosages include those with conditions that cause abnormal medication distribution from the GI tract or from parenteral sites to the sites of action. Premature infants and patients with low serum protein levels or severe liver or kidney disease who can't metabolize or excrete medications as readily as normal patients also require special medication dosages. Nurses help individualize medication regimens for these patients by assessing and monitoring their kidney or liver function, monitoring blood levels of medications, and calculating exact dosages.

Formula (desired over have) methods will be used for illustrations purposes in the following chapters.

The following section reviews these mathematical concepts and shows incredibly easy step-by-step calculations.

Advice from the experts

Helpful hints to minimize math mistakes

To avoid math mistakes when computing dosages, use these helpful hints:

- Write out all calculations, using the proper formula.
- Recheck calculations with another nurse or the pharmacist. This should be an independent evaluation of the calculation. Compare results after.

Four rules for calculating medication dosages

To help prevent calculation and medication errors and simplify calculations, remember these four rules. (See *Helpful hints to minimize math mistakes*.)

Rule 1: Use correct units of measure

Using the incorrect unit of measure is one of the most common dosage calculation errors. When calculating doses, match units of measure in the numerator and the denominator so that they cancel each other leaving the correct unit of measure in the answer. Here's an example:

How many milligrams (mg) of medication are in two tablets if one tablet contains 5 mg of the medication?

Step 1: State the problem as a proportion:

$$5 \text{ mg} : 1 \text{ tablet} :: X : 2 \text{ tablets}$$

Step 2: Remember that the product of the means equals the product of the extremes:

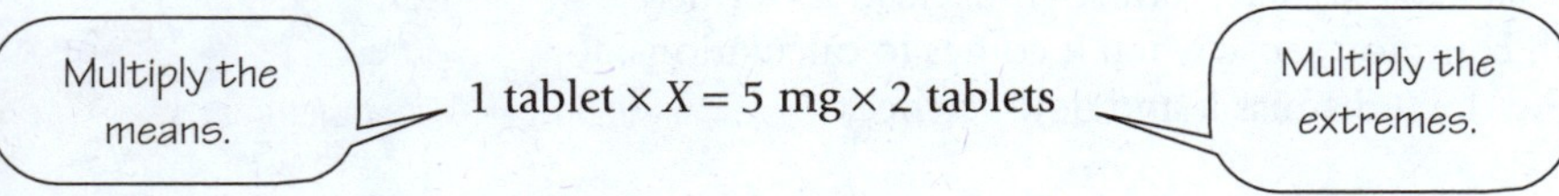
Multiply the means.
1 tablet × X = 5 mg × 2 tablets
Multiply the extremes.

Step 3: Solve for *X*. Divide each side of the equation by the known value, 1 tablet, and cancel units that appear in both the numerator and the denominator:

$$\frac{\cancel{1 \text{ tablet}} \times X}{\cancel{1 \text{ tablet}}} = \frac{5 \text{ mg} \times 2 \cancel{\text{ tablets}}}{1 \cancel{\text{ tablet}}}$$

$$X = 10 \text{ mg}$$

Rule 2: Double-check decimals and zeros

An error in the number of decimal places or zeros in a dosage calculation can cause a 10-fold or greater dosage error. Here's an example using decimals and zeros: The licensed practitioner orders *0.05 mg Synthroid by mouth,* but the only Synthroid on hand is in tablets that contain 0.025 mg each. How many tablets should the nurse give?

Step 1: State the problem as a proportion:

$$0.025 \text{ mg} : 1 \text{ tablet} :: 0.05 \text{ mg} : X$$

Step 2: The product of the means equals the product of the extremes:

$$1 \text{ tablet} \times 0.05 \text{ mg} = 0.025 \text{ mg} \times X$$

Step 3: Solve for *X*. Divide each side of the equation by 0.025 mg and cancel units that appear in both the numerator and the denominator. Be careful with decimal placement:

$$\frac{1 \text{ tablet} \times 0.05 \cancel{\text{mg}}}{0.025 \cancel{\text{mg}}} = \frac{\cancel{0.025 \text{ mg}} \times X}{\cancel{0.025 \text{ mg}}}$$

$$X = 2 \text{ tablet}$$

The nurse should administer 2 tablets.

Rule 3: Question strange answers

Nurses should question and recheck suspicious-looking calculations. For example, if a dosage calculation suggests giving 15 tablets or 200 mL of a suspension liquid, assume that there is an error and recheck the calculation. If still unsure of the results, have another nurse double-check the calculations.

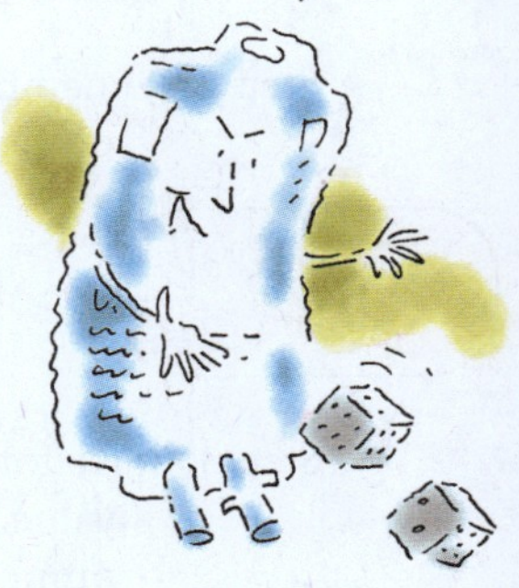
Don't roll the dice when it comes to medication calculations. If the answer seems odd, double-check the numbers!

Rule 4: Get out the calculator

A handheld calculator can improve the accuracy and speed of calculations, *but it can't guarantee accuracy*. Nurses must also use critical thinking along with common sense when it comes to calculations. If it doesn't seem right, don't dismiss it and double-check!

Special considerations

Occasionally when administering oral medications, nurses may come across unusual situations that require extra steps to be taken.

Divided doses

Most tablets, capsules, and similar dose forms are available in only a few strengths. On occasion, scored tablets may have to be split in half to administer the proper dosage. For example, a patient has a stat order for 0.5 mg PO alprazolam (Xanax) but is only available in a 1 mg scored tablet. The nurse will have to break (split) the scored tablet to provide the correct dose.

When a medication dose requires needing only a half of a tablet or a smaller portion, the tablet should be scored. Scored tablets provide for more accurate dosing. Nurses should contact the pharmacist if half of a tablet is needed but the medication is not scored.

Before you give that medication!

Be cautious with tablets and capsules

For patients who have difficulty swallowing, a common solution is to crush tablets or open capsules but in doing so, can alter how the medication is absorbed and cause patient harm. Nurses need to consult their available resources to verify if a tablet can be crushed or capsule opened. Also, the pharmacy may be to offer smaller dosage strengths or in liquid form for those patients who have difficulty swallowing. As a reference, these medications shouldn't be broken or crushed:

- Sustained-release medications can also be called *extended-release, delayed-release, timed-release*, or *controlled-release. These types of medications usually have s*uffixes in the name such as "SR," "CR," "DUR," "XR," "CD," and "LA."
- Capsules contain tiny beads of medication surrounded by a gelatin-based shell (hard or soft). Most capsules should not be opened or crushed, however, there are a few that can be opened and served with applesauce or pudding for patients with difficulty in swallowing.
- Enteric-coated (EC) tablets are tablets which have a hard coating (usually shiny or glossy) that's designed to protect the upper GI tract from irritation. Aspirin is often prescribed in EC form to patients needing to take it over a long period of time to prevent stomach irritation.
- Buccal and sublingual tablets are designed to be absorbed in the cheek or under the tongue and should not be crushed.

Tips for crushing and breaking

There are several different methods nurses can use to crush tablets. One method is to crush the tablet while it's still in its package, using a type of pill crusher. Another method is to remove it from the package and crush it with a mortar and pestle or a different commercial product for crushing medication.

As described earlier, tablets needing to be split (broken) should already come scored. Using a pill cutter, carefully cut the tablet on the score line. If a smaller dose is needed and is not scored, consult the pharmacist for assistance.

Breaking a scored tablet in portions smaller than one-half is not recommended as it usually creates inaccurate doses. If a smaller dose is needed, the nurse should contact the pharmacy for a possible substitution.

On the other hand, some oral preparations shouldn't be opened, broken, scored, or crushed because those actions change the medication's effect. (See *Be cautious with tablets and capsules*.)

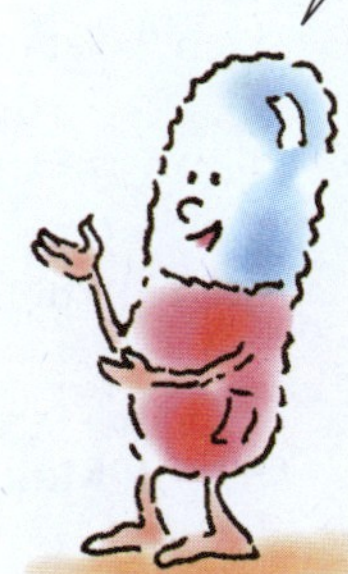

It is best to check with a medication book or pharmacist before I am opened!

Real-world problems

When using the Ratio Proportion method to calculate the number of tablets to administer, set up the first ratio or fraction with the known tablet strength. Set up the second ratio or fraction with the prescribed dose and the unknown quantity of tablets or capsules, then solve for X to determine the correct dose. Here are some typical patient situations.

The acetaminophen answer

The licensed practitioner orders *650 mg acetaminophen PO × 1 now,* for a patient, but the medication is available only in 325-mg tablets. How many tablets should the nurse give?

Here's the calculation using ratios.

Step 1: Set up the first ratio with the known tablet strength:

$$325 \text{ mg}:1 \text{ tablet}$$

Step 2: Set up the second ratio with the desired dose and the unknown number of tablets:

$$650 \text{ mg}:X$$

Step 3: Put these ratios into a proportion:

$$325 \text{ mg}:1 \text{ tablet}::650 \text{ mg}:X$$

Step 4: Set up the equation by multiplying the means and extremes:

$$1 \text{ tablet} \times 650 \text{ mg} = 325 \text{ mg} \times X$$

Step 5: Solve for *X*. Divide both sides of the equation by 325 mg and cancel units that appear in both the numerator and the denominator:

$$\frac{1 \text{ tablet} \times 650 \cancel{\text{mg}}}{325 \cancel{\text{mg}}} = \frac{\cancel{325 \text{ mg}} \times X}{\cancel{325 \text{ mg}}}$$

$$X = 2 \text{ tablets}$$

The nurse should administer 2 tablets to the patient.

The clozapine clue

A patient is prescribed *250 mg clozapine PO daily.* The medication is available in 100 mg per tablet. How many tablets should the nurse administer?

Here's the calculation using ratios.

Step 1: Set up the first ratio with the known tablet strength:

$$100 \text{ mg}:1 \text{ tablet}$$

Step 2: Set up the second ratio with the desired dose and the unknown number of tablets:

$$250 \text{ mg}:X$$

Step 3: Put these ratios into a proportion:

$$100 \text{ mg}:1 \text{ tablet}::250 \text{ mg}:X$$

Step 4: Multiply the means and the extremes:

$$1 \text{ tablet} \times 250 \text{ mg} = 100 \text{ mg} \times X$$

Step 5: Solve for X. Divide each side of the equation by 100 mg and cancel units that appear in both the numerator and the denominator:

$$\frac{1 \text{ tablet} \times 250 \cancel{\text{ mg}}}{100 \cancel{\text{ mg}}} = \frac{\cancel{100 \text{ mg}} \times X}{\cancel{100 \text{ mg}}}$$

$$X = \frac{250 \text{ tablet}}{100}$$

$$X = 2.5, \text{ or } 2\tfrac{1}{2} \text{ tablets}$$

The nurse should administer 2.5 or 2½ tablets to the patient. Since the tablets need to be split, the tablets should be scored.

Dosage drill

Test your math skills with this drill

A patient has been taking 500-mg tablets of acetaminophen (Tylenol) by mouth for postoperative pain after an inguinal hernia repair. If the patient took a total of 1,500 mg in 24 hours, how many tablets did the patient take?

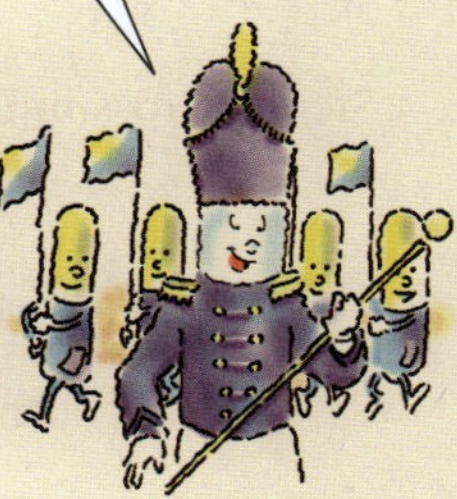
Be sure to show how you arrive at your answer.

Your answer: ____________

To find the answer, set up ratios and a proportion and solve for X.

$$500 \text{ mg} : 1 \text{ tab} :: 1{,}500 \text{ mg} : X \text{ tab}$$

$$500 \text{ mg} \times X = 1 \times 1{,}500 \text{ mg}$$

$$500X = 1{,}500$$

$$X = \frac{1{,}500}{500}$$

$$X = 3 \text{ tablets}$$

The patient took 3 tablets.

Gliding through glyburide

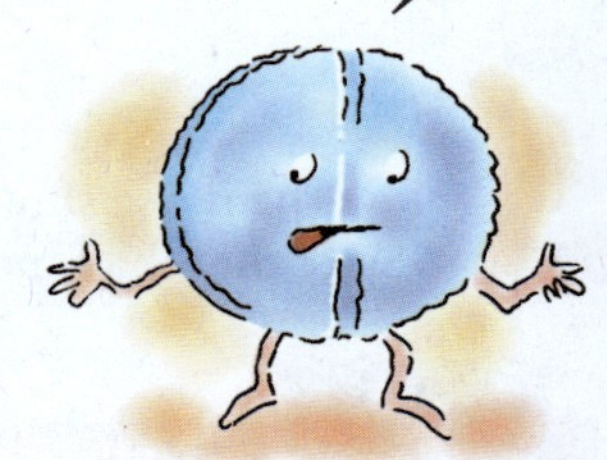

Don't forget to check the expiration dates on all medications!

An order reads *Give 3 tablets of glyburide 1.5-mg tablets PO daily*. How many milligrams (mg) will the patient receive daily?

Here's the solution using fractions.

Step 1: Set up the first fraction with the known tablet strength:

$$\frac{1.5 \text{ mg}}{1 \text{ tablet}}$$

Step 2: Set up the second fraction with the desired dose and the unknown number of mg:

$$\frac{X}{3 \text{ tablets}}$$

Step 3: Put these fractions into a proportion:

$$\frac{X}{3 \text{ tablets}} = \frac{1.5 \text{ mg}}{1 \text{ tablet}}$$

Step 4: Cross-multiply the fractions:

$$X \times 1 \text{ tablet} = 3 \text{ tablets} \times 1.5 \text{ mg}$$

Step 5: Solve for X. Divide both sides of the equation by 1 tablet and cancel units that appear in both the numerator and the denominator:

$$\frac{X \times \cancel{1 \text{ tablet}}}{\cancel{1 \text{ tablet}}} = \frac{3 \cancel{\text{ tablets}} \times 1.5 \text{ mg}}{1 \cancel{\text{ tablet}}}$$

$$X = 4.5 \text{ mg}$$

The patient will receive 4.5 mg of glyburide daily.

Calculating liquid dosages

In addition to tablets, patients can also receive liquid medications in suspension or elixir form. To calculate a dosage in liquid form, carefully read the label to identify the dose strength that is available in the specified amount of solution.

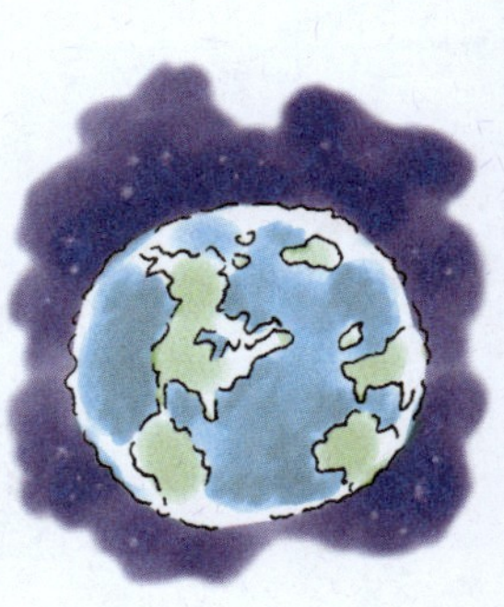

More real-world problems

Use the Ratio Proportion Method to solve each of the following problems.

Step 1: Set up the first ratio or fraction with the known solution strength.

Step 2: Set up the second ratio or fraction with the desired dose and the unknown quantity.

Step 3: Solve for X to find the correct dose.

Here are some typical patient situations.

Pay attention to the suspension

A patient is receiving 500 mg of cefaclor oral suspension by mouth every 8 hours for pneumonia. The label reads *cefaclor 250 mg/5 mL*, and the bottle contains 100 mL. How many mL of cefaclor should the patient take for each dose? *Remember not to be confused by the medication being ordered three times daily. The question is asking for the amount of mL of medication per dose, not for the daily amount.

Here's the solution using fractions.

Step 1: Set up the first fraction with the known solution strength:

$$\frac{5\text{ mL}}{250\text{ mg}}$$

Step 2: Set up the second fraction with the desired dose and the unknown number of mL:

$$\frac{X}{500\text{ mg}}$$

Step 3: Put these fractions into a proportion:

$$\frac{X}{500\text{ mg}} = \frac{5\text{ mL}}{250\text{ mg}}$$

Step 4: Cross-multiply the fractions:

$$X \times 250\text{ mg} = 5\text{ mL} \times 500\text{ mg}$$

Step 5: Solve for X. Divide both sides of the equation by 250 mg and cancel units that appear in both the numerator and the denominator:

$$\frac{X \times \cancel{250\text{ mg}}}{\cancel{250\text{ mg}}} = \frac{5\text{ mL} \times 500\ \cancel{\text{mg}}}{250\ \cancel{\text{mg}}}$$

$$X = \frac{2{,}500\text{ mL}}{250}$$

$$X = 10\text{ mL}$$

The patient should take 10 mL of cefaclor per dose.

Note this: If the problem asked for the *daily total* of the medication in mL in the problem above, how would this answer be calculated? (Hint: It's ordered *three* times a *day*.)

Answer: 30 mL daily

Dosage drill

Test your math skills with this drill

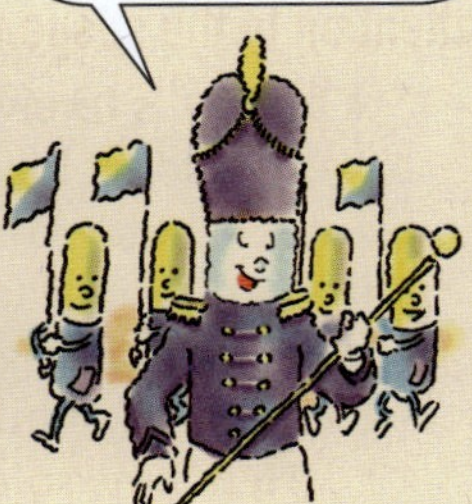
Be sure to show how you arrive at your answer.

The licensed practitioner orders 0.125 mg of digoxin (Lanoxin) elixir PO daily for a patient developing heart failure and pulmonary edema. The bottle is labeled 0.05 mg/mL. How many mL should the nurse administer?

Your answer: ________________

To find the answer, set up ratios and a proportion and solve for *X*.

$$0.05\text{ mg}:1\text{ mL}::0.125\text{ mg}:X\text{ mL}$$

$$0.05\text{ mg} \times X\text{ mL} = 0.125\text{ mg} \times 1\text{ mL}$$

$$\frac{\cancel{0.05\text{ mg}} \times X\text{ mL}}{\cancel{0.05\text{ mg}}} = \frac{0.125\ \cancel{\text{mg}} \times 1\text{ mL}}{0.05\ \cancel{\text{mg}}}$$

$$X = \frac{0.125\text{ mL}}{0.05}$$

$$X = 2.5\text{ mL}$$

The nurse should administer 2.5 mL of digoxin.

Erythromycin enigma

A patient has an order for 400 mg of erythromycin oral suspension PO twice daily for an active infection. The label reads *erythromycin 200 mg/5 mL*. How many mL should the nurse give to the patient? *Remember not to be confused by the medication being ordered three times daily. The question is asking how much per dose and not the daily total!

Here's the calculation using ratios.

Step 1: Set up the first ratio with the known solution strength:

$$5 \text{ mL:}200 \text{ mg}$$

Step 2: Set up the second ratio with the unknown number of mL and the desired dose:

$$X\text{:}400 \text{ mg}$$

Step 3: Put these ratios into a proportion:

$$5 \text{ mL:}200 \text{ mg::}X\text{:}400 \text{ mg}$$

Step 4: Set up an equation by multiplying the means and extremes:

$$X \times 200 \text{ mg} = 5 \text{ mL} \times 400 \text{ mg}$$

Step 5: Solve for *X*. Divide both sides of the equation by 200 mg and canceling units that appear in both the numerator and the denominator:

$$\frac{X \times 200 \cancel{\text{mg}}}{200 \cancel{\text{mg}}} = \frac{5 \text{ mL} \times 400 \cancel{\text{mg}}}{200 \cancel{\text{mg}}}$$

$$X = \frac{2{,}000 \text{ mL}}{200}$$

$$X = 10 \text{ mL}$$

The nurse should give 10 mL of erythromycin.

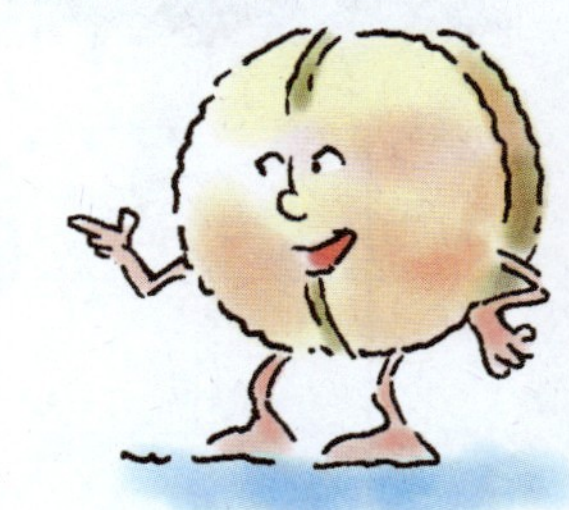

Once the proportion is set up, it's all about multiplication and division! Use a calculator to help with accuracy!

Don't dally over dilantin doses

The licensed practitioner orders *100 mg phenytoin sodium (Dilantin) oral suspension PO TID* (three times a day) for a patient with a history of seizures. The label reads *Dilantin (phenytoin sodium) 125 mg/5 mL*. How many mL should the nurse give to the patient?

Here's the calculation using ratios.

Step 1: Set up the first fraction with the known solution strength:

$$5 \text{ mL:}125 \text{ mg}$$

Step 2: Set up the second fraction with the unknown number of mL and the desired dose:

$$X\text{:}100 \text{ mg}$$

Dosage drill

Test your math skills with this drill

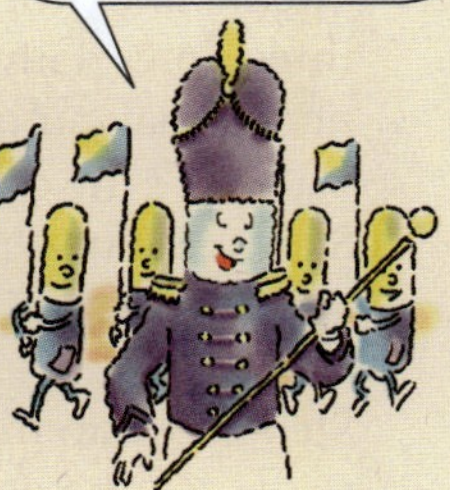
Be sure to show how you arrive at your answer.

A licensed practitioner orders 25 g of lactulose (Cephulac) PO once for a patient in liver failure. The bottle is labeled lactulose 10 g/15 mL. How many mL of lactulose should the patient receive?

Your answer: ______________

To find the answer, set up ratios and a proportion and solve for X.

$$10 \text{ g}:15 \text{ mL}::25 \text{ g}:X \text{ mL}$$

$$10 \text{ mg} \times X \text{ mL} = 15 \text{ mL} \times 25 \text{ mg}$$

$$\frac{\cancel{10 \text{ mg}} \times X \text{ mL}}{\cancel{10 \text{ mg}}} = \frac{15 \text{ mL} \times 25 \cancel{\text{ mg}}}{10 \cancel{\text{ mg}}}$$

$$X = \frac{375 \text{ mL}}{10}$$

$$X = 37.5 \text{ mL}$$

The patient should receive 37.5 mL of the lactulose.

Step 3: Put these ratios into a proportion:

$$X:100 \text{ mg}::5 \text{ mL}:125 \text{ mg}$$

Step 4: Set up an equation by multiplying the means and extremes:

$$100 \text{ mg} \times 5 \text{ mL} = 125 \text{ mg} \times X$$

Step 5: Solve for X. Divide each side of the equation by 125 mg and cancel units that appear in both the numerator and the denominator:

$$\frac{100\ \cancel{\text{mg}} \times 5\ \text{mL}}{125\ \cancel{\text{mg}}} = \frac{\cancel{125\ \text{mg}} \times X}{\cancel{125\ \text{mg}}}$$

$$X = \frac{500\ \text{mL}}{125}$$

$$X = 4\ \text{mL}$$

The nurse should give 4 mL of phenytoin sodium (Dilantin).

To set up a proportion, the nurse needs to know what is needed, what is available, and what isn't known.

Diluting powders

Some medications become unstable when they're stored as liquids, therefore they're supplied in powder form. Before giving these medications, they need to be diluted or mixed with the appropriate diluent, according to the manufacturer's directions. Read the medication label carefully to see what type and how much diluent to add to the powder.

After adding the diluent and mixing thoroughly, read the label again to determine what the final concentration of the medication is available.

Weighing in

The dose concentration in oral solutions is expressed as the weight—or dose strength—of the medication contained in a volume of solution. For example, a furosemide (Lasix) oral solution is provided as 10 mg/mL. Therefore, the solution contains 10 mg of furosemide (Lasix) (medication strength) in 1 mL (solution volume).

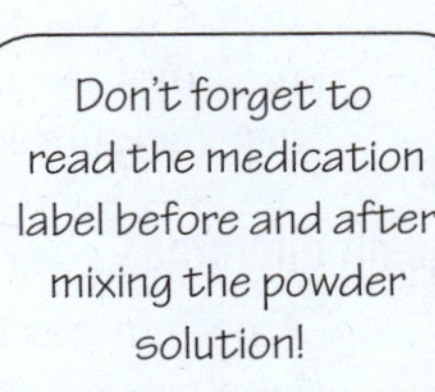

Don't forget to read the medication label before and after mixing the powder solution!

Measuring oral solutions

To administer an oral solution accurately, measure it with a medicine cup, dropper, or syringe.

Good to the last drop

Medicine cups are calibrated to measure solutions in milliliters, tablespoons, teaspoons, drams, and ounces. For accuracy, hold the cup at eye level while pouring the solution. Also, hold the solution container with the medication label turned toward the palm of your hand so that the solution doesn't drip over the label when poured.

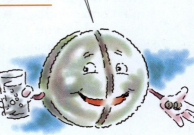

For good measure

Medications that are prescribed in drops are usually packaged with a dropper. If a dropper was not included, use a standard dropper as it can be used to measure solutions in milliliters or teaspoons. After measuring and administering a medication from a multiple-dose container, store it as directed on the medication label.

Syringe cringe

Syringes are handy for drawing up and measuring solutions accurately. However, never use an IV syringe to administer an oral medication. Use only an oral or enteral syringe for oral medication administration. This type of syringe has FOR ORAL USE ONLY written on the syringe and does not have the ability to attach to an IV hub/site. In addition, some oral or enteral syringes are amber in color to make them stand out from IV syringes. Nurse must also not forget to remove the plastic tip before administering the medication to prevent the aspiration of it.

Advice from the experts

When you need a new measure

When needing to convert measurements, remember these tips:

- Read the medication order thoroughly, paying close attention to decimal places and zeros.
- Convert the dose from the system in which it's ordered to the system in which it's available.
- Calculate the number of capsules or tablets or the amount of solution needed to obtain the desired dose.

Two-step dosage calculations

Most dosage calculations require more than one equation. For example, a licensed practitioner may order a medication in grams, but is only available in milligrams. When this happens, the nurse needs to convert from one measurement to another before determining how much medication to administer. (See *When you need a new measure*.)

Digoxin dilemma

A patient has an order for *62.5 mcg of digoxin elixir PO daily.* The elixir label reads *0.05 mg/mL.* How many mL of digoxin should the nurse give?

Here's how to solve this problem using ratios.

Step 1: Convert micrograms to milligrams. Recall that 1,000 mcg equals 1 mg.

Step 2: Set up the first ratio with the standard equivalent value:

$$1 \text{ mg}:1{,}000 \text{ mcg}$$

Step 3: Set up the second ratio with the unknown quantity in the appropriate position:

$$X:62.5 \text{ mcg}$$

Step 4: Put these ratios into a proportion:

$$1 \text{ mg}:1{,}000 \text{ mcg}::X:62.5 \text{ mcg}$$

Step 5: Multiply the means and the extremes:

$$X \times 1{,}000 \text{ mcg} = 1 \text{ mg} \times 62.5 \text{ mcg}$$

Step 6: Solve for X. Divide both sides of the equation by 1,000 mcg and cancel units that appear in both the numerator and the denominator:

$$\frac{X \times 1{,}000\ \cancel{\text{mcg}}}{1{,}000\ \cancel{\text{mcg}}} = \frac{1\ \text{mg} \times 62.5\ \cancel{\text{mcg}}}{1{,}000\ \cancel{\text{mcg}}}$$

$$X = \frac{62.5\ \text{mg}}{1{,}000}$$

$$X = 0.0625\ \text{mg}$$

Dosage drill

Test your math skills with this drill

A patient is to receive 0.25 mg of Synthroid PO daily. The medication is only available in tablets that contain 125 mcg each. How many tablets should the nurse administer?

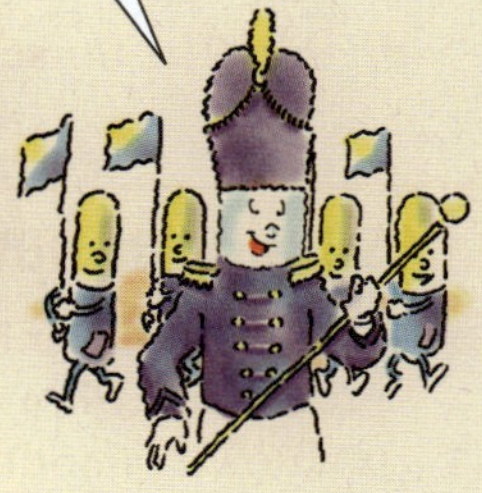
Be sure to show how you arrive at your answer.

Your answer: ____________

To find the answer, remember to convert first (keep in mind that 1 mg equals 1,000 mcg). Then use ratios and a proportion to solve for X.

$$1\ \text{mg}:1{,}000\ \text{mcg}::0.25\ \text{mg}:X\ \text{mcg}$$

$$1\ \text{mg} \times X\ \text{mcg} = 1{,}000\ \text{mcg} \times 0.25\ \text{mg}$$

$$X = 250\ \text{mcg}$$

$$250\ \text{mcg}:X\ \text{tablets}::125\ \text{mcg}:X\ \text{tablets}$$

$$250 = 125X$$

$$X = \frac{250}{125}$$

$$X = 2\ \text{tablets}$$

The nurse should administer 2 tablets.

Step 7: The prescribed dose is 62.5 mcg, or 0.0625 mg. Calculate the number of mL to be given by setting up a proportion:

$$0.0625 \text{ mg}:X::0.05 \text{ mg}:1 \text{ mL}$$

Step 8: Set up an equation by multiplying the means and extremes:

$$X \times 0.05 \text{ mg} = 1 \text{ mL} \times 0.0625 \text{ mg}$$

Step 9: Solve for X. Divide each side of the equation by 0.05 mg and cancel units that appear in both the numerator and the denominator:

$$\frac{X \times \cancel{0.05 \text{ mg}}}{\cancel{0.05 \text{ mg}}} = \frac{1 \text{ mL} \times 0.0625 \ \cancel{\text{mg}}}{0.05 \ \cancel{\text{mg}}}$$

$$X = \frac{0.0625 \text{ mL}}{0.05}$$

$$X = 1.25 \text{ mL}$$

The nurse should give 1.25 mL of the elixir.

The desired over have or formula method

Nurses overall prefer using the "desired over have method" to perform their dosage calculations.

The desired over have method is another way to solve two-step problems. This method uses fractions to express the known and unknown quantities:

$$X = \frac{\text{Desired dose (D)}}{\text{Have on hand (H)}} \times \text{Quantity (Q)}$$

D/H × Q = X, or desired dose (amount) = ordered dose amount/amount on hand × quantity.

D = Desired dose or ordered dose

H = Have on hand or what is available

Q = Quantity—the form and amount in which the medication is supplied

X = answer

The following three problems show how to use the desired over have method.

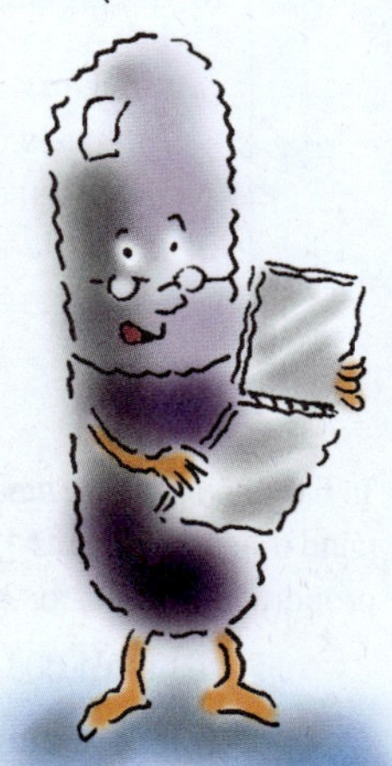

Acetaminophen alley

The order reads *acetaminophen elixir 650 mg PO × 1 now*. The pharmacy sends *acetaminophen* (Tylenol) 325 mg/5 mL. How many mL does the nurse give?

Here's the calculation.

Step 1: Set up the formula with the information provided:

- Desired dose: 650 mg
- Have on hand: 325 mg
- Quantity: 5 mL

*Note that both the desired amount (D) and the available amount (H) are the same units of measure and do not need converting.

$$X = \frac{650 \text{ mg}}{325 \text{ mg}} \times 5 \text{ mL}$$

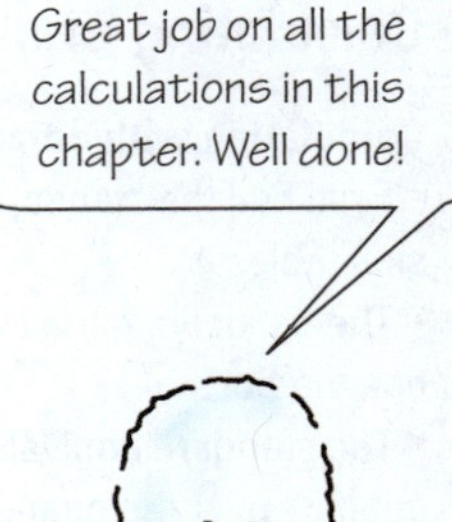

Great job on all the calculations in this chapter. Well done!

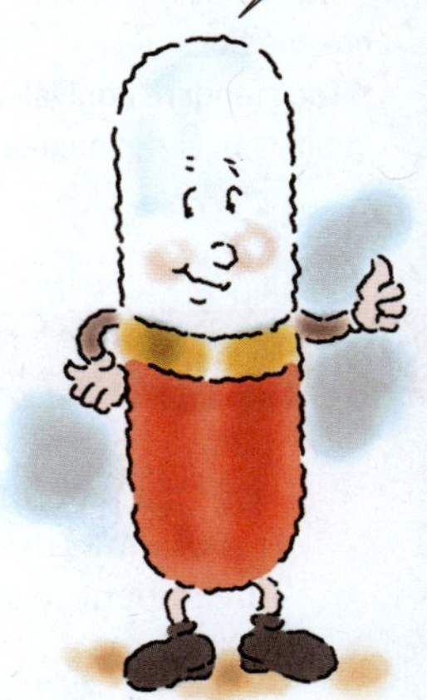

Step 2: Cancel the units that appear in both the numerator and the denominator:

$$X = \frac{650 \cancel{\text{mg}}}{325 \cancel{\text{mg}}} \times 5 \text{ mL}$$

Step 3: Multiply the desired dose by quantity (650×5):

$$X = \frac{3{,}250 \text{ mL}}{325}$$

Step 4: Solve for X. Divide the numerator by the denominator ($3{,}250 \div 325$):

$$X = 10 \text{ mL}$$

The dose to be given is 10 mL of acetaminophen elixir.

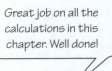

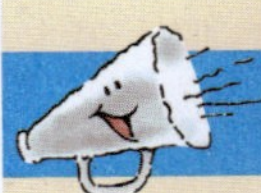

That's a wrap!

Calculating oral medication dosages review

Keep these important facts in mind when calculating doses of oral medications.

Reading oral medication labels

- First, check the medication's generic name and, if available, trade name. Remember that combination medications are usually ordered using the trade name.
- Then, check the dose strength and verify the route.
- Last, check the expiration date.

Safe oral medication administration

- Check the six "rights" of medication administration.
- Compare medication names, the dose, and route from the label to the MAR or eMAR
- Review and note any special considerations.
- Check orders and labels three times.

Dosage calculation key

- Use correct units of measure.
- Double-check units of measure and decimal places.
- Check answers that seem wrong.
- Use a calculator.

Liquid dosages

- Read medication labels carefully: the medication concentration is expressed as the dose strength contained in a volume of solution.
- Dilute powders with the appropriate diluent according to the manufacturer's directions.
- Measure oral solutions with a medicine cup, dropper, or syringe.

(continued)

Calculating oral medication dosages review (*continued*)

Calculating with different systems

- First, find the standard equivalent value with a conversion table.
- Then, calculate the dosage using the ratio and proportion method.
- The standard equivalent values equal the unknown quantity over the quantity ordered.

Desired over have method

- The amount desired (D) over the amount available on hand (H) multiplied by the quantity (Q) equals the amount to be given (X).
- Verify that the units of measure in the numerator and the denominator correspond to one another.

Quick quiz

1. If a patient is ordered 100 mcg of levothyroxine (Synthroid) by mouth and the available dose is 25 mcg/tablet, how many tablets will the patient receive?

A. 2
B. 3
C. 4
D. 6

Answer: C. If 1 tablet provides 25 mcg, divide 100 by 25 to get the answer: 4 tablets.

2. If 250 mg of clozapine (Clozaril) is ordered for a patient to be given orally, but only 100-mg tablets are available, how many tablets should the nurse administer?

A. 2 tablets
B. 2½ tablets
C. 3 tablets
D. 3½ tablets

Answer: B. By dividing 250 by 100, you get 2.5, or 2½ tablets.

3. A patient has an order for potassium chloride 75 mEq PO daily in three equally divided doses. Available: potassium chloride 20 mEq/15 mL. How many mL of potassium will the patient receive in one of the divided doses?

A. 56.25 mL
B. 50.8 mL
C. 18.75 mL
D. 17 mL

Answer: C. The patient needs 18.75 mL per dose. By using the ratio and proportion set-up of X mL:25 mEq::15 mL:20 mEq or Formula Method: D = 25 mEq; H = 20 mEq; Q = 15 mL; 25/20 = 1.25 × 15 = 18.75

4. A patient has an order for 50 mg of Benadryl elixir PO × 1 to be given now. The bottle label reads *Benadryl 12.5 mg/5 mL*. How many mL will the nurse administer?

A. 15 mL
B. 18 mL
C. 20 mL
D. 25 mL

Answer: C. Use fractions to solve for X. The known factor is 12.5 mg equals 5 mL or use the formula method: D = 50 mg; H = 12.5 mg; Q = 5 mL. Therefore 50/12.5 × 50 = 20 mL

Scoring

☆☆☆ If you answered all four items correctly, excellent! Expressed as a ratio, it's 10:10::100:100 (in other words, perfect).

☆☆ If you answered three items correctly, good job! Your calculation skills are almost perfect! (But, remember, a good calculator never hurt anybody).

☆ If you answered fewer than three items correctly, don't worry! Keep on calculatin' (a little practice goes a long way).

Suggested References

Center for Drug Evaluation and Research. (2017, November 24). The FDA's Drug Review process: ensuring drugs are safe and effective. U.S. Food and Drug Administration. https://www.fda.gov/drugs/information-consumers-and-patients-drugs/fdas-drug-review-process-ensuring-drugs-are-safe-and-effective

Center for Drug Evaluation and Research. (2021, November 1). Generic Drug Facts. U.S. Food and Drug Administration. https://www.fda.gov/drugs/generic-drugs/generic-drug-facts

Crushing or splitting the wrong tablet can be a deadly error. (2017). *ISMP Long-Term Care AdviseERR*, *5*(4), 1–5. https://www.ismp.org/sites/default/files/attachments/2018-04/LTC201704.pdf

FDA. (2020, May 7). CPG SEC 430.100 unit dose labeling for solid and liquid oral dosage fo. U.S. Food and Drug Administration. https://www.fda.gov/regulatory-information/search-fda-guidance-documents/cpg-sec-430100-unit-dose-labeling-solid-and-liquid-oral-dosage-forms

Hanson, A., & Haddad, L. M. Nursing rights of medication administration. [Updated 2022 Sep 5]. In: *StatPearls [Internet]*. StatPearls Publishing; 2023 Jan. https://www.ncbi.nlm.nih.gov/books/NBK560654/

Toney-Butler, T. J., Nicolas, S., & Wilcox, L. Dose calculation desired over have formula method. [Updated 2023 Jun 20]. In: *StatPearls [Internet]*. StatPearls Publishing; 2023 Jan. https://www.ncbi.nlm.nih.gov/books/NBK493162/

U.S. Department of Health and Human Services. (2021, December 20). How are drugs approved for use in the United States? Eunice Kennedy Shriver National Institute of Child Health and Human Development. https://www.nichd.nih.gov/health/topics/pharma/conditioninfo/approval

Chapter 11

Calculating topical and rectal medication dosages

Just the facts

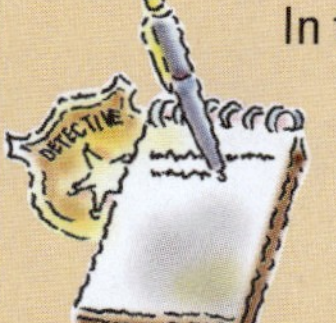

In this chapter, you'll learn how to:

- interpret topical and rectal medication labels
- determine what types of medications are given topically and rectally and how they work
- perform dosage calculations for topical and rectal medications

A look at topical and rectal medications

Some types of medications must be administered by the topical or dermal route. These medications include creams, lotions, ointments, and powders which are commonly used for dermatologic treatment or wound care. Topical patches can also be used to treat angina, localized pain, nicotine withdrawal, or high blood pressure. Topical medications are applied to the skin and slowly absorbed through the epidermis into the dermis.

Medications may also be given rectally. This route may be best for patients who aren't able to take medications orally, such as in cases where a patient has an order to have nothing by mouth (NPO) and has a nasogastric tube, is experiencing nausea or vomiting, or may not be able to swallow safely. The rectal method is especially helpful to achieve specific local and systemic effects. Rectal medications include enemas and suppositories.

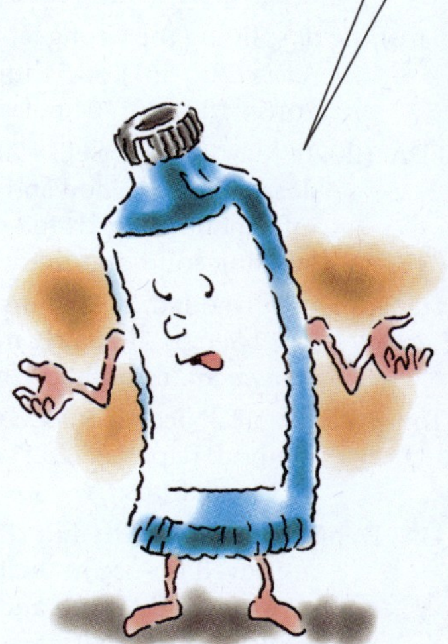
Ointments like me are applied topically to the skin and absorbed through the epidermis into the dermal layer. Pretty deep stuff, huh?

Are you label able?

When reading the labels on topical and rectal medications, look for the same information found on oral and parenteral medication labels. (See *Labeling a successful administration*, p. 199.)

The trade name appears first, followed by the generic name, the dose strength and form, and the total volume of the package. Labels may also contain special administration instructions. Sometimes the print on the labels can be quite small, so look carefully. (See *Combination product alert*, p. 199.)

Before you give that medication!

Labeling a successful administration

There are three rules for administering medication: Read the label, read the label, and read the label.

A topical topic

When reading a topical ointment label, note the following information as shown on the box label below:

- generic name (mupirocin)
- trade name (Bactroban)
- dose strength and form (2% ointment)
- total package volume (22 g)
- special instructions (not included on this label).

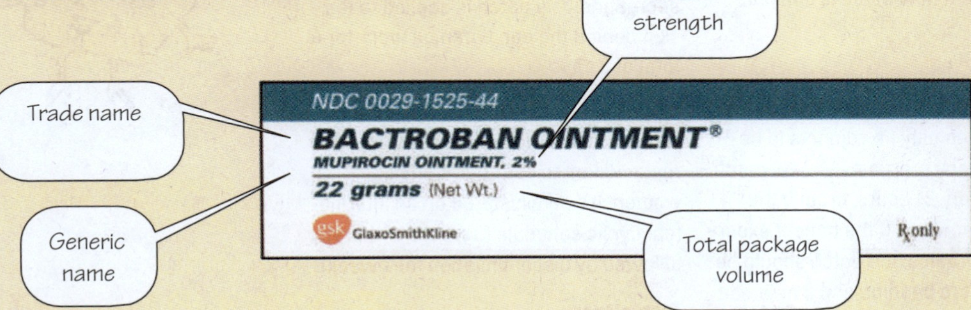

Dose strength
Trade name
Generic name
Total package volume
NDC 0029-1525-44
BACTROBAN OINTMENT®
MUPIROCIN OINTMENT, 2%
22 grams (Net Wt.)
gsk GlaxoSmithKline
℞ only

Transdermal patches

In the past, topical medications were used almost solely for their local effects. Today, however, several topical medications, such as transdermal patches, are used for their systemic effects as well.

Note this: It is important, sometimes *vital*, to cleanse the skin of any leftover medication after removing any medication patch. Doing this ensures that leftover medication does not continue to absorb and raise medication levels.

I've got you under my skin

Transdermal patch medications penetrate the outer layers of the skin by way of passive diffusion at a constant rate; then the medication is absorbed into the circulation. Patches are a good way to administer medications that aren't absorbed well in the GI tract as well as those that are metabolized and eliminated too quickly to be effective by mouth.

Patches are convenient and easy to use, and they maintain consistent blood levels of the medication. They also have disadvantages. Their onset of action is slow, and so a therapeutic blood level takes hours or

Before you give that medication

Combination product alert

Topical preparations may contain more than one medication. For example, Neosporin ointment contains bacitracin, neomycin, and polymyxin B. Carefully note all ingredients when checking labels and make sure that a patient isn't allergic to any of them.

Prescribed patches

Transdermal medications can be applied topically but have a systemic effect.

Nitroglycerin
Transdermal nitroglycerin provides prophylactic treatment of chronic angina. A new patch is applied daily (usually in the morning) and removed after 12 to 14 hours to prevent the patient from developing a tolerance to the medication. It is important to remove any residual medication before a new patch is applied.

Nicotine
Transdermal nicotine is used to treat smoking addiction. These medications should be used only as adjuncts to behavioral therapy programs. A new patch is applied every 24 hours, around the same time each day. If the patient experiences vivid dreams, the patch should be removed before bedtime and a new one applied in the morning.

Fentanyl
Transdermal fentanyl is administered to treat severe chronic pain. These patches may be worn for up to 72 hours. To reduce the chances of an overdose, it is very important that all old patches are removed before a new one is applied.

Clonidine
Clonidine is used to treat hypertension. Unlike the other transdermal patches, this one is removed and applied every 7 days.

Scopolamine
Scopolamine is used to treat nausea, vomiting, vertigo, and often used with hospice patients to decrease respiratory secretions. The patch is applied to the skin behind the ear. It can be worn for a total of 3 days.

Estradiol
Transdermal estradiol provides hormone replacement to estrogen-deficient women. It's administered on an intermittent cyclic schedule (3 weeks of therapy followed by discontinuation for 1 week).

Testosterone
Transdermal testosterone provides hormone replacement for men with testosterone deficiency. The testosterone patch is applied once daily to clean intact, nonscrotal skin (back, abdomen, thighs, or upper arm).

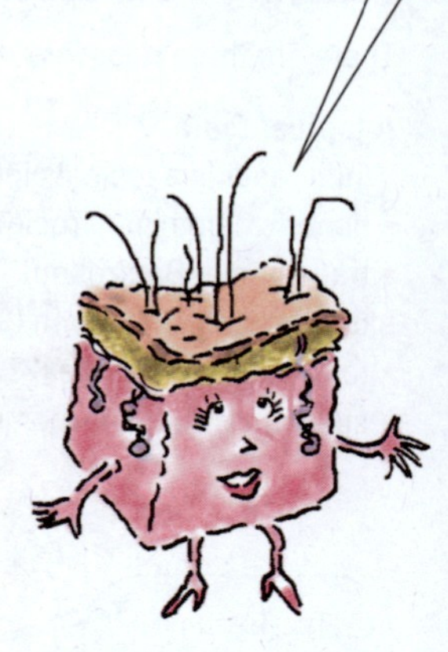

Every time they order a patch, I end up having a bad hair day.

even days to achieve. Patches must also be checked frequently, especially if the patient is active, because they may become displaced. In addition, reversing the toxic effects of patches can be difficult because the medication takes so long to be metabolized. Upon a new patch placement, nurses and/or patients should date and time the patches to help reduce the chance of removing a patch too early or too late.

Release me

Medication concentrations in transdermal patches vary depending on the design of the patch, but the concentration isn't as important as the medication's rate of release. Two patches containing the same medication in different concentrations may actually release the same amount of medication per hour. (See *Prescribed patches.*) In addition, site locations should be rotated each time a new patch is applied.

Batches of patches

Patches are available for many conditions, including a nitroglycerin patch to prevent angina, a clonidine patch to control hypertension, and a fentanyl patch to manage chronic pain.

The fentanyl (Duragesic) transdermal patch is an example of a transdermal medication used for systemic distribution of the medication. The medication is held in a reservoir behind a membrane that allows controlled absorption of the medication through the skin. These patches are available in doses of 12.5, 25, 50, 75, and 100 mcg/hr with the higher doses for use with opioid-resistant patients. To ensure that the patient receives the correct dose, patches need to be changed every 72 hours and check the label to verify the fentanyl dosage. Remember to cleanse the skin where the old patch was when placing a new patch!

Topical medication dosages

Determining topical medication dosages requires very little calculating. As previously discussed, transdermal patches are changed at regular intervals to ensure that the patient receives the correct dose. To apply a patch, simply remove the old patch and replace it with a new one at the appropriate time, following the manufacturer's guidelines. Be sure to alternate administration sites to avoid skin irritation and possibly more severe side effects. Don't forget to write the date and time on the patch in addition to documenting where the patch was placed.

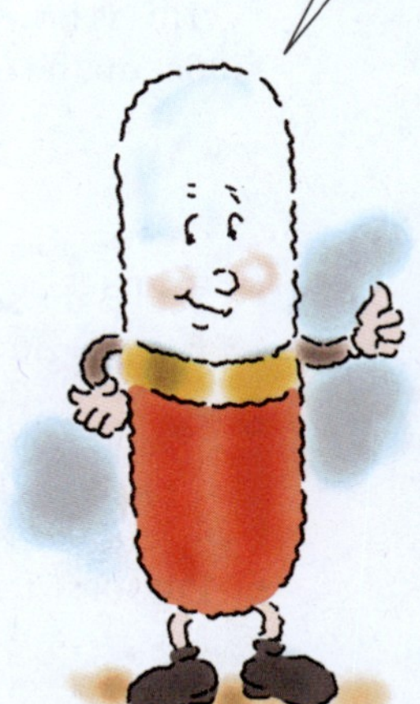
Good news! Topical medication dosages require very little calculating, if at all.

Applying your judgment (along with the ointment)

When the licensed practitioner prescribes an ointment as part of wound care or dermatologic treatment, administration guidelines may not state the amount to apply. There may be general guidance, such as "use a thin layer" or "apply thickly." When an ointment contains a medication intended for a systemic effect, more specific administration guidelines are necessary. If the nurse is not sure whether the medication is intended for a systemic effect, the nurse should ask!

Many ointments, including nitroglycerin, are available in tubes or individual packages. To apply ointment from a tube, use a paper ruler applicator, if available to measure the correct dose. (See *Measuring a topical dose*, p. 202.)

Measuring a topical dose

To measure a specified amount of ointment from a tube, squeeze the prescribed length of ointment in inches or centimeters onto a paper ruler. Then use the ruler to apply the ointment to the patient's skin at the appropriate time, following the manufacturer's guidelines for administration.

Rectal medication dosages

Rectal medications include enemas and suppositories. Suppositories are the most common form of rectal medications, whereas acetaminophen and laxatives are some of the most common medications ordered rectally. Antibiotic enemas may also be ordered, and nurses should follow a facility's policy and protocol for proper administration.

Having a rectal suppository insertion can be an uncomfortable situation for a patient. Nurses should provide an opportunity for the patient to self-administer if they are able. In either case, providing patient privacy is essential. The nurse should also have the patient lay on their left side and provide a generous amount of lubrication before insertion.

Dealing with a Dulcolax dilemma

The patient has a medication order that states *bisacodyl (Dulcolax) 10 mg per rectum at 6 AM daily*. The pharmacy provides 5-mg suppositories. How many suppositories should the nurse give this patient?

This is how to solve this problem using fractions.

- Set up the first fraction with the known suppository dose:

$$\frac{1 \text{ supp}}{5 \text{ mg}}$$

- Set up the second fraction with the desired dose and the unknown number of suppositories:

$$\frac{X}{10 \text{ mg}}$$

- Put these fractions into a proportion:

$$\frac{1 \text{ supp}}{5 \text{ mg}} = \frac{X}{10 \text{ mg}}$$

- Cross-multiply the fractions:

$$1 \text{ supp} \times 10 \text{ mg} = X \times 5 \text{ mg}$$

- Solve for X by dividing each side of the equation by 5 mg and canceling units that appear in both the numerator and the denominator:

$$\frac{1 \text{ supp} \times 10 \cancel{\text{mg}}}{5 \cancel{\text{mg}}} = \frac{X \times \cancel{5 \text{ mg}}}{\cancel{5 \text{ mg}}}$$

$$X = 2 \text{ suppositories}$$

Don't compro–mize your calculations

In this scenario, let's solve the problem by using ratios instead.

The licensed practitioner orders a 10-mg prochlorperazine (Compro) suppository for a patient. The pharmacy is closed, and the only Compro on hand contains 5 mg per suppository. How many suppositories should the nurse give?

- Set up the first ratio with the known suppository dose:

$$1 \text{ supp:}5 \text{ mg}$$

- Set up the second ratio with the desired dose and the unknown number of suppositories:

$$X\text{:}10 \text{ mg}$$

- Put these ratios into a proportion:

$$1 \text{ supp:}5 \text{ mg::}X\text{:}10 \text{ mg}$$

- Multiply the means and the extremes:

$$5 \text{ mg} \times X = 10 \text{ mg} \times 1 \text{ supp}$$

- Solve for X by dividing each side of the equation by 5 mg and canceling units that appear in both the numerator and the denominator:

$$\frac{\cancel{5 \text{ mg}} \times X}{\cancel{5 \text{ mg}}} = \frac{10 \cancel{\text{mg}} \times 1 \text{ supp}}{5 \cancel{\text{mg}}}$$

$$X = 2 \text{ suppositories}$$

Dosage drill

Test your math skills with this drill

A patient has a medication order for a 300-mg aspirin suppository to be given rectally daily. The pharmacy is closed and the only aspirin on hand contains 600-mg per suppository. How many suppositories should the patient receive?

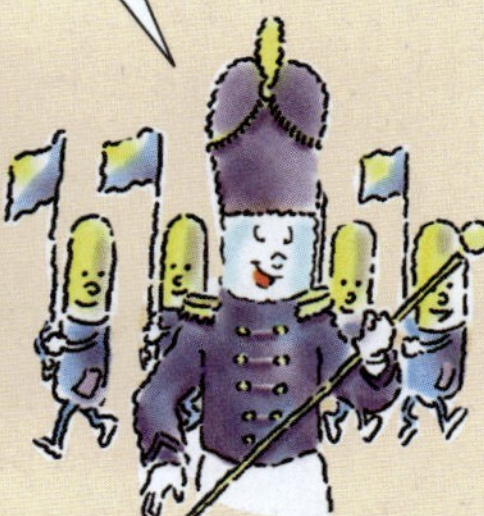
Use this drill to work out the problems.

Your answer: ____________________

To find the answer, set up the equation using ratios and a proportion. Then solve for *X*.

$$1 \text{ supp:600 mg}$$

$$X \text{ supp:300 mg}$$

$$1 \text{ supp:600 mg::}X \text{ supp:300 mg}$$

$$600 \text{ mg} \times X \text{ supp} = 300 \text{ mg} \times 1 \text{ supp}$$

$$\frac{\cancel{600 \text{ mg}} \times X \text{ supp}}{\cancel{600 \text{ mg}}} = \frac{300 \cancel{\text{ mg}} \times 1 \text{ supp}}{600 \cancel{\text{ mg}}}$$

$$X = 0.5 \text{ suppository}$$

The nurse should give a half (1/2) of a suppository to the patient.

Dosage drill

Test your math skills with this drill

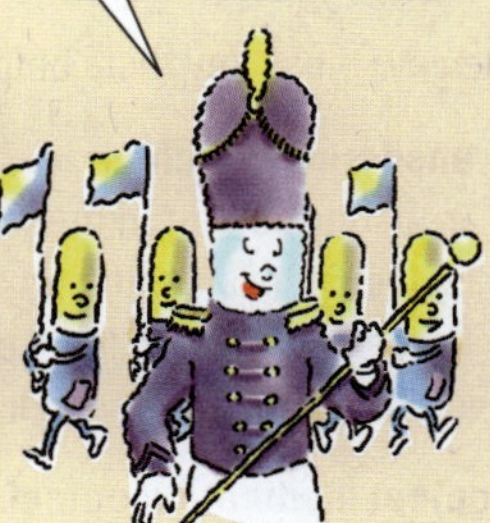
Use this drill
to work out the
problems.

A licensed practitioner orders a bisacodyl suppository 10 mg per rectum prn for constipation for a patient. The only available dosage is 5 mg per suppository. How many suppositories should the nurse administer?

Your answer: ____________

To find the answer, remember to use ratios and a proportion. Then solve for *X*.

$$10 \text{ mg}:X \text{ supp}::5 \text{ mg}:1 \text{ supp}$$

$$10 \text{ mg} \times 1 \text{ supp} = 5 \text{ mg} \times X \text{ supp}$$

$$10 = 5X$$

$$X = \frac{10}{5}$$

$$X = 2 \text{ supp}$$

The nurse should give two suppositories.

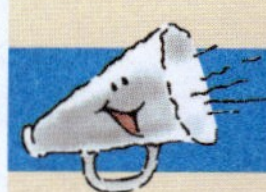

That's a wrap!

Topical and rectal medication dosages review

Review these key facts before giving topical and rectal medications.

Transdermal patches

- Transdermal patch medications penetrate the outer layers of the skin by passive diffusion and then are absorbed into the circulation.
- These medications have a slow onset of action, and so it may take hours or even days to achieve a therapeutic medication level.

Topical medication calculations

- Generalized instructions may be given where nurses must use their own judgment in applying the medication.
- Follow specific guidelines for medications prescribed for a systemic effect.

Rectal medication calculations

- To calculate, use the proportion method with ratios or fractions.
- A dose is typically prescribed to be provided in one suppository (occasionally two).

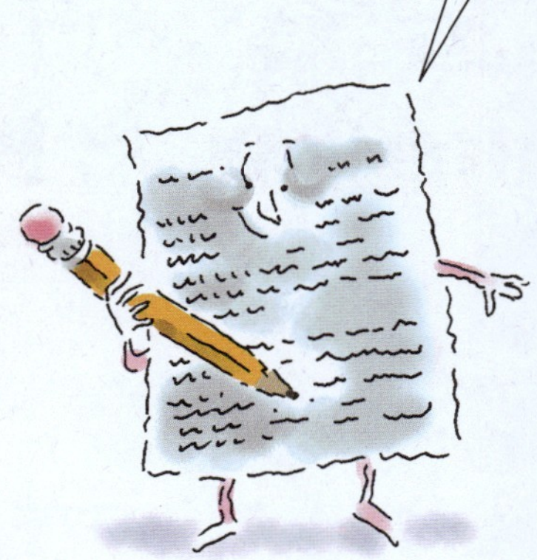

According to my calculations, you've handled this chapter just fine!

Quick quiz

1. A patient asks the nurse how a transdermal patch will help relieve their chronic pain. How should the nurse respond?

A. Since it has controlled absorption through the skin, pain relief lasts for hours.
B. The patches have an enhanced effect on local tissue.
C. Pain relief happens rapidly but then has a slow release of analgesics.
D. The patches have sustained-release dosing to control pain

Answer: A. These medications are slowly released and absorbed through the skin over time.

2. Which medication is commonly used as a transdermal medication?

A. Anectine
B. Nitroglycerin
C. MS Contin
D. Morphine

Answer: B. Nitroglycerin patches are used to prevent angina.

3. The medication label reads as follows: *prochlorperazine (Compro) suppositories 5 mg, Paddock Laboratories, for rectal use only*. What is the medication's proprietary name?

A. Compro
B. Prochlorperazine
C. Paddock Laboratories
D. Suppositories

Answer: A. The proprietary name, or trade name, begins with a capital letter and usually appears before or just above the generic name.

4. A licensed practitioner writes an order for nitroglycerin (nitropaste) *1″ topical q6h prn for chest pain*. How will the nurse properly measure this dose?

A. By using a paper ruler applicator to measure the medication
B. By using their judgment to approximate 1″ of ointment on the skin
C. By holding a wooden ruler to the patient's skin to measure the ointment
D. By dispensing the ointment into a syringe

Answer: A. Nitroglycerin ointment comes with its own paper ruler. Squeeze the prescribed length of ointment onto the ruler and then use the ruler to apply the ointment to the patient's skin.

5. A patient needs 500 mg of aminophylline by suppository. Only 250-mg suppositories are available. How many suppositories should be administered?

A. 1 suppository
B. 2 suppositories
C. 3 suppositories
D. 4 suppositories

Answer: B. Using simple calculation, the patient needs two suppositories. However, because more than one suppository is needed, the nurse should check the calculations, have another nurse do the same, and then call the pharmacy to see if a 500-mg dose is available.

6. The licensed practitioner prescribes an antibiotic ointment for a finger laceration. What should the nurse do?

A. Ask the licensed practitioner to prescribe a specific amount.
B. Use a paper applicator to apply the ointment.
C. The nurse should apply an amount based on their judgment.
D. Call the pharmacist for the recommended amount of ointment to apply.

Answer: C. Unless the ointment has a systemic effect, the licensed practitioner will usually leave the amount to apply up to the nurse.

7. A child needs 2.5 mg of prochlorperazine (Compro). The package label reads *Compro suppositories 5 mg.* How many suppositories should be administered?

A. Two suppositories
B. 1½ suppositories
C. One suppository
D. ½ suppository

Answer: D. By setting up a proportion and solving for *X*, you'll find that the child needs ½ of a 5-mg suppository. The nurse could also call the pharmacist to see if this dose is available in one suppository to ensure the most accurate dose.

8. A patient has an order for a clonidine patch to treat hypertension. How often should the nurse anticipate removing and replacing this patch?

A. Every 7 days
B. Every 72 hours
C. Every 12 to 14 hours
D. Every 24 hours

Answer: A. Transdermal clonidine patches should be removed every 7 days.

Scoring

☆☆☆ If you answered all eight items correctly, wow! You know your routes better than AAA!

☆☆ If you answered six or seven items correctly, all right! You'll soon be top dog in topical medication administration.

☆ If you answered fewer than six items correctly, keep at it! You're absorbing information at an incredible rate.

Suggested Reference

Hua, S. (2019). Physiological and pharmaceutical considerations for rectal drug formulations. *Frontiers in pharmacology, 10*, 1196.

Part V

Parenteral administration

Chapter 12

Calculating parenteral injections

Just the facts

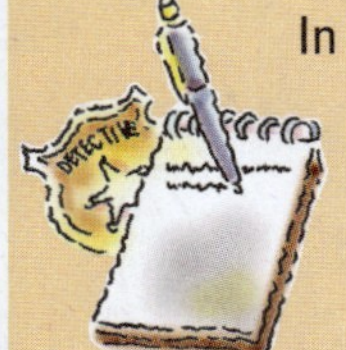

In this chapter, you'll learn how to:

- calculate intradermal, subcutaneous, and intramuscular injections
- distinguish between different types of syringes and needles
- interpret parenteral medication labels
- reconstitute powdered medications

A look at parenteral injections

Parenteral is a term that refers to medications placed into the tissues and the circulatory system by injection. More simply stated, parental medications are those placed "outside the intestines." Medications may be administered parenterally through direct injection into the skin, subcutaneous (subcut) tissue, or muscle using proper syringe and needle combination. Another parenteral option is intravenous (IV) injections, which is covered in Chapters 13 and 16. Medications may be supplied as liquids or as powders which require reconstitution. When using either form, nurses need to perform calculations to determine the correct amount of liquid medication to inject as ordered.

This chapter shows how to use the ratio or fraction and proportion method to calculate liquid parenteral dosages as well as how to reconstitute powdered medications. Dimensional analysis may be used to calculate these dosages as well. Refer to Chapter 4 of this book if needed.

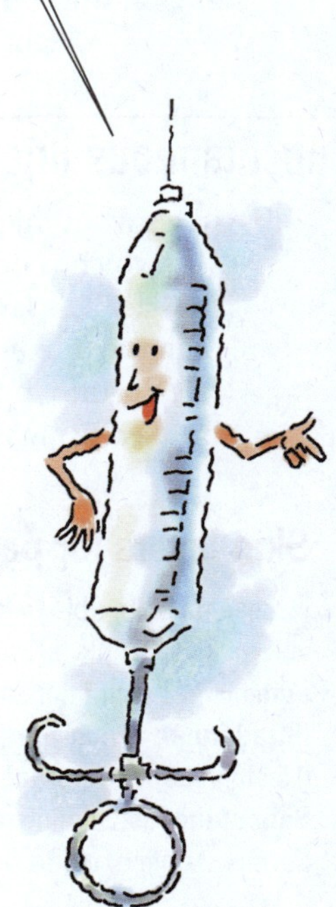

My point is... nurses need to stay sharp and focused when giving parenteral medications. (Just trying to inject a little humor into the situation!)

Types of injections

Parenteral medications are administered by four types of injections:

- Intradermal
- Subcutaneous (Subcut)
- Intramuscular (IM)
- Intravenous (IV) (See Chapters 13 and 16.)

Giving parenteral medications safely depends heavily on choosing the right syringe and needle size for the type of injection ordered.

Appropriate syringe and needle size is based on the purpose, patient's age, and body composition. One size does not fit all!

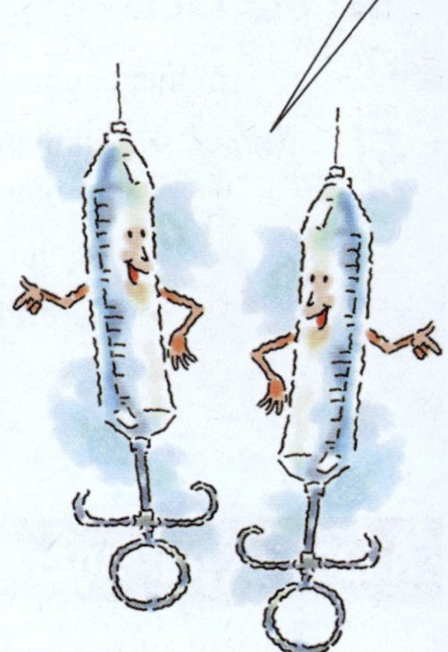

Always choose the right syringe and needle size for the specific type of injection ordered.

Intradermal injections

In an intradermal injection, medication is injected into the dermis—the layer of skin beneath the epidermis, or the outermost layer of skin. This type of injection is commonly used to anesthetize the skin for invasive procedures and to test for allergies, tuberculosis, histoplasmosis, and other diseases.

I've got you intra my skin

Intradermal injections are less than 0.5 mL by volume. A 1-mL syringe, calibrated in 0.01-mL increments, is usually used, along with a 25- to 27-gauge needle that's ⅜″ to ⅝″ long. Always check the facility's protocol on intradermal injections before choosing a particular needle size.

To perform an intradermal injection, follow these incredibly easy steps:

Step 1: Cleanse the skin thoroughly using an antiseptic swab.

Step 2: Stretch the skin taut with one hand.

Step 3: With the other hand, insert the needle at a 10- to 15-degree angle with the bevel of the needle faced up to a depth of about 0.5 cm.

Step 4: Inject the medication making a small wheal (what looks like a tight bubble under the skin), which forms at the injection site.

Subcutaneous injections

In a subcut injection, the medication is injected into the subcut tissue, which is beneath the epidermis and dermis layers but above the muscle. This layer of tissue contains fewer capillaries than muscle; therefore medications administered by this route have a slow, sustained rate. Insulin, heparin, tetanus toxoid, and some opioid analgesics are injected using this route.

Skin layers for parenteral injections

Nurses must be able to identify not only the appropriate needle size/gauge and volume for parenteral injections, but they also need to know the injection angle to administer medication in the appropriate skin layer.

Intradermal: administered in the dermis layer just under the epidermis layer about 0.5 cm in depth. Approach the needle almost parallel to skin at a 5 to 15 degree angle.

Subcutaneous: administered into the loose connective tissue located just below the dermis. Angle of insertion is typically between 45 and 90 degrees.

Skin layers for parenteral injections (*continued*)

Intramuscular: administered into the muscle below the subcutaneous tissue. Angle insertion ranges from 75 to a 90 degree angle with the majority at 90 degrees.

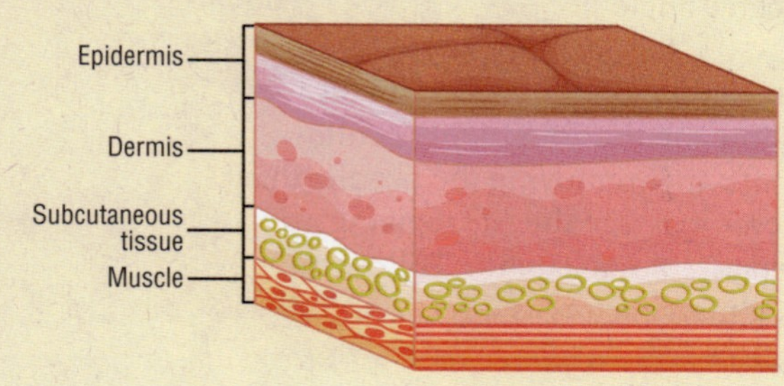

More than skin deep

Only 0.5 to 1 mL of a medication can be injected into subcut tissue at one time. The most common needle size used for these injections are 23 to 25 gauge and ½″ to ⅝″ long. Always check the facility's protocol on subcut injections before choosing a needle size. Subcut injection sites include:

- Anterior aspect of the thighs
- Lateral areas of the upper arms and thighs
- Abdomen (above, below, and lateral to the umbilicus)
- Upper gluteal (backside) area

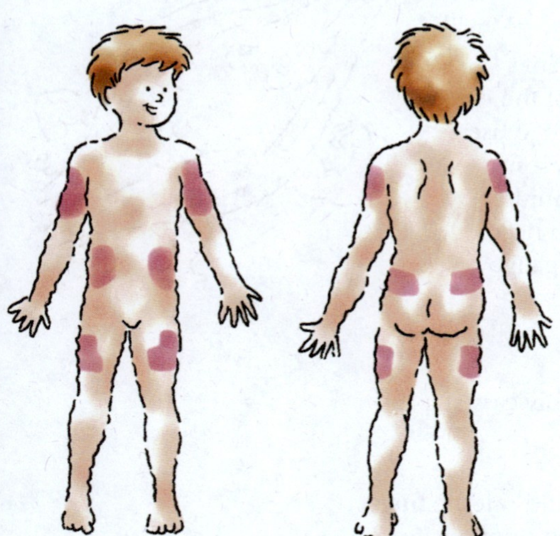

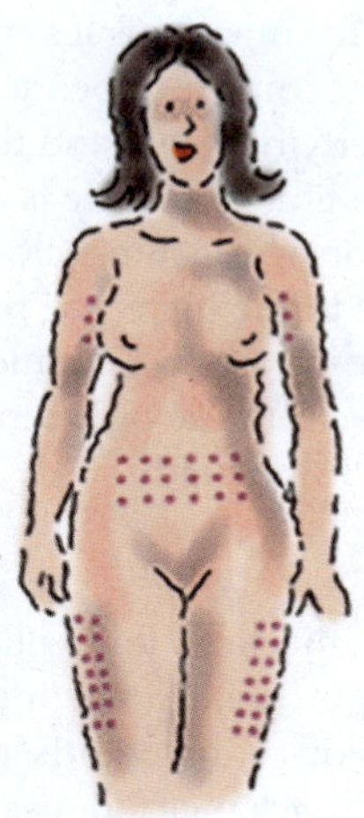

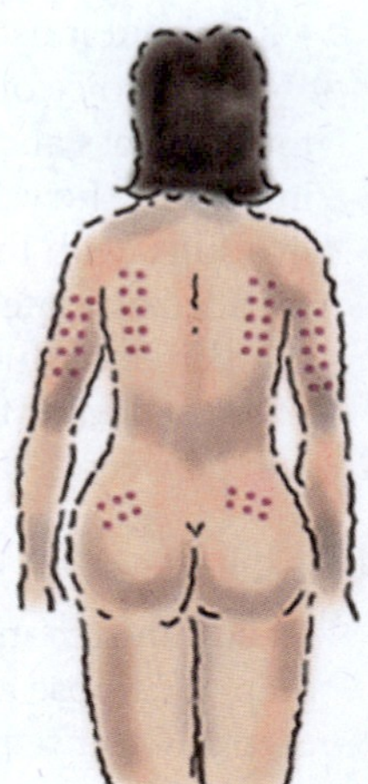

To perform a subcut injection, follow these incredibly easy steps:

Step 1: Choose an appropriate injection site.

Step 2: Cleanse the skin with an antiseptic swab.

Step 3: If the patient does not have adequate tissue mass, pinch the skin between the index finger and thumb, and insert the needle at a 45-degree angle.

Step 4: If the patient has adequate tissue mass, insert the needle into the fatty tissue at a 90-degree angle.

Step 5: Administer the injection.

Step 6: This next step may differ depending on the type of medication administered. For some medications, apply gentle pressure or massage the site after removing the needle; this enhances absorption. Never massage the site if giving an anticoagulant such as heparin or enoxaparin. Follow the facility's policies and drug manufacturer's directions for best administration practices.

Step 7: Document site location and patient tolerance. Site locations should be rotated between injections.

Intramuscular injections

IM injections, injections into a muscle, are used for medications that need to be absorbed quickly and/or may be irritating to tissues. The volume for these injections ranges from 0.5 to 3 mL. IM injection sites include:

- Ventral gluteal muscle
- Vastus lateralis muscle (primarily used in infants and children)
- Deltoid muscle (for injections less than 2 mL)

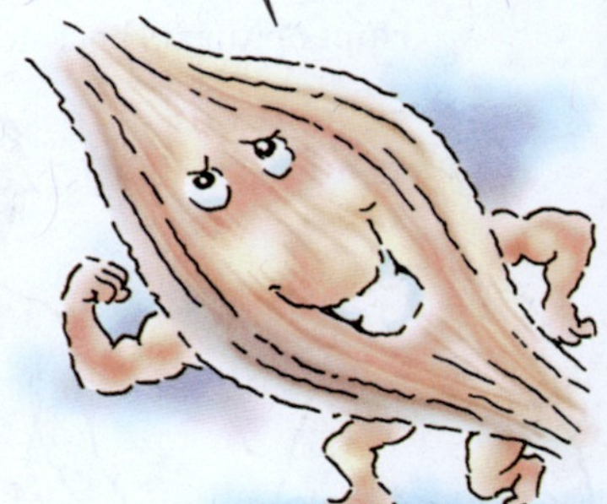
The choice of IM injection site depends on the patient's muscle mass, among other things.

The choice of injection site depends on the patient's muscle mass and overlying tissue and the volume of the injection. The ventral gluteal muscle is the safest site to use in adults, with the dorsogluteal muscle no longer recommended as a site due to the increased risk of nerve injury (Gutierrez & Munakomi, 2023). The most common needle sizes used for IM injections are between 18 and 25 gauge and between 1″ and 3″ in length.

Use a little muscle

To administer an IM injection, follow these incredibly easy steps:

Step 1: Choose an appropriate injection site.

Step 2: Cleanse the skin with an antiseptic swab.

Step 3: If using the *Z-track* method, use the index and middle finger to pull the skin surrounding the injection in opposite directions. This helps reduce any potential leakage into the surrounding tissue. Always check the facility's protocol and drug manufacturer's recommendations for best administration practices before administering.

Step 4: Use a quick, dart-like action to insert the needle at a 90-degree angle.

Step 5: Aspirate for blood before injecting the medication to verify that the needle isn't in a vein. Aspirate by pulling back on the plunger to see if blood returns in the syringe. If blood is present, remove the needle immediately and do not inject the medication. Start the process over by discarding the medication and obtaining new supplies. Aspiration is not necessary for the administration of vaccines (Centers for Disease Control and Prevention, 2023).

Step 6: If no blood is aspirated, then push the plunger to administer the medication. Be sure to keep the syringe steady.

Step 7: After the medication is injected, pull the needle straight out. Check with the facility's protocols and/or the drug manufacturer's recommendations to see if pressure should be applied at the site of injection.

Syringes and needles

The many types of syringes and needles used to administer parenteral medications are designed for specific purposes.

Types of syringes

To measure and administer parenteral medications, three basic types of syringes are used. These include:

- Standard syringes
- Tuberculin syringes
- Prefilled syringes
- Insulin syringes (discussed in Chapter 17)

Although these syringes are sometimes calibrated in cubic centimeters (cc), the medications they're used to measure are commonly ordered in milliliters (mL). Recall that these are equal measurements.

Standard syringes

Standard syringes are available in 1, 3, 5, 10, 20, 30, 50, and 60 mL. Each syringe consists of a plunger, a barrel, and a hub. (See *Anatomy of a syringe,* p. 216.) The most commonly used syringe size for parenteral medication administration includes the 1-, 3-, and 5-mL syringes. Syringes may come prepackaged with a predetermined gauge and needle size, but more often, the nurse chooses the appropriate size needle to use. Several different size and gauge needles are available and must be chosen according to the purpose (i.e., intradermal, subcut, or IM) and while taking a patient's age and tissue composition into consideration.

Anatomy of a syringe

Standard syringes come in many different sizes, but each syringe has the same components. This illustration shows the parts of a standard syringe.

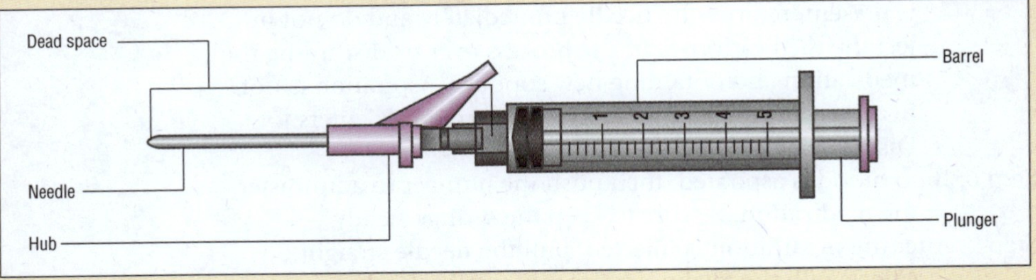

Marked for good measure

The calibration marks on a syringe allows accurate medication dose measurements. The 3-mL syringe, most commonly used, is calibrated in tenths of a mL on the right and minims on the left. It has large marks for every 0.5 mL on the right. The larger-volume syringes are calibrated in 2- to 10-mL increments.

To draw up a medication in a syringe, follow these incredibly easy steps:

Step 1: Calculate the medication dose.
Step 2: Using aseptic technique, remove the vial cap, and scrub the top of the vial.
Step 3: Insert needle and draw up the medication into the syringe by pulling the plunger back on the syringe until the top ring of the plunger's black portion aligns with the correct calibration mark.
Step 4: Double-check the dose measurement.

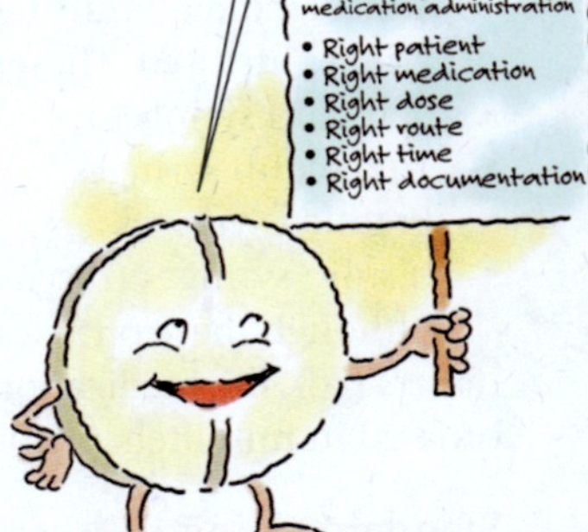

Don't forget to use the six "rights" of medication administration!
6 rights of medication administration
• Right patient
• Right medication
• Right dose
• Right route
• Right time
• Right documentation

Double the fun (well, not exactly fun)

Parenteral medications come in various strengths or concentrations in which the usual adult dose can be contained in 1 to 3 mL of solution. If a patient needs a dose larger than 3 mL, split the medication into two separate injections and give at two different sites (at least 1-inch apart) to ensure proper medication absorption.

Tuberculin syringes

Tuberculin syringes are commonly used for intradermal injections and to administer small amounts of medications such as those given to pediatric patients or those in intensive care settings. Each syringe is calibrated

Touring a tuberculin syringe

A tuberculin syringe has the same components as a standard syringe; however, size and calibration of the syringe are distinct. Take extra care when reading the dose, because the measurements on this type of syringe are so small.

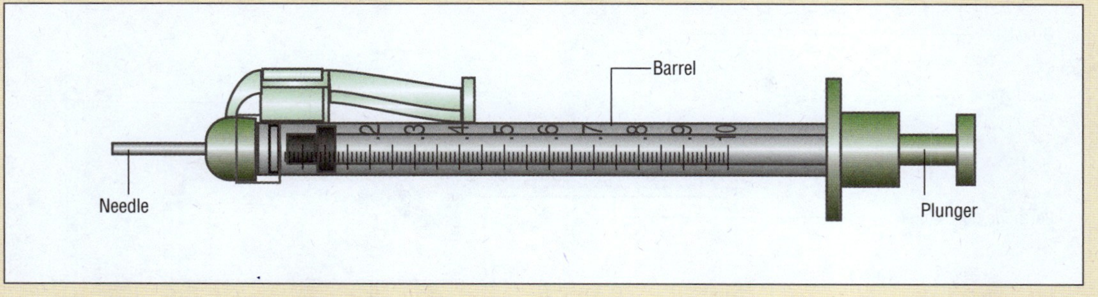
Barrel
Needle
Plunger
.1
.2
.3
.4
.5
.6
.7
.8
.9
.10

in hundredths of a mL, allowing accurate measurement of smaller doses as little as 0.25 mL. (See *Touring a tuberculin syringe*.)

Prefilled syringes

A sterile syringe filled with a premeasured dose of medication is called a *prefilled syringe*. These syringes usually come with a cartridge-needle unit and require a special holder called a *Carpuject* to release the medication from the cartridge. Each cartridge is calibrated in tenths of a mL and has larger marks for half and full mL. (See *Perusing a prefilled syringe*, p. 218.)

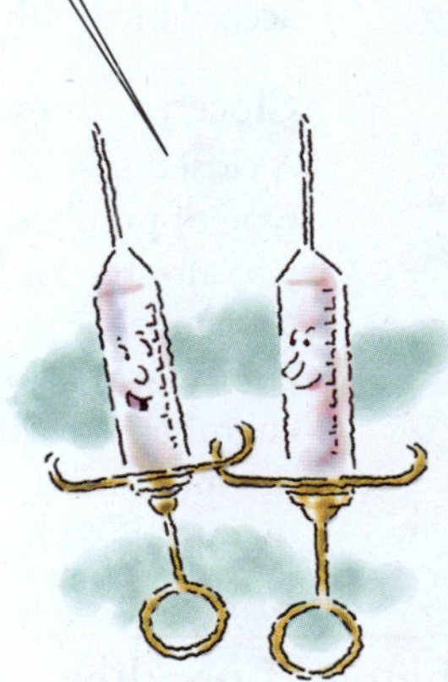
If a patient needs a dose larger than 3 mL, split the medication into two separate injections and give at two different sites to ensure proper medication absorption.

Room for one more

Some cartridges are designed so that a diluent or a second medication can be added when a combined dose is ordered. For example, one manufacturer of the antianxiety medication lorazepam (Ativan) comes in prefilled syringes. Lorazepam requires the addition of a diluent, so these cartridges come with this additional space to allow for the second solution. Remember to always check compatibility before adding a diluent or mixing more than one medication in a syringe.

First, the good news…

Prefilled syringes have many advantages over multiple-dose vials. Prefilled syringes come prelabeled with the medication's name and dose, which reduces medication errors and preparation time. Controlled substances that are provided in prefilled syringes makes witnessing, wasting, and documenting much easier for both nurses involved in this process.

Perusing a prefilled syringe

This illustration shows the parts of a prefilled syringe. *Carpuject* is the brand name of one type of prefilled syringe that requires the use of a holder as pictured.

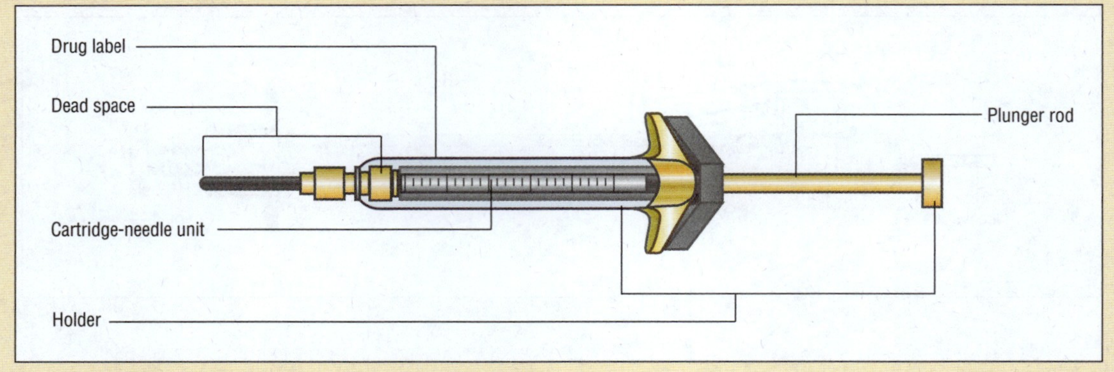

...Now, the bad news

Unfortunately, not all medications come prepared in prefilled syringes, nor do they all come in all the ordered dose amounts. When the ordered dose doesn't match the amount in the prefilled syringe, the nurse will need to calculate the correct amount of medication needed.

Before giving the injection, expel the air and discard any extra medication from the syringe per the facility's policy. Remember, if the medication is a controlled substance, such as an opioid, the discard needs to be witnessed by another nurse and documented carefully in accordance with the facility's protocol.

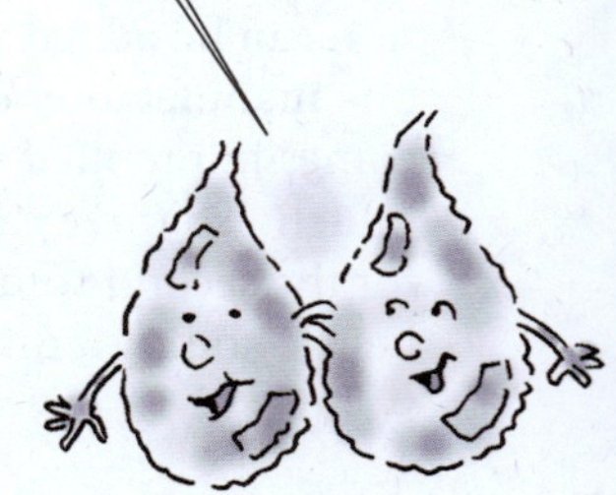

Most manufacturers add a little extra medication to their prefilled syringes to account for what is wasted when purging the syringe of air.

Closed-system devices

A closed-system device is yet another type of prefilled syringe. This type of prefilled syringe already comes with a predetermined needle size along with the prefilled medication chamber. Enoxaparin (Lovenox) is an example of this type of prefilled syringe. Uniquely, enoxaparin also comes with an air bubble within the medication chamber. This air bubble should not be expelled as it helps push the medication into the subcut tissue (Lovenox for anticoagulant therapy, 2021).

Types of needles

As mentioned, some syringes come with a preattached needle, but most often, nurses have to choose which needle to use.

There are several different gauge and needle lengths available as different needle sizes are designed for different purposes.

When choosing a needle, consider the gauge, bevel, and length:

- Gauge refers to the inside diameter of the needle; the smaller the gauge, the larger the diameter. For example, a 14-gauge needle has a larger diameter than a 25-gauge needle.
- Bevel refers to the angle at which the needle tip is opened. The bevel may be short, medium, or long.
- Length describes the distance from needle tip to needle hub. It ranges from ⅜″ to 3″.

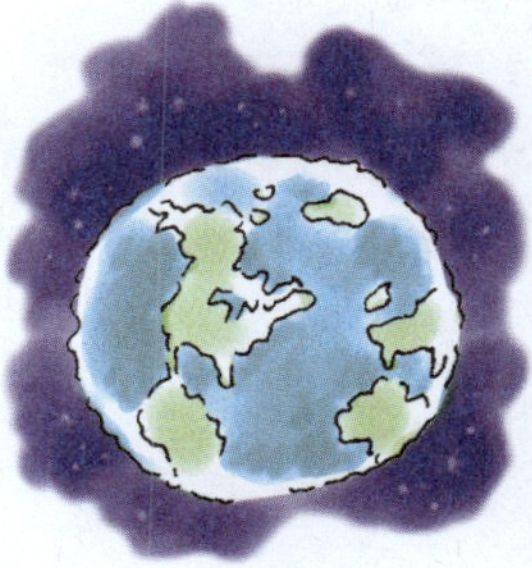

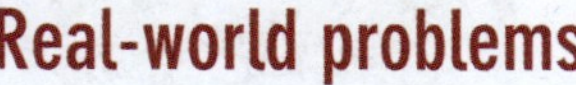

Real-world problems

Now that we covered the basics of parenteral medications, let's move on to working with the calculations! The following examples show how to use the ratio proportion method to calculate doses given by injection.

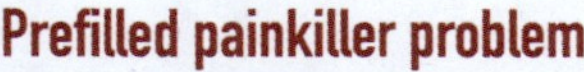

Prefilled painkiller problem

The licensed practitioner prescribes *4 mg of IM morphine q3h* to a patient for moderate pain (scale of 4 to 7). The medication is available in a prefilled syringe containing 10 mg of morphine per 1 mL (10 mg/mL). How many mL of morphine does the nurse need to discard from the prefilled syringe?

Follow these incredibly easy steps to solve this problem using fractions.

Step 1: Set up the first fraction using the known morphine concentration:

$$\frac{10 \text{ mg}}{1 \text{ mL}}$$

Step 2: Set up the second fraction with the desired dose and the unknown amount of morphine:

$$\frac{4 \text{ mg}}{X}$$

Step 3: Put these fractions into a proportion:

$$\frac{10 \text{ mg}}{1 \text{ mL}} = \frac{4 \text{ mg}}{X}$$

Step 4: Cross-multiply the fractions:

$$10 \text{ mg} \times X = 4 \text{ mg} \times 1 \text{ mL}$$

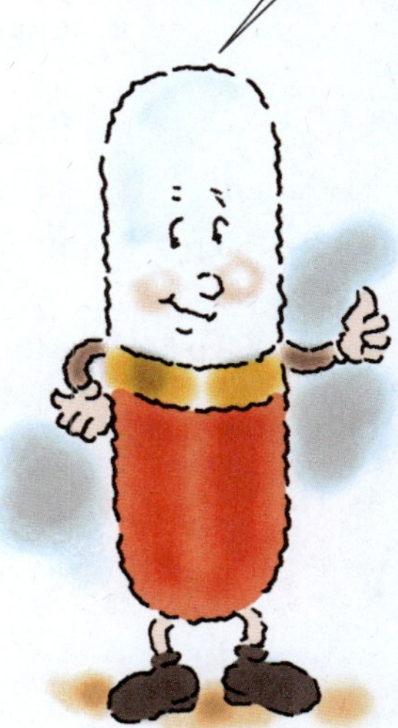

When disposing of an opioid or another type of controlled substance, remember that it requires two nurses to be involved in the process—one to discard or waste and the other to witness this action.

Step 5: Solve for X. Divide each side of the equation by 10 mg and cancel units that appear in both the numerator and the denominator:

$$\frac{\cancel{10\text{ mg}} \times X}{\cancel{10\text{ mg}}} = \frac{4\ \cancel{\text{mg}} \times 1\text{ mL}}{10\ \cancel{\text{mg}}}$$

$$X = \frac{4\text{ mL}}{10}$$

$$X = 0.4\text{ mL}$$

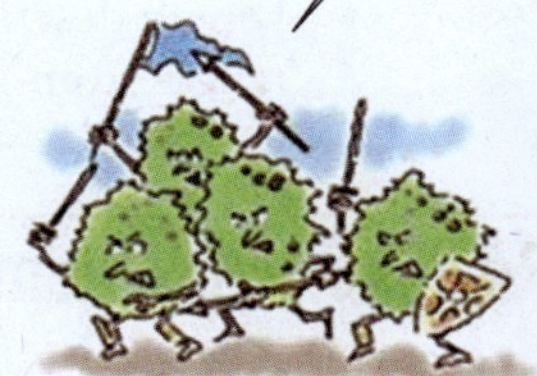

Divide and conquer...oops, I mean, cancel. Sounds like a good plan!

Step 6: The amount of morphine to give the patient is 0.4 mL. Now, calculate the amount to be wasted by subtracting the ordered dose from the entire contents of the syringe:

$$\begin{array}{r} 1.0\text{ mL} = 10\text{ mg morphine} \\ -0.4\text{ mL} = 4\text{ mg morphine} \\ \hline 0.6\text{ mL} = 6\text{ mg morphine} \end{array}$$

The amount of morphine to be discarded is 0.6 mL. (Remember to have another nurse witness the waste and cosign following the facility's protocol.)

Medrol milligram mystery

A patient has an order for *100 mg methylprednisolone (Solu-Medrol) IM q4h* for a patient with asthma. The vial contains 120 mg/mL. How much methylprednisolone should the nurse give?

Here's how to solve this problem using the ratios proportion method.

Step 1: Set up the first ratio with the known concentration:

$$120\text{ mg:1 mL}$$

Step 2: Set up the second ratio with the desired dose and the unknown amount of *methylprednisolone*:

$$100\text{ mg:}X$$

Step 3: Put these ratios into a proportion:

$$120\text{ mg:1 mL::100 mg:}X$$

Step 4: Set up an equation by multiplying the means and extremes:

$$100\text{ mg} \times 1\text{ mL} = 120\text{ mg} \times X$$

Step 5: Solve for X. Divide each side of the equation by 120 mg and cancel units that appear in both the numerator and the denominator:

$$\frac{100\ \cancel{\text{mg}} \times 1\text{ mL}}{120\ \cancel{\text{mg}}} = \frac{\cancel{120\text{ mg}} \times X}{\cancel{120\text{ mg}}}$$

$$\frac{100\text{ mL}}{120} = X$$

$$X = 0.83\text{ mL}$$

The nurse should give the patient 0.83 mL of methylprednisolone.

Vial trial

The licensed practitioner prescribes *100 mg of gentamicin IM* for an infection. The vial available contains 40 mg/mL. How much gentamicin should the nurse administer?

Here's how to solve this problem using ratios:

Step 1: Set up the first ratio with the known gentamicin concentration:

$$40\text{ mg}:1\text{ mL}$$

Step 2: Set up the second ratio with the desired dose and the unknown amount of gentamicin:

$$100\text{ mg}:X$$

Step 3: Put these ratios into a proportion:

$$40\text{ mg}:1\text{ mL}::100\text{ mg}:X\text{ mL}$$

Step 4: Set up an equation by multiplying the means and extremes:

$$1\text{ mL}\times 100\text{ mg} = 40\text{ mg}\times X\text{ mL}$$

Step 5: Solve for X. Divide each side of the equation by 40 mg and cancel units that appear in both the numerator and the denominator:

$$\frac{1\text{ mL}\times 100\ \cancel{\text{mg}}}{40\ \cancel{\text{mg}}} = \frac{\cancel{40\text{ mg}}\times X}{\cancel{40\text{ mg}}}$$

$$\frac{100\text{ mL}}{40} = X$$

$$X = 2.5\text{ mL}$$

The nurse should administer 2.5 mL of gentamicin.

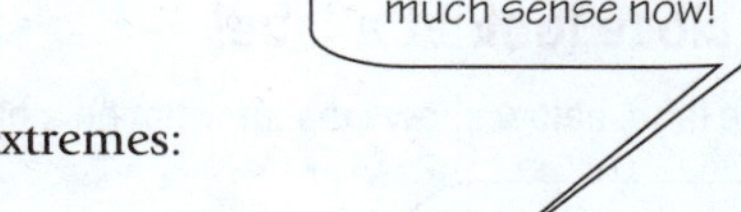
This makes so much sense now!

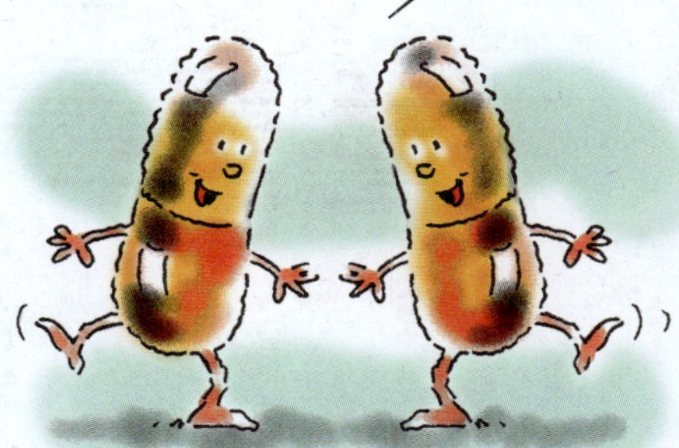

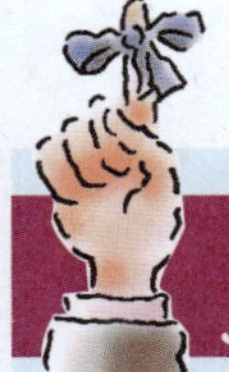

Memory jogger

When working with ratios and proportions, the trick is to keep like units of measure in the same position on both sides of the proportion:

120 **mg**:1 **mL**::100 **mg**:*X* **mL**

Remember to multiply the means and extremes:

means = **m**iddle numbers

extremes = **e**nd numbers.

Finally, isolate *X* to solve the problem:

Divide each side of the equation by the number to be eliminated so that *X* is by itself, and then cancel the units that appear in both the numerator and the denominator.

Interpreting medication labels

Nurses must know how to read and interpret medication labels before they can safely administer them. (See *A close look at a label*.) Parenteral medications come packaged in glass ampules, in single- or multiple-dose vials with rubber stoppers, and in prefilled syringes and cartridges. The packaging will clearly state that the medications are used for injection.

A close look at a label

The label below shows the information a nurse needs to safely administer a parenteral medication.

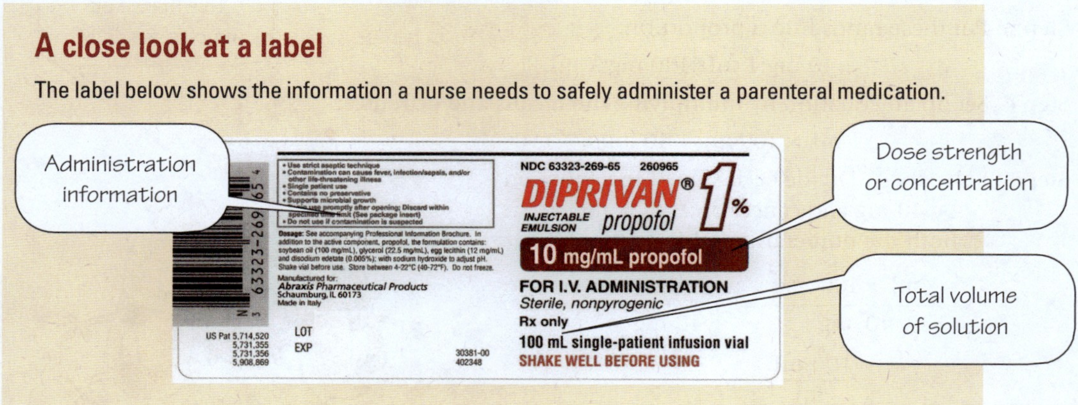

Looking at labels

Labels of parenteral solutions look very similar to those found with oral solutions. These labels should contain the following information:

- trade name, generic name, or both
- total volume of solution in the container
- dose strength or concentration (medication dose present in a volume of solution)
- approved routes of administration
- expiration date
- special instructions, as needed

Solution components

A solute is a liquid or solid form of a medication. A solution is a liquid that contains a solute dissolved in a diluent or solvent, most commonly sterile water. Normal saline solution is a solution of salt (the solute) in purified water (the solvent).

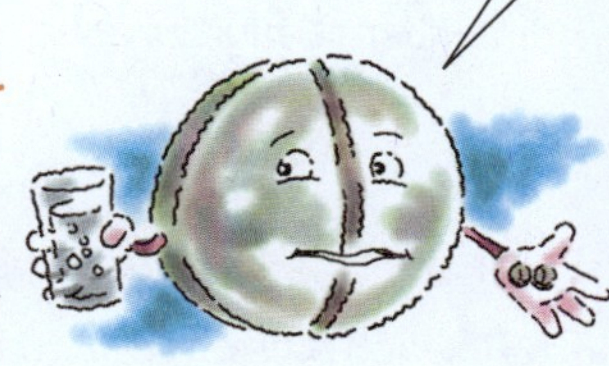

Here's the problem…how to fit a large medication like me into this tiny glass of sterile water… sure hope the solution presents itself quickly.

Reconstituting powders

Some medications—such as levothyroxine sodium (Synthroid) and penicillin antibiotics—are manufactured and packaged in powder form because they become unstable quickly when in solution form. Therefore, this type of medication requires reconstitution before it can be administered.

The strength of one or many

Powdered medications come in single-strength or multiple-strength formulations. A single-strength powder—such as levothyroxine sodium—may be reconstituted to only one dose strength per administration route, as specified by the manufacturer. A multiple-strength powder—such as penicillin—can be reconstituted to various dose strengths by adjusting the amounts of diluent.

When reconstituting a multiple-strength powder, check the medication label or package insert for the dose-strength options and choose the one that's closest to the ordered dose strength.

How to reconstitute

Follow the general guidelines described here when reconstituting a powder for injection.

Learn from the label

Begin by checking the label of the powder container. The label states the quantity of medication in a vial, the amount and type of diluent to add to the powder, and the strength and expiration date of the resulting solution.

Fluid out exceeds fluid in

When a diluent is added to a powder, the fluid volume increases. That's why the label calls for less diluent than the total volume of the prepared solution. For example, the instructions may state to add 1.7 mL of diluent to a vial of powdered medication to obtain 2 mL of prepared solution.

Check out the chambers

Some medications come packaged in vials with two chambers separated by a rubber stopper. The upper chamber contains the diluent, and the lower chamber contains the powdered medication. (See *Two chambers [one's a powder room!]*.)

Two chambers (one's a powder room!)

Some medications that require reconstitution are packaged in vials with two chambers separated by a rubber stopper. In the illustration below, note that the upper chamber contains the diluent and the lower chamber contains the powder. The plunger is depressed to inject the diluent into the powder.

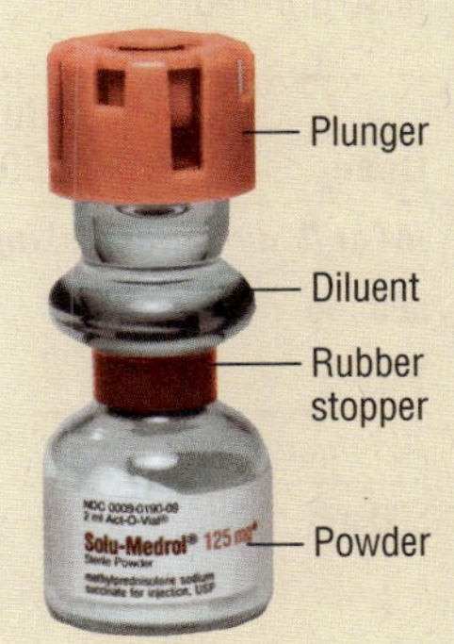

When the top of the vial is depressed, the stopper dislodges, allowing the diluent to flow into the lower chamber, where it mixes with the powdered medication. The nurse can then remove the correct amount of solution needed from the vial using a syringe.

Say it with an equation

To determine how much solution to give, refer to the medication label for information about the dose strength of the prepared solution. For example, an order states to give a patient 500 mg of a medication when the dose strength of the solution is 1 g (or 1,000 mg)/10 mL. Set up a proportion with fractions as follows:

$$\frac{X}{500 \text{ mg}} = \frac{10 \text{ mL}}{1{,}000 \text{ mg}}$$

If information about a medication's dose strength isn't on the label, check the package insert. The label or insert will also list the type and amount of diluent needed, the dose strength after reconstitution, and special instructions about administration and storage after reconstitution. (See *Inspect the insert*.)

Before you give that medication!

Inspect the insert

Package inserts provided with medications commonly contain a great deal of information that may not be on the outer label. For example, the medication label for ceftazidime provides no information about reconstitution, but the package insert does. Listed below are the possible diluent combinations as they appear in the package insert that comes with this medication. Notice that different dilution amounts that need to be added to provide the correct solution depending on the route and dose ordered.

Dose	Diluent to be added (mL)	Approximate available (mL)	Approximate average concentration (mg/mL)
IM or IV direct (bolus) injection			
500 mg	1.5	1.8	280
1 g	3	3.6	280
IV infusion			
500 mg	5.3	5.7	100
1 g	10	10.8	100
2 g	10	11.5	170

Special considerations

When reconstituting a powder that comes in multiple strengths, the nurse must be especially careful in choosing how much diluent to add for the correct dose prescribed.

Label logic

Once a medication has been reconstituted, the nurse must label the syringe with the following information:

- reconstitution date and time
- dose strength
- expiration date
- the nurse's initials

Real-world problems

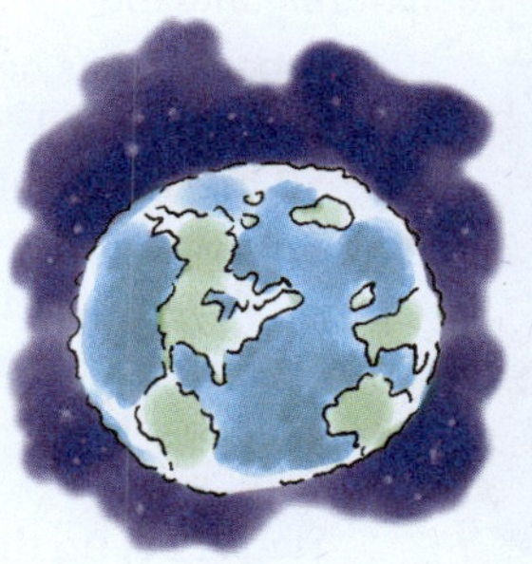

The following problems show how to calculate the amount of reconstituted medication to give a patient.

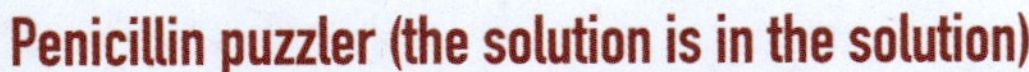

Penicillin puzzler (the solution is in the solution)

The licensed practitioner prescribes *100,000 units penicillin* IM for a patient with an infection, but the only available vial holds 1 million units. The medication label says to add 4.5 mL of normal saline to yield 1 million units/5 mL. After reconstitution, how much of the penicillin solution should the nurse administer?

Here's how to solve this problem using fractions.

Step 1: Dilute the powder according to the instructions on the label.

Step 2: Set up the first fraction with the known penicillin concentration:

$$\frac{1{,}000{,}000 \text{ units}}{5 \text{ mL}}$$

Step 3: Set up the second fraction with the desired dose and the unknown amount of solution:

$$\frac{100{,}000 \text{ units}}{X}$$

Step 4: Put these fractions into a proportion:

$$\frac{1{,}000{,}000 \text{ units}}{5 \text{ mL}} = \frac{100{,}000 \text{ units}}{X}$$

Step 5: Cross-multiply the fractions:

$$5 \text{ mL} \times 100{,}000 \text{ units} = X \times 1{,}000{,}000 \text{ units}$$

Step 6: Solve for X. Divide each side of the equation by 1 million units and cancel units that appear in both the numerator and the denominator:

$$\frac{5\text{ mL} \times 100{,}000\ \cancel{\text{units}}}{1{,}000{,}000\ \cancel{\text{units}}} = \frac{X \times \cancel{1{,}000{,}000\text{ units}}}{\cancel{1{,}000{,}000\text{ units}}}$$

$$X = \frac{500{,}000\text{ mL}}{1{,}000{,}000}$$

$$X = 0.5\text{ mL}$$

The amount of solution that yields 100,000 units of penicillin after reconstitution is 0.5 mL.

The nurse should administer 0.5 mL of the penicillin solution.

Deciphering diluents

A patient has been ordered 25 mg of gentamicin IM daily. The label states to add 1.3 mL of sterile 0.9% sodium chloride to yield 50 mg/1.5 mL. How many mL of reconstituted solution should the nurse administer?

Here's how to solve this problem using ratios.

Step 1: Set up the first ratio with the known gentamicin concentration:

$$50\text{ mg:}1.5\text{ mL}$$

Step 2: Set up the second ratio with the desired dose and the unknown amount of solution:

$$25\text{ mg:}X$$

Step 3: Put these ratios into a proportion:

$$50\text{ mg:}1.5\text{ mL::}25\text{ mg:}X$$

Step 4: Set up an equation by multiplying the means and extremes:

$$1.5\text{ mL} \times 25\text{ mg} = X \times 50\text{ mg}$$

Step 5: Solve for X. Divide each side of the equation by 50 mg and cancel the units that appear in both the numerator and the denominator:

$$\frac{1.5\text{ mL} \times 25\ \cancel{\text{mg}}}{50\ \cancel{\text{mg}}} = \frac{X \times \cancel{50\text{ mg}}}{\cancel{50\text{ mg}}}$$

$$X = \frac{37.5\text{ mL}}{50}$$

$$X = 0.75\text{ mL}$$

The patient should receive 0.75 mL of the gentamicin solution.

Attaining the ampicillin answer

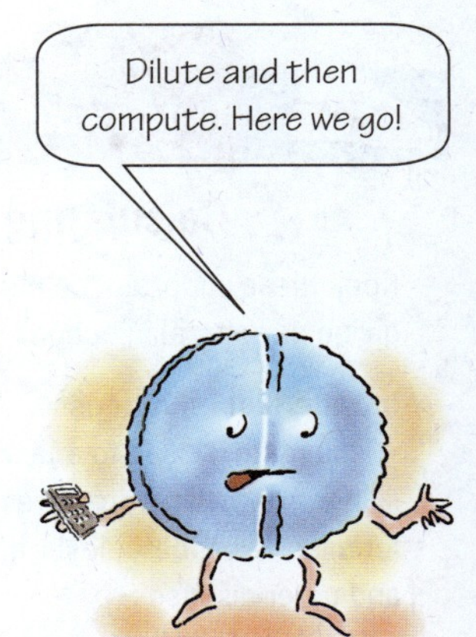
Dilute and then compute. Here we go!

The licensed practitioner orders *500 mg ampicillin* IM daily for a patient. A 1-g vial of powdered ampicillin is available. The label states to add 4.5 mL of sterile water to yield 1 g/5 mL. How many mL of reconstituted ampicillin should the nurse administer?

Here's how to solve this problem using fractions.

Step 1: Set up the first fraction with the known ampicillin concentration (recall that 1 g equals 1,000 mg):

$$\frac{1{,}000 \text{ mg}}{5 \text{ mL}}$$

Step 2: Set up the second fraction with the desired dose and the unknown amount of solution:

$$\frac{500 \text{ mg}}{X}$$

Step 3: Put these fractions into a proportion, making sure the same units of measure appear in both numerators. In this case, the units of measure must be grams or mg. If using mg, the proportion would be:

$$\frac{1{,}000 \text{ mg}}{5 \text{ mL}} = \frac{500 \text{ mg}}{X}$$

Step 4: Cross-multiply the fractions:

$$1{,}000 \text{ mg} \times X = 500 \text{ mg} \times 5 \text{ mL}$$

Step 5: Solve for X by dividing each side of the equation by 1,000 mg and cancel the units that appear in both the numerator and the denominator:

$$\frac{\cancel{1{,}000 \text{ mg}} \times X}{\cancel{1{,}000 \text{ mg}}} = \frac{500 \cancel{\text{ mg}} \times 5 \text{ mL}}{1{,}000 \cancel{\text{ mg}}}$$

$$X = \frac{2{,}500 \text{ mL}}{1{,}000}$$

$$X = 2.5 \text{ mL}$$

The nurse should administer 2.5 mL of the ampicillin solution.

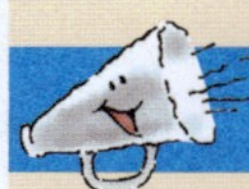

That's a wrap!

Calculating parenteral injections review

Keep these important points in mind when giving parenteral injections.

Intradermal injections

- This route is used to anesthetize the skin for invasive procedures and to test for allergies, tuberculosis, histoplasmosis, and other diseases.
- Amount of medication injected is less than 0.5 mL.
- Syringe and needle, respectively: 1-mL syringe with a 25- to 27-gauge needle that's 3/8″ to 5/8″ long.
- 5–15 degree angle for injection.

Subcutaneous injections

- Medications commonly given subcutaneously include insulin, heparin, tetanus toxoid, and some opioids.
- Amount of medication injected ranges from 0.5 to 1 mL.
- Needle is 23- to 28-gauge and 1/2″ to 5/8″ long.
- 45–90 degree angle for injection.

Intramuscular (IM) injections

- This route is used for medications that require quick absorption or those that are irritating to tissue.
- Amount of medication injected ranges from 0.5 to 3 mL.
- Needles are 18 to 25 gauge and 1″ to 3″ long.
- Follow the facility's protocols regarding the Z track technique and the need for aspiration.
- 75–90 degree angle for injection.

Syringe types

- Standard syringes come in a variety of sizes (1, 3, 5, 10, 20, 30, 50, and 60 mL).
- Tuberculin syringes (commonly used for intradermal injections) are 1-mL syringes marked to hundredths of a mL allowing for accurate measurement of very small doses.
- Prefilled syringes—sterile syringes that contain a premeasured medication dose—some require the use of a special holder (Carpuject) to release the medication from the cartridge while others come prepackaged with a needle already in place.

Needle terminology

- Gauge: inside diameter of the needle (the smaller the gauge, the larger the diameter)
- Bevel: angle at which the needle tip is open (may be short, medium, or long)
- Length: distance from needle tip to hub (ranges from 3/8″ to 3″)

Important parts of a parenteral medication label

- Trade name, generic name, or both
- Total volume of solution in the container
- Dose strength or concentration
- Approved routes of administration
- Expiration date
- Special instructions, if applicable

Solution strengths

- Solute is a medication in liquid or solid form that's added to a solvent (diluent) to make a solution.
- Solution is a liquid (usually sterile water) containing a dissolved solute.

Powders for reconstitution

- The fluid volume increases with the added diluent.
- Single-strength powders are reconstituted to one dose strength per administration route.
- Multiple-strength powders are reconstituted to appropriate strengths by adjusting the amount of diluent.

Quick quiz

1. What is needed to administer a medication provided in a prefilled syringe?
   A. A Carpuject
   B. A standard syringe
   C. Dead space
   D. A tuberculin syringe

Answer: A. Prefilled syringes come with a cartridge-needle unit and requires a special holder like a Carpuject to release the medication from the cartridge.

2. The nurse is preparing to administer a medication in a prefilled syringe. What action should the nurse perform before administering the medication?
   A. Empty the prefilled syringe into a medicine cup.
   B. Expel the air out of the syringe.
   C. Remove the medication using a standard syringe.
   D. Shake to mix the prefilled syringe.

Answer: B. The nurse must expel or purge the air from a prefilled syringe. Since a small amount of medication is wasted during purging, most manufacturers add a little extra medication to prefilled syringes.

3. Which needle is used to administer an intradermal injection?
   A. 25 to 27 gauge and ⅜″ to ⅝″ long.
   B. 14 to 18 gauge and 1″ to 1½″ long.
   C. 22 gauge and ¾″ long.
   D. 18 to 23 gauge and 1″ to 3″ long.

Answer: A. This type of needle is used for intradermal injections along with a 1-mL syringe calibrated in 0.01-mL increments.

4. When administering a subcutaneous injection, where is the medication injected?
   A. In the muscle tissue.
   B. In the tissue in the vastus lateralis.
   C. In the tissue above the dermis.
   D. In the tissue below the dermis.

Answer: D. A subcutaneous injection delivers the medication into the subcutaneous tissue, located below the dermis but above the muscle.

5. When a diluent is added to a powder for injection, what happens to the fluid volume?

A. The fluid volume increases.
B. The fluid volume decreases.
C. The fluid volume stays the same.
D. The fluid volume always doubles.

Answer: A. When a diluent is added to a powder, the fluid volume increases. That's why the label calls for less diluent than the total volume of the prepared solution.

6. What action should the nurse take if the information about a medication's dose strength is not included on the medication label?

A. Call the physician.
B. Check the package insert.
C. Mix it with 5 mL of normal saline solution.
D. Administer the medication without the information.

Answer: B. The package insert includes information about the medication's dose strength, the amount of diluent needed, the dose strength after reconstitution, and any special instructions.

Scoring

☆☆☆ If you answered all nine items correctly, bravo! You've earned the right to say to anyone, "This won't hurt a bit."

☆☆ If you answered six to eight items correctly, you're almost a parenteral powerhouse!

☆ If you answered fewer than six items correctly, okay! Remember the golden rule of dosage calculations: Keep things in proportion.

Suggested References

Centers for Disease Control and Prevention. (2023, June 20). ACIP Vaccine Administration Guidelines for Immunization. *Centers for Disease Control and Prevention*. https://www.cdc.gov/vaccines/hcp/acip-recs/general-recs/administration.html

Open Resources for Nursing (Open RN); Ernstmeyer, K., & Christman, E. (Eds). (2021). Chapter 18: Administration of parenteral medications. *Nursing skills [Internet]*. Chippewa Valley Technical College. https://www.ncbi.nlm.nih.gov/books/NBK593214

Polania Gutierrez, J. J., & Munakomi, S. (2023). Intramuscular injection. [Updated August 13, 2023]. In *StatPearls [Internet]*. StatPearls Publishing. https://www.ncbi.nlm.nih.gov/books/NBK556121/

Winthrop U.S. (2021). Lovenox® for anticoagulant therapy. Lovenox enoxaparin sodium injection. https://www.lovenox.com/enoxaparin-sodium

Chapter 13

Calculating intravenous infusions

Just the facts

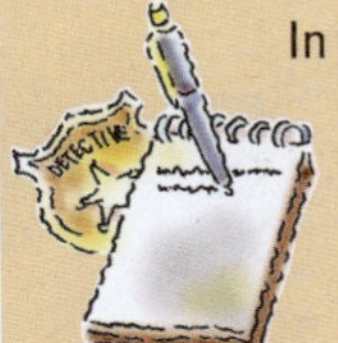

In this chapter, you'll learn how to:

- calculate drip rates and flow rates
- regulate an infusion manually and electronically
- calculate infusion times
- calculate, monitor, and regulate infusions of substances like electrolytes, blood, and parenteral nutrition

A look at intravenous infusions

Intravenous (IV) is yet another route used to administer fluids and medications especially when immediate onset is required. Although the safest and most convenient route is by administering medications orally, it may be necessary for patients hospitalized in acute care facilities to receive treatment utilizing the IV route for correction of fluid and electrolyte imbalances. Additionally, IV therapy is also used for the administration of medications to patients who may need acute treatment and management of conditions such as severe infections and cardiovascular complications. Errors can occur with all routes of medication administration; however, IV therapy is invasive and poses an increased risk of patient complications requiring nurses to be extra diligent in the medication administration process.

Nurses working with IV medications must have specific knowledge and skills to provide safe patient care. Following state laws and regulations in addition to all policies and procedures set by an institution will help the nurse provide safe practice.

Work from the outside in

To begin the process of safe IV therapy, the nurse must first be familiar with working with IV medications and infusions. The nurse needs to know specific information about the IV solution (which is provided in an order) that includes the solution's name, how much to give and/or over what time period. However, the nurse also is responsible for knowing the components of the solution, the compatibility (what can be added), and the tonicity (osmotic pulling power), which will not be covered in this book.

IV fluid comes in an assortment of volumes with 50 mL, 100 mL, 250 mL, 500 mL, and 1 L solution bags being the most common. The nurse begins by choosing the appropriate IV bag that was ordered. Take a look at the outside of a 1-L IV bag and its components in the section *Read the bag*.

Next, the nurse needs to select proper tubing, calculate drip and flow rates, and become comfortable working with equipment such as electronic infusion devices. (See *Checking an IV*, p. 233.)

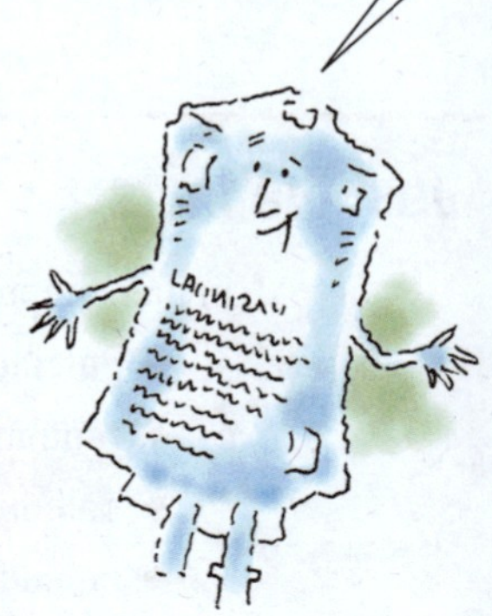

Don't forget to inspect me for any leaks or discoloration before you hang me up!

Before you give that medication!

Read the bag

The outside of an IV bag contains important information used for calculating infusion rates and times. Read it carefully!

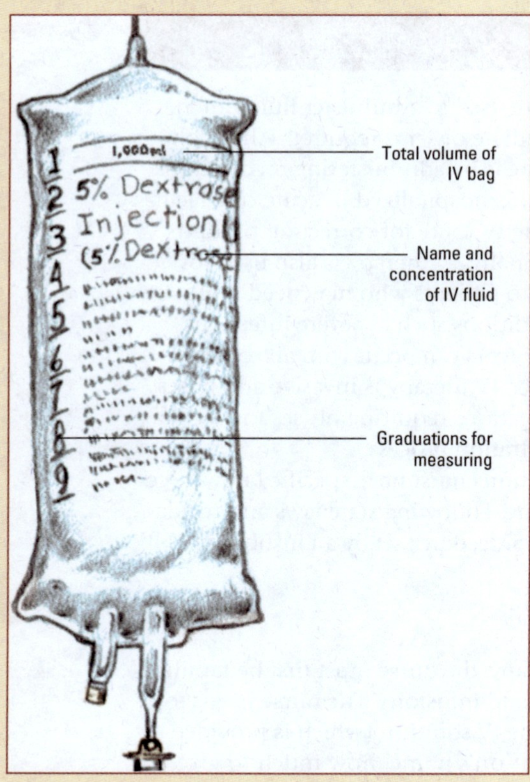

Advice from the experts

Checking an IV

Not only is it best practice, but nurses can save time by assessing a patient's IV infusion at the beginning of their shift. Save time by assessing the IV site for any potential complications and verify what is currently running through the IV site. Being proactive saves time and reduces errors and confusion when things get busy! Here is what the nurse should be assessing:

Continuous IV fluid infusions:

- Verifying that the hanging IV solution bag matches the order including any additives such as electrolytes. When certain additives are prepared and added by pharmacy or possibly a nurse, a label must be added to the IV bag with the additive name, date and time added, and expiration date. If an additive is present, verify that the solution is labeled with this required information.
- Checking the time and amount of volume remaining in the bag. Calculate the amount of time the IV bag will be completed and/or needs to be replaced.
- Checking the programming of electronic infusion devices. Verify that it's programmed correctly. (See the *Electronic Infusion Pumps* section in this chapter, p. 243.)
- Verify the drop factor being used with gravity infusion sets is appropriate and is infusing at the calculated drip rate.

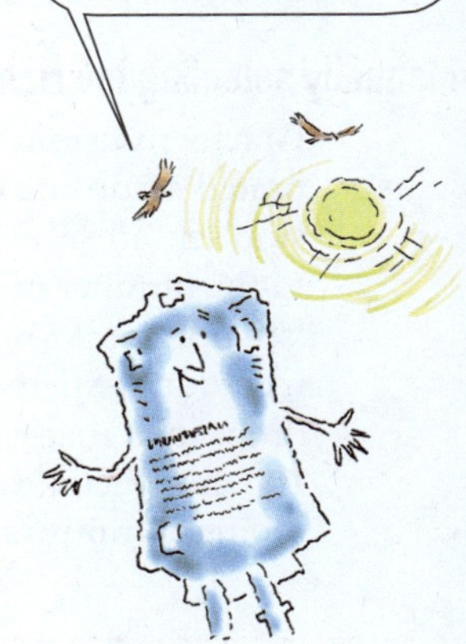

Getting to know me, getting to know all about me… (and my components!)

Administering IV fluids

IV therapy may be used to infuse continuous or intermittent fluids, electrolytes, or medications. IV therapy infusions are regulated in one of two methods:

- Gravity (manual): infusions regulated by using a clamp on the IV tubing, which the rate of infusion can be increased or decreased. Infusions with gravity infusion sets are calculated in drops/minutes (gtt/min).
- Electronic infusion device: infusions are regulated by an electronic pump (referred to as an IV pump) for more precise and accurate rates and volume delivery to a patient. IV pumps regulate the rate of fluids in mL/hr. Using an IV pump is the safest method to infuse IV therapy as it ensures specific amounts of fluid are being administered.

The method the nurse chooses is dependent on several different variables including what is being infused and what equipment is available. Follow a facility's policy and protocols for guidance on which solutions must be infused using an electronic infusion device.

Depending on the regulation method used for infusion, the nurse will need to determine how the flow rate is going to be regulated: either by gravity or by using an IV pump. Therefore, the method the nurse chooses plays an important role in how the nurse calculates IV infusion rates.

Manually selecting the right tube

Gravity infusions utilizes administration infusion sets which are calibrated according to a drop (gtt) factor. Different gravity tubing infusion sets are available with various drop factors. The drop factor refers to the number of milliliter (mL) of solution calibrated for an administration set. Most facilities stock IV tubing in two sizes: microdrip and macrodrip. Microdrip tubing, as its name implies, delivers smaller drops than macrodrip. Microdrip also delivers more drops per minute. The drop factor can be found listed on the package containing the IV tubing administration set.

Calculating drip rates

To infuse IV fluids and medication using a gravity infusion set, the nurse must calculate the number of drops of solution needed to infuse per minute (gtt/min) also known as the *drip rate*. Since a partial drop cannot be calculated, all drip rates are rounded to the nearest whole number.

Advice from the experts

Gravity tubing sizes

Gravity tubing comes in different drop factor sizes. The nurse chooses an appropriate size based on availability, the purpose, and the desired infusion rate. (See *Tube tips,* p. 235.) Here is a quick reference of administration sets:

Macrodrip tubing • Used for more rapid infusing such as 125 mL/hr	Available calibration size: 10 gtt/mL 15 gtt/mL 20 gtt/mL
Microdrip tubing • Used for slow and more precise infusions such as 40 mL/hr	Available calibration size: 60 gtt/mL

Advice from the experts

Tube tips

Follow these general guidelines* when working with IV tubing:

- Use macrodrip tubing for infusions with a flow rate of 80 mL/hr or greater.
- Use microdrip tubing for infusions with a flow rate of 80 mL/hr or less.
- With electronic infusion devices, select the tubing specifically made to work with those devices.
- Continuous infusion tubing should be replaced every 72 to 96 hours.
- Intermittent infusions, such as used for IV piggyback (IVPB) infusions, should be replaced every 24 hours.
- When a patient has multiple lines infusing, each line needs to be labeled with the corresponding medication infusing in that line.
- When hanging new tubing, label the tubing with the date, time, and nurse's initials.

*Always refer to a facility's policies and procedures.

A formula dripping with success

One way to calculate drip rates is to use the formula below:

$$\text{Drip rate (gtts/min)} = \frac{\text{Volume to be infused (in mL)}}{\text{Time (in minutes)}} \times \text{Drop factor (gtts/mL)}$$

The following two examples show how to calculate drip rates using this formula.

Doing the dextrose drip

A patient has an order for an infusion of dextrose 5% in water (D_5W) at 125 mL/hr. If the tubing set available is calibrated with a drop factor of 15 gtt/mL, what's the drip rate?

Step 1: Convert 1 hour to 60 minutes to fit the formula.

Step 2: Set up the formula with the information provided:

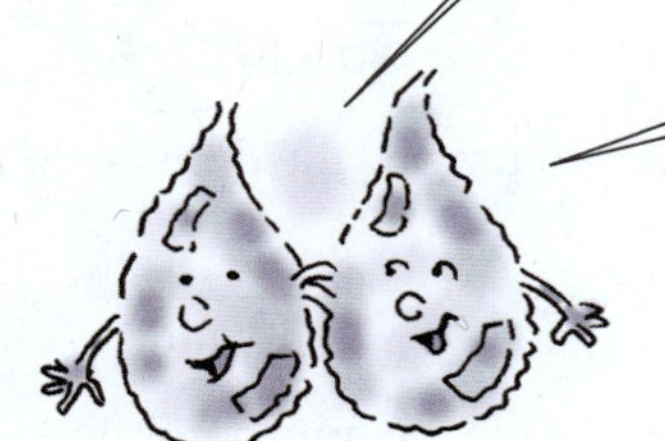
To determine the drip rate—the number of drops of solution to infuse per minute (gtt/min)—the nurse needs to know the drop factor for the specific administration set being used.
The drop factor is listed on the package containing the IV tubing administration set.

$$\text{Drip rate (gtts/min)} = \frac{\text{Volume to be infused (in mL)}}{\text{Time (in minutes)}} \times \text{Drop factor (gtts/mL)}$$

$$X = \frac{125 \text{ mL}}{60 \text{ min}} \times \frac{15 \text{ gtt}}{1 \text{ mL}}$$

Step 3: Cancel the units that appear in both the numerator and the denominator:

$$X = \frac{125 \cancel{mL}}{60 \text{ min}} \times \frac{15 \text{ gtt}}{1 \cancel{mL}}$$

Step 4: Multiply the volume by the drop factor (125 by 15):

$$X = \frac{125 \times 15 \text{ gtt}}{60 \text{ min}}$$

Step 5: Solve for *X*. Divide the numerator by the denominator (1,875 ÷ 60):

$$X = \frac{1{,}875 \text{ gtt}}{60 \text{ min}}$$

$$X = 31.25 \text{ gtt/min}$$

Round the drip rate to the nearest whole number. The drip rate is 31 gtt/min.

Note this: Dimensional Analysis can also be used to calculate drip rates. Refer back to Chapter 4 for assistance!

Thirst quencher

A patient's order reads Infuse *0.9% Normal Saline (NS) 500 mL over 30 minutes*. The nurse chooses a macrodrip infusion set with a drop factor of 10 gtt/mL. What's the drip rate?

Step 1: Set up the formula with the information provided:

$$X = \frac{500 \text{ mL}}{30 \text{ min}} \times \frac{10 \text{ gtt}}{\text{mL}}$$

Step 2: Cancel the units that appear in both the numerator and the denominator:

$$X = \frac{500 \cancel{mL}}{30 \text{ min}} \times \frac{10 \text{ gtt}}{\cancel{mL}}$$

Step 3: Multiply the volume by the drop factor (500 by 10):

$$X = \frac{500 \times 10 \text{ gtt}}{30 \text{ min}}$$

Step 4: Solve for *X*. Divide the numerator by the denominator (5,000 by 30):

$$X = \frac{5{,}000 \text{ gtt}}{30 \text{ min}}$$

$$X = 166.6666 \text{ gtt/min}$$

Round the drip rate to the nearest whole number. The drip rate is 167 gtt/min.

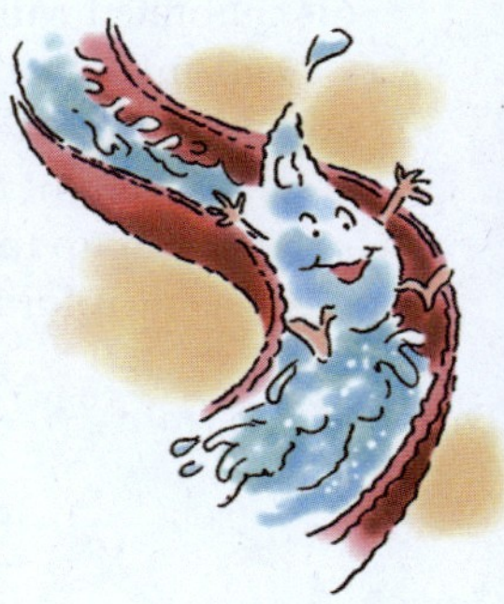
When you're a little drop like me, you drip mighty fast. Wheee!!!

Dosage drill

Test your math skills with this drill

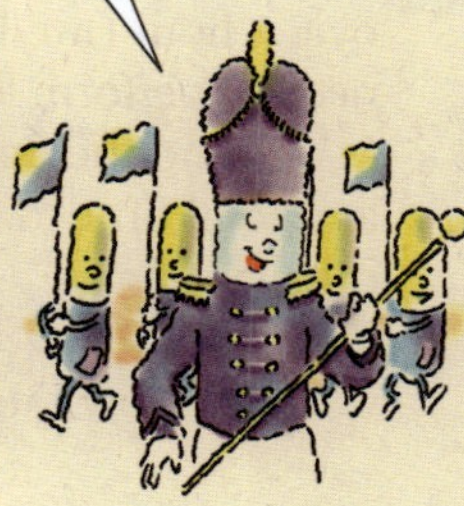
Be sure to show how you arrive at your answer.

A licensed practitioner orders 2 g of ceftriaxone sodium (Rocephin) in 50 mL 0.9% sodium chloride to infuse over 30 minutes. What's the drip rate for this medication if the microdrip administration set delivers 60 gtt/mL?

Your answer: ______________

To find the answer, change mL/hr to drops using the drip rate formula.

Step 1: Set up the formula with the information provided:

$$X \text{ (drip rate)} = \frac{50 \text{ mL (total volume)}}{30 \text{ min (time in min)}} \times 60 \text{ gtt/mL (drop factor)}$$

Step 2: Cancel the units appearing in both the numerator and the denominator:

$$X = \frac{50 \cancel{\text{mL}}}{30 \text{ min}} \times \frac{60 \text{ gtt}}{1 \cancel{\text{mL}}}$$

Step 3: Multiply the volume by the drop factor (50 × 60):

$$X = \frac{50 \times 60 \text{ gtt}}{30 \text{ min}} = \frac{3{,}000 \text{ gtt}}{30 \text{ min}}$$

Step 4: Solve for *X*. Divide the numerator by the denominator (3,000 by 30):

$$X = 100 \text{ gtt/min}$$

The drip rate is 100 gtt/min.

Calculating the flow rate

IV fluids may also be ordered by the total volume to be given over a certain amount of time. In these cases, the nurse will need to calculate the flow rate. The *flow rate* is the number of mL of fluid to administer over 1 hour (mL/hr). If using gravity infusion sets, the nurse would need to perform further calculations to find out the drip rate (gtt/min).

To find the flow rate, the nurse needs to know the total volume and total time to be infused. Use the flow rate formula to perform the calculation:

$$\text{Flow rate (mL/hr)} = \frac{\text{Total volume ordered (in mL)}}{\text{Total time (in hours)}}$$

The next two examples outline how to determine the correct flow rate.

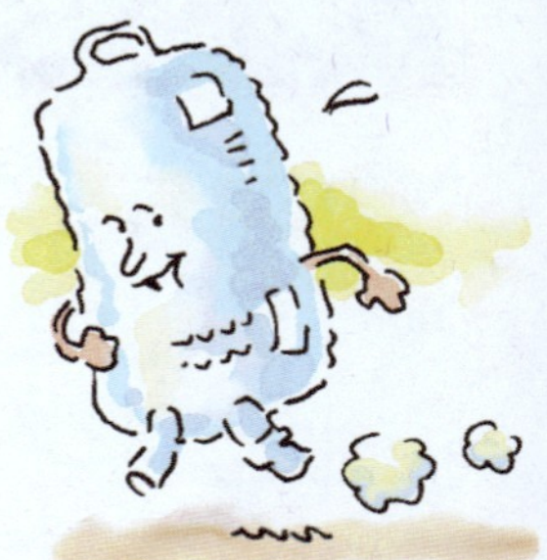
How fast can I run? Flow rates refer to the number of mL of fluid to administer over the course of 1 hour (mL/hr).

So, how flows it?

A patient has an order for an infusion of 1,000 mL of 0.45% normal saline over 8 hours. Find the flow rate by dividing the volume by the number of hours.

- Set up the formula with the information provided. Solve for *X*:

$$\text{Flow rate} = \frac{1{,}000 \text{ mL}}{8 \text{ hr}} = 125 \text{ mL/hr}$$

The flow rate is 125 mL/hr.

Salient saline solution

A patient has an order for 250 mL of normal saline (NS) solution to infuse over 2 hours. Find the flow rate by dividing the volume by the number of hours.

- Set up the formula with the information provided. Solve for *X*:

$$\text{Flow rate} = \frac{250 \text{ mL}}{2 \text{ hr}} = 125 \text{ mL/hr}$$

The flow rate is 125 mL/hr.

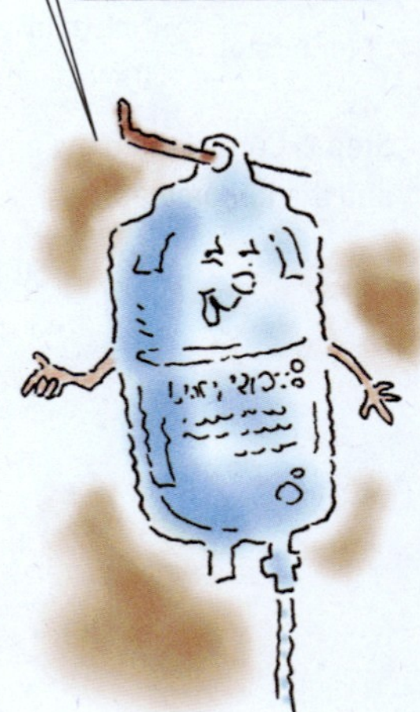

Quick calculation of drip rates

Here's a shortcut for converting flow rates to drip rates. It's based on the premise that all drop factors can be evenly divided into 60.

For macrodrip sets, use these rules to calculate drip rates:

- For sets that deliver **10 gtt/mL**, divide the hourly flow rate by **6**.
- For sets that deliver **15 gtt/mL**, divide the hourly flow rate by **4**.
- For sets that deliver **20 gtt/mL**, divide the hourly flow rate by **3**.

For a microdrip set with a drop factor of 60 gtt/mL, simply remember that the drip rate is the same as the flow rate.

Take the shortcut

The licensed practitioner prescribes *1,000 mL of normal saline to be infused over 12 hours*. The available administration set delivers 15 gtt/mL. Using the shortcut method, determine the drip rate.

Step 1: Find the flow rate. Set up the formula with the information provided:

$$X \text{ (Flow rate)} = \frac{1{,}000 \text{ mL}}{12 \text{ hours}} = 83.3333 \text{ mL/hr}$$

For accuracy, do not round within the problem itself, only round the final answer.

The flow rate is 83.3333 mL/hr.

Step 2: Find the drip rate using the shortcut method:

Remember the rule: for sets that deliver 15 gtt/mL, divide the flow rate by 4:

$$X = \frac{83.3333}{4}$$

Step 3: Solve for *X*. Divide the numerator by the denominator (83.3333 by 4):

$$X = 20.833325 \text{ gtt/min}$$

Rounded to the nearest whole number, the drip factor is 21 gtt/min.

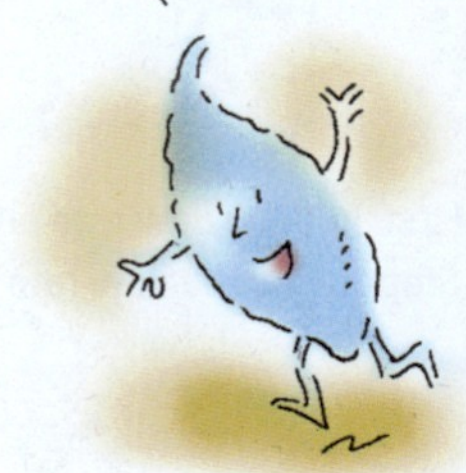
With a microdrip infusion set (60 gtt/mL), simply remember that the drip rate is the same as the flow rate!

Follow the golden microdrip rule

Solve the following problem without using a pencil and paper or a calculator.

A patient has an order for an IV infusion of LR at 150 mL/hr. The nurse uses a microdrip infusion set with a drop factor of 60 gtt/mL. What's the drip rate?

Remember the golden rule: Since the flow rate is 150 mL/hr, the drip rate would also be 150 gtt/min!

Calculating infusion times

Knowing the time it takes for an infusion to be completed allows nurses to anticipate and manage their time when it comes to replacing fluids and hanging medications. To determine infusion time, the nurse

Dosage drill

Test your math skills with this drill

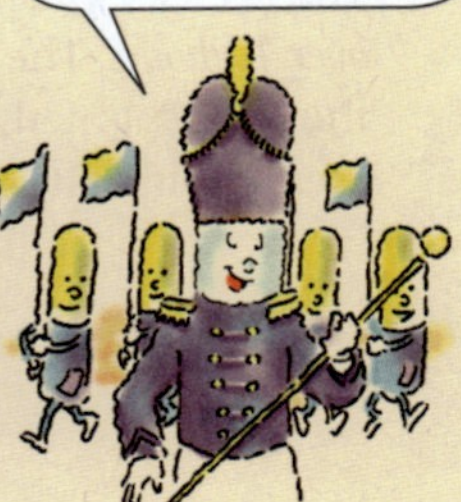
Be sure to show how you arrive at your answer.

A fluid bolus has been ordered for a patient presenting with dehydration. The order reads 0.9% NS 500 mL bolus over 2 hours. An IV pump is not available, so the nurses choose an infusion set calibrated to 15 gtt/mL. Using the shortcut method, determine the drip factor for the fluid bolus:

Your answer: ____________

First, find the flow rate and then find the drip rate.

Step 1: Find the flow rate using the information provided:

$$X \text{ (Flow rate)} = \frac{500 \text{ mL}}{2 \text{ hours}} = 250 \text{ mL/hr}$$

The flow rate is 250 mL/hr.

Step 2: Use the flow rate to determine the drip factor using the shortcut method:

$$X \text{ (drip factor)} = \frac{250}{4} = X = 62.5 \text{ gtt/min}$$

Rounding to the nearest whole number, the nurse should set the drip rate at 63 gtt/min.

must know the flow rate and volume to be infused. The formula to determine the infusion time is:

$$\text{Infusion Time} = \frac{\text{Total volume ordered (in mL)}}{\text{Flow rate (mL/hr)}}$$

Be back in ______ minutes!

The following examples break down how to use this formula to calculate infusion times.

The nurse has an order to infuse 1 L of D_5W at 50 mL/hr. Calculate the total infusion time.

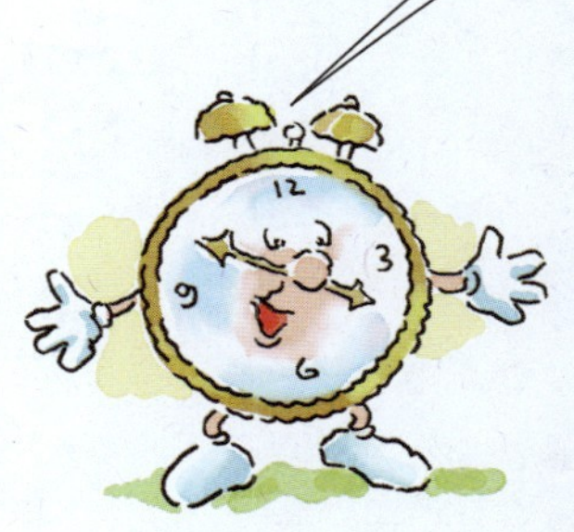

Keep the infusion
on schedule. Know
your formula!

Step 1: Convert 1 L to 1,000 mL to make units of measure equivalent.

Step 2: Set up the formula with the information provided:

$$X = \frac{1{,}000 \text{ mL}}{50 \text{ mL/hr}}$$

Step 3: Cancel the units appearing in both the numerator and the denominator:

$$X = \frac{1{,}000 \cancel{\text{mL}}}{50 \cancel{\text{mL}}\text{/hr}}$$

Step 4: Solve for X. Divide the numerator by the denominator (1,000 by 50):

$$X = 20 \text{ hr}$$

The 1 L of D_5W will infuse in 20 hours.

The bag will be empty at ______ o'clock

A patient has an order for 500 mL of normal saline solution to infuse at 80 mL/hr. What's the total infusion time? If the normal saline solution is hung at 0500, at what time will the infusion end?

Step 1: Find the infusion time. Set up the formula with the information provided:

$$X = \frac{500 \text{ mL}}{80 \text{ mL/hr}}$$

Step 2: Cancel the units appearing in both the numerator and the denominator:

$$X = \frac{500 \cancel{\text{mL}}}{80 \cancel{\text{mL}}\text{/hr}}$$

Step 3: Solve for X. Divide the numerator by the denominator (500 by 80):

$$X = 6.25 \text{ hr}$$

Dosage drill

Test your math skills with this drill

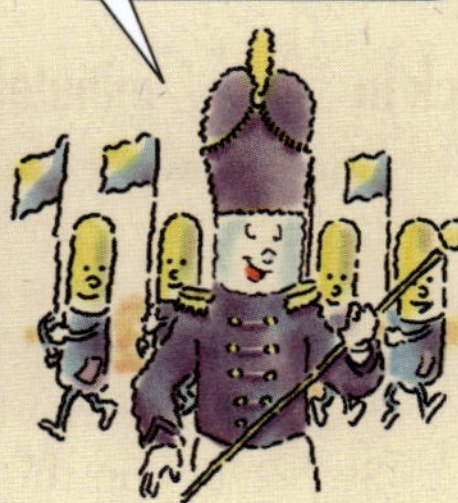
Be sure to show how you arrive at your answer.

At 0600, a patient received a preoperative infusion of 1,000 mL of dextrose 5% in 0.45% normal saline (D5 and ½ NS) at 125 mL/hr, followed by 1,000 mL of dextrose 5% in water (D_5W) at 100 mL/hr. How long did it take to infuse both solutions?

Your answer: ______________

Step 1: Find the infusion time of the first solution. Set up the formula with the information provided:

$$X = \frac{1{,}000\text{ mL}}{125\text{ mL/hr}}$$

Step 2: Cancel the units appearing in both the numerator and the denominator:

$$X = \frac{1{,}000\ \cancel{\text{mL}}}{125\ \cancel{\text{mL}}\text{/hr}}$$

Step 3: Solve for *X*. Divide the numerator by the denominator (1,000 by 125):

$$X = 8\text{ hr}$$

Total infusion time for the first infusion is 8 hours

Step 4: Find the infusion time of the second solution. Set up the formula with the information provided:

$$X = \frac{1{,}000\text{ mL}}{100\text{ mL/hr}}$$

Step 5: Cancel the units appearing in both the numerator and the denominator:

$$X = \frac{1{,}000\ \cancel{\text{mL}}}{100\ \cancel{\text{mL}}\text{/hr}}$$

Step 6: Solve for *X*. Divide the numerator by the denominator (1,000 by 100):

$$X = 10\text{ hr}$$

Total infusion time for the second infusion is 10 hours

Step 7: Add the times of both infusions together:

$$8\text{ hr} + 10\text{ hr} = 18\text{ hr}$$

The total infusion time for both solutions was 18 hours.

The normal saline solution will infuse in 6.25 hours (6 hours and 15 minutes).

Step 4: Determine at what time the infusion will be completed:

$$0500 + 6.25 = 1115$$

The infusion will end at 1115.

Regulating infusions

There are two primary methods of regulating infusions that include gravity and an IV pump. The use of patient-controlled analgesia (PCA) pumps is yet another way to regulate infusion, although it is not as commonly used.

Regulating IV flow manually

Nurses may manually regulate IV flow with gravity-calibrated infusion sets. The infusion is regulated by counting the number of drops going into the drip chamber over a 1-minute timeframe. To adjust the infusion rate, nurses use the roller clamp until the fluid is infusing at the appropriate number of drops per minute (gtt/min).

Fifteen seconds works fine

To save time, don't count the drops for a full minute. Instead, count the drops for only 15 seconds. The nurse will need to calculate the drip rate and divide by 4 (15 seconds is ¼ of a minute). For example, if the drip rate is 31 gtt/min, divide 31 by 4 to get 8 (rounded up from 7.75). The nurse then adjusts the roller clamp until the drip chamber shows 8 drops in a 15 second time frame.

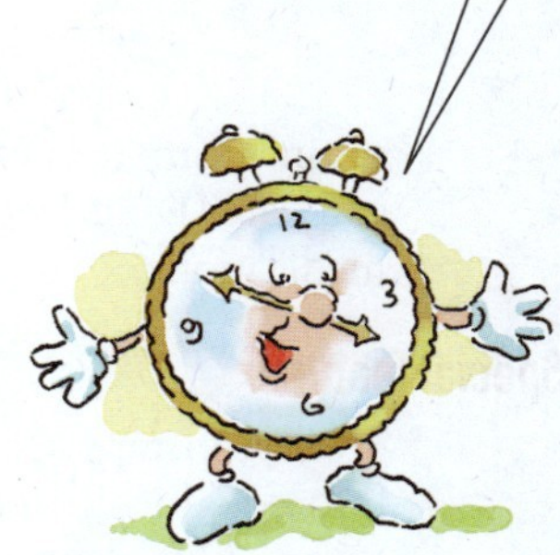
Save time! Divide the drip rate by 4 and count the drops for only 15 seconds instead of a full minute!
12
3
9
6

Tape it up!

Time taping is a patient safety strategy nurses can use when administering low-risk gravity drip IV infusions. (See *Taped up and ready to drip,* p. 244.)

Electronic infusion pumps

Electronic infusion pumps, often referred to as IV pumps, facilitate IV therapy administration. These pumps administer fluid under positive pressure and are calibrated by volume and flow rate. Nurses program the pumps to deliver a set rate (mL/hr) and volume (mL) as ordered by a licensed practitioner. Furthermore, "smart" infusion pumps are the most common type of IV pump used in acute care

Advice from the experts

Taped up and ready to drip

Time-taping an IV bag can be used with gravity calibration infusion sets to help ensure that an IV solution is administered at the prescribed rate. It also helps facilitate the recording of fluid intake.

To time-tape an IV bag, place a strip of adhesive tape from the top to the bottom of the bag, next to the fluid level markings. (This illustration shows a bag time-taped for a rate of 100 mL/hr beginning at 1000.)

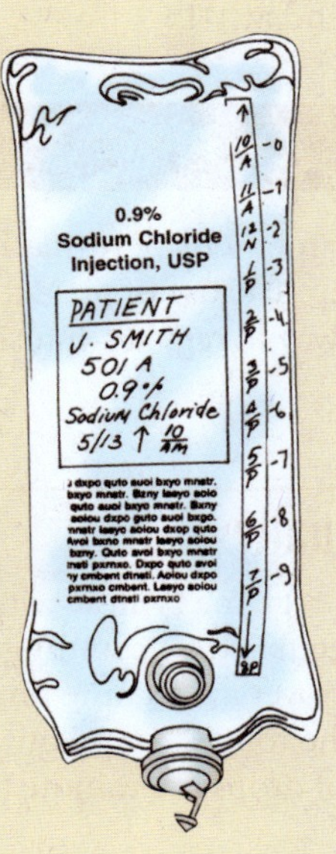

0 marks the spot

Next to the "0" marking, record the time that the infusion was started. Then, knowing the hourly rate, mark each hour on the tape next to the corresponding fluid marking. At the bottom of the tape, mark the time at which the solution will be completely infused. This allows nurses to have a visual indicator of the flow rate of the infusion. The tape marking will indicate to the nurse if the infusion is going too fast or too slow.

Ink alert

Don't write directly on the bag with a felt tip marker because the ink may seep into the fluid. Some manufacturers provide printed time tapes for use with their solutions.

settings. Smart pumps can be programmed with dose-error reduction software (DERS) which allows facilities to create a tailored library of medications.

Special features

Most IV pumps keep track of the amount of fluid that has been infused which helps maintain accurate intake and output records. Many of the pumps also have alarms that signal when the fluid container is empty or when a mechanical problem occurs. Some devices have variable pressure limits that prevent them from pumping fluids into infiltrated sites.

Regulating IV flow with pumps

When using an IV pump to administer fluids and medications, nurses regulate IV flow by programming the device using mL/hr. Some pumps can be programmed with specific flow rates that are calculated to the tenth space. An example of this would be programming the flow rate

The edge on electronic pumps

Using an IV pump is the safest method of IV administration. Not only do these pumps deliver precise and accurate amounts of fluids, but they also have other advantages as well including:

- allowing easy control of the rate and/or volume by programming data directly into the pump.
- detecting dosing and programming errors that may harm patients.
- having alert systems to notify nurses when the IV pump needs attention including air bubbles in lines, high pressures detected, completed infusions, and battery depletion.
- shortening the time needed to perform calculations for infusion rates.

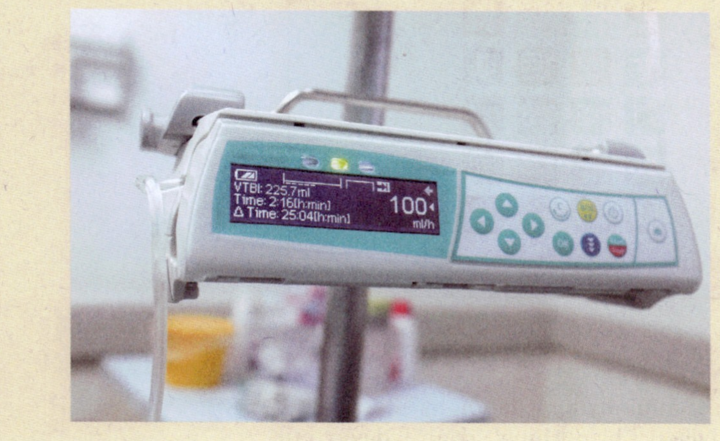

at 83.3 mL/hr. If this is not an available option, round flow rates to the nearest whole number. Check with manufacturer directions for device programming options.

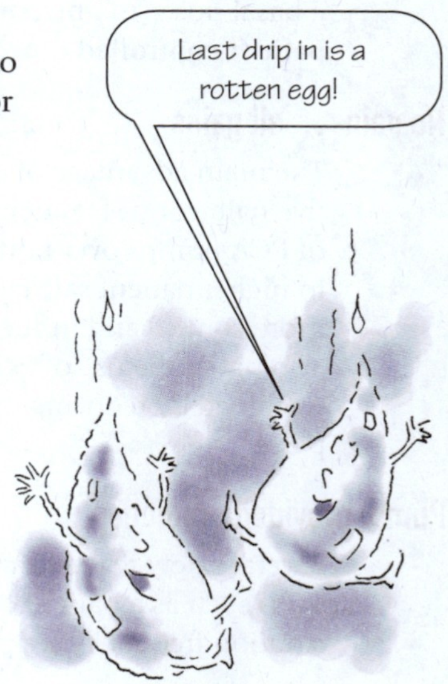

Programming the pump

To determine pump settings, consider the volume of fluid to be given and the total infusion time. With most devices, both the amount of fluid to be infused and the hourly flow rate need to be programmed. Mistakes still can be made using an IV pump as they don't eliminate the need for careful calculations and assessment of infusion rates.

Patient-controlled analgesia pumps

Another type of infusion device is the PCA pump that is used to treat acute, chronic, postoperative, and labor pain. Patients

Advice from the experts

Putting your patient in control

A patient-controlled analgesia (PCA) pump contains a programmable screen, such as the one shown here, allowing patients to self-administer pain medication with the push of a button. Although there are different varieties of PCA pumps available, all contain the essential components of a locking device, medication chamber, programming screen, and patient button.

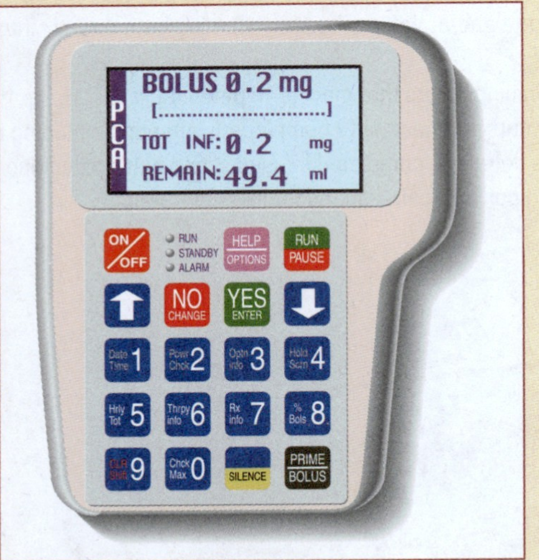

receive optimal analgesia while minimizing sedation by allowing patients to self-administer analgesics by pushing a control device button. Additionally, these pumps can also be programmed to deliver a basal dose (maintenance dose) of medication in addition to the patient-controlled dose. (See *Putting your patient in control*.)

No pains . . . all gains

The main advantage of using a PCA pump is to provide more effective pain control. Patients experience better pain control with the use of PCA pumps over non–patient-controlled opioid injections leading to higher patient satisfaction. Additionally, patients feel they have more control and influence around their pain control care. Nurses also prefer the use of PCA pumps for pain control as it decreases their workload by reducing the amount of scheduled or unscheduled med passes.

Pump-provided protection

Several safety features are built into PCA pumps to avoid complications such as a patient overdosing. Medication dose and administration frequency are programmed, preventing the patient from self-medicating too often. If the patient tries to overmedicate, the medical device simply ignores the request. Also, some pumps record the number of requests and the number of times the patient actually receives medication, which helps evaluate whether the prescriber needs to increase or decrease the medication dosing.

And the password is...

PCA pumps require an access code or the use of a key before entering medication dose and frequency information into the system. This prevents unauthorized users from tampering with or accidentally resetting the pump.

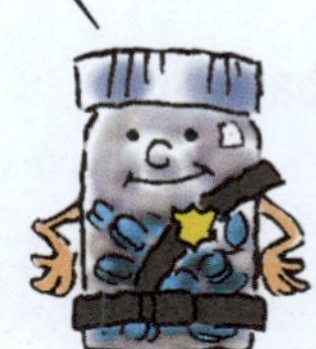

Don't worry. PCA pumps have safety features built into them to prevent patients from overmedicating themselves.

Recording medication dosage with a PCA

Every 4 hours, the nurse needs to document information obtained from the PCA. This data includes how much medication the patient has received during a 4-hour period and depending on the PCA pump, may include how many attempts and how many doses the patient actually received. The time frame is typically every 4 hours but is dependent on a facility's policy.

A double dose of accuracy

Most facilities require two nurses to verify the medication, the setup, and that the PCA settings matching the order. Each nurse who checks the PCA settings, double-checks and records this information.

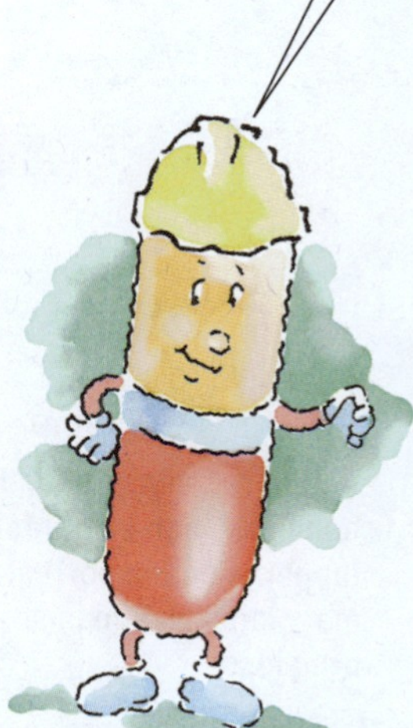

For safety sakes! Checking and double-checking the MAR or eMAR helps ensure the accuracy of the PCA programming.

Advice from the experts

PCA preparation

When preparing a PCA pump for a patient, follow these incredibly easy guidelines:

- Obtain the correct amount and concentration of medication—like morphine—and insert it into the PCA pump. Prefilled cartridges are more commonly used but is dependent on the type of PCA pump.
- Unlock the PCA keypad with an access code and/or use a PCA key to unlock the medication chamber.
- Program the pump according to the PCA order. An example of an order:
  - *Start morphine sulfate PCA. Give 2 mg/hr basal rate and 1 mg/q15 minute on demand, with a lock-out time of 6 mg/4 hr.*
- Based on a facility's policy, have a second nurse witness this information ensuring to match the order. Document accordingly.

Electrolyte and nutrient infusions

IV fluids can be mixed with electrolytes and other nutrients to be delivered directly into a patient's bloodstream.

Adding up the additives

Large-volume infusions with additives can maintain and restore a patient's electrolyte status or supply additional electrolytes, vitamins, or other nutrients. Common additives include potassium chloride, vitamins B and C, and trace elements.

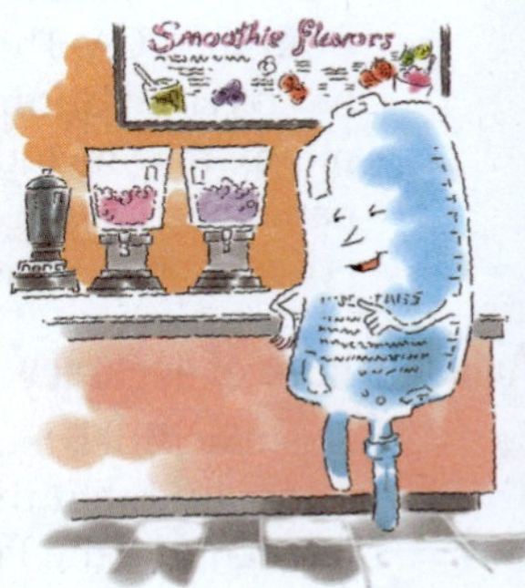
Make that a large decaf potassium chloride with a vitamin B on the side please.
Smoothie flavors

Piggyback ride

Electrolytes and antibiotics are usually supplied in small volume bags with 50 mL or 100 mL solutions being the most common. These

Two methods of administering small-volume intermittent IV infusions

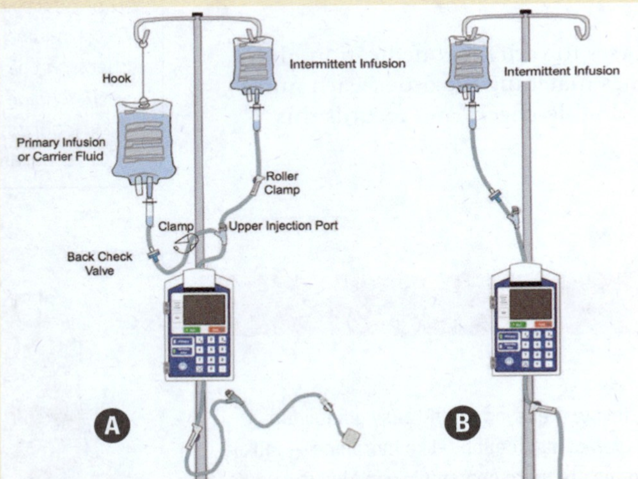

A (left, recommended): Using a secondary administration set attached at the Y-site (upper injection port) of a carrier fluid or primary infusion administration set (minimizes drug loss)

B (right, NOT recommended): Using a primary administration set connected directly to the patient's vascular access device (leads to significant drug loss)

Reprinted with permission from Institute for Safe Medication Practices. Hidden medication loss when using a primary administration set for small-volume intermittent infusions. *ISMP Medication Safety Alert!® Acute Care.* 2020;25(24):1–6.

medications may be infused intermittingly through primary infusion administration sets or given via IV piggyback (IVPB) in which the small-volume solution is connected to a primary IV line through a secondary administration set. Nurses can choose to either hang an IVPB medication using primary tubing alone or to use both primary and secondary infusion sets together. According to the Institute for Safe Medication Practices (2020), it is recommended to use the IVPB setup to reduce medication loss that occurs with using a primary line only. In either method, the flow rate is calculated in the same manner. (See *Calculating piggyback infusions*, p. 250.)

Prepare to prepare

Commonly, additives come already prepared in premixed solutions. However, on a rare occasion, nurses may have to add the additive themselves. In this case, the nurse will need to perform a calculation on how much additive to add to the solution. Here's an example.

Thinking about thiamine

A patient has an order for 1,000 mL of D_5W with an additive of 150 mg of thiamine/L to be infused over 12 hours. The nurse must add the thiamine to the solution. The thiamine is available in a prepared syringe of 100 mg/mL. How many mL of thiamine must the nurse add to the solution?

Step 1: Write the first ratio to describe the known solution strength (amount of medication per 1 mL):

$$100 \text{ mg:} 1 \text{ mL}$$

Step 2: Set up the second ratio. Write the amount of thiamine ordered on one side and the unknown amount to be added to the solution on the other side:

$$150 \text{ mg:} X$$

Step 3: Put these ratios into a proportion:

$$100 \text{ mg:} 1 \text{ mL} :: 150 \text{ mg:} X$$

Step 4: Solve for X. Multiply the extremes and the means:

$$X \times 100 \text{ mg} = 150 \text{ mg} \times 1 \text{ mL}$$

Step 5: Divide each side of the equation by 100 mg and cancel units that appear in both the numerator and denominator:

$$\frac{X \times \cancel{100 \text{ mg}}}{\cancel{100 \text{ mg}}} = \frac{150 \cancel{\text{ mg}} \times 1 \text{ mL}}{100 \cancel{\text{ mg}}}$$

$$X = \frac{150 \text{ mL}}{100}$$

$$X = 1.5 \text{ mL}$$

The nurse must add 1.5 mL of thiamine to the solution.

Calculating piggyback infusions

An IV piggyback (IVPB) is a small-volume, intermittent infusion that connects to an existing IV line containing maintenance fluid. Antibiotics and electrolytes are the most common form of IVPB. The following is an example of how to determine how much medication to mix in a small infusion bag to create an IVPB.

Piggyback problem

A patient has an order for 500 mg of imipenem IV in 100 mL of normal saline solution to be infused over 1 hour. The imipenem vial contains 1,000 mg (1 g). The insert says to reconstitute the powder with 5 mL of normal saline solution.

- How many mL of the reconstituted solution should the nurse remove from the vial?
- Determine the flow rate of the IVPB.

Solution solution

Step 1: Write the first ratio to describe the known solution strength (amount of medication compared to the known amount of solution):

$$1{,}000 \text{ mg:}5 \text{ mL}$$

Step 2: Write the second ratio, which compares the desired dose of imipenem and the unknown amount of solution:

$$500 \text{ mg:}X$$

Step 3: Put these ratios into a proportion:

$$1{,}000 \text{ mg:}5 \text{ mL::}500 \text{ mg:}X$$

Step 4: Multiply the extremes and the means:

$$1{,}000 \text{ mg} \times X = 500 \text{ mg} \times 5 \text{ mL}$$

Step 5: Solve for *X*. Divide each side of the equation by 1,000 mg and cancel units that appear in both the numerator and the denominator:

$$\frac{\cancel{1{,}000 \text{ mg}} \times X}{\cancel{1{,}000 \text{ mg}}} = \frac{500 \cancel{\text{ mg}} \times 5 \text{ mL}}{1{,}000 \cancel{\text{ mg}}}$$

$$X = \frac{500 \times 5 \text{ mL}}{1{,}000}$$

$$X = \frac{2{,}500 \text{ mL}}{1{,}000}$$

$$X = 2.5 \text{ mL}$$

The nurse should remove 2.5 mL from the vial of imipenem to add to the 100 mL of normal saline to make an IVPB solution.

Flow rate

Recall that the flow rate is the number of mL to administer over 1 hour. Therefore, 100 mL divided by 1 hour equals 100 mL/hr.

The flow rate is 100 mL/hr.

Compatibility counts

The nurse must check compatibility with the medication or solution contained in an IVPB with the primary IV fluid being administered. The same goes for medications mixed in the same syringe or IV bag. Some facilities have medication compatibility charts available in a unit's medication room. More often, since medications are continuously added and updated, nurses use medication handbooks or on-line drug libraries to check for compatibility. Pharmacists are also a great resource!

Step 6: Find the flow rate by using the information provided:

Recall the formula:

$$\text{Flow rate (mL/hr)} = \frac{\text{Total volume ordered (in mL)}}{\text{Total time (in hours)}}$$

If the volume is 1,000 mL and the time is 12 hours, divide 1,000 by 12 to find the flow rate for 1 hour:

$$\frac{1{,}000 \text{ mL}}{12 \text{ hr}} = 83.3 \text{ mL/hr}$$

If rounding to the whole number, the flow rate would be 83 mL/hr.

Blood and blood product infusions

The process of blood administration can be complex as many necessary steps need to be taken before the actual transfusion takes place. These steps range from having a signed consent, having proper IV access (18, 20, or 22 gauge IV), gathering special tubing and supplies, obtaining vital signs, and having another nurse available to be a witness for double verification. Timing is especially important in the process such as when to take vital signs and the time limit of blood transfusion. In general, clinical practice guidelines of whole blood and packed red blood cells (PRBCs) recommend infusion times no longer than 4 hours. This timeframe is also determinate on different factors including age, the patient's diagnosis, and the stability of the patient's condition. Nurses need to follow their facility's protocols and policies regarding blood administration.

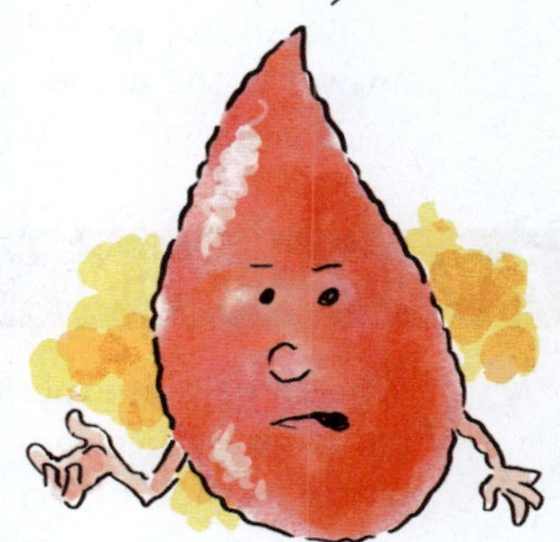

Be especially careful when infusing or transfusing blood. Use the right equipment, watch the time, and always follow a facility's protocol.

Written in blood

Most blood products require special blood administration sets that have specialized tubing and contain filters to prevent cell damage. These administration sets are generally available for infusion by gravity or by an IV pump. Again, nurses need to follow the facility's policy for blood administration guidelines.

Blood cell brain teaser

The following is an example of a dosage calculation problem involving PRBCs:

A patient has an order to receive 250 mL of PRBCs over 4 hours. The nurse chooses a gravity infusion set with a drop factor of 10 gtt/mL. At what drip rate will the nurse infuse the PRBCs?

Recall the formula for drip rate:

$$\text{Drip rate (gtts/min)} = \frac{\text{Volume to be infused (in mL)}}{\text{Time (in minutes)}} \times \text{Drop factor (gtts/mL)}$$

Step 1: Convert the hours to minutes to make units of measure equivalent (4×60).

Step 2: Set up the formula with the information provided:

$$X = \frac{250 \text{ mL}}{240 \text{ min}} \times \frac{10 \text{ gtt}}{1 \text{ mL}}$$

Step 3: Cancel units that appear in both the numerator and the denominator:

$$X = \frac{250 \cancel{\text{mL}}}{240 \text{ min}} \times \frac{10 \text{ gtt}}{1 \cancel{\text{mL}}}$$

Step 4: Multiply the volume by the drop rate (250 by 10):

$$X = \frac{250 \times 10 \text{ gtt}}{240 \text{ min}}$$

Step 5: Solve for *X*. Divide 2,500 by 240:

$$X = \frac{2{,}500 \text{ gtt}}{240 \text{ min}}$$

$$X = 10.416 \text{ gtt/min}$$

Recall that partial drops can't be counted; therefore, round the answer to the newest whole number.

The drip rate is 10 gtt/min.

Parenteral nutrition

When a patient experiences impaired gastrointestinal function and has contraindications to enteral nutrition, they may need an alternative method of receiving nutrition. This alternative method is referred to as parenteral nutrition (PN) available as total parenteral nutrition (TPN) or partial parenteral nutrition (PPN). Both methods have a common goal of correcting a patient's malnutrition status.

One of the primary differences between TPN and PPN is PPN is intended to only partially fulfill a patient's daily nutrition requirements. PPN is primarily used to supplement nutrition for those patients who are able to consume some nutrition while TPN provides a patient's full daily caloric requirement. Another difference between the two is that PPN can be infused through a peripheral line, unlike TPN which must be infused through a central venous catheter (CVC) due to high osmolarity.

Both TPN and PPN are available as commercially prepared products or individually formulated solutions from the pharmacy. Orders for TPN or PPN are only valid for a 24-hour period requiring the prescriber to review the patient's nutritional needs daily.

Since most PN require refrigeration, nurses should look in the refrigerator for their patient's prepared solution. Before administration, most facilities require two nurses to verify the contents of the PPN or TPN solution.

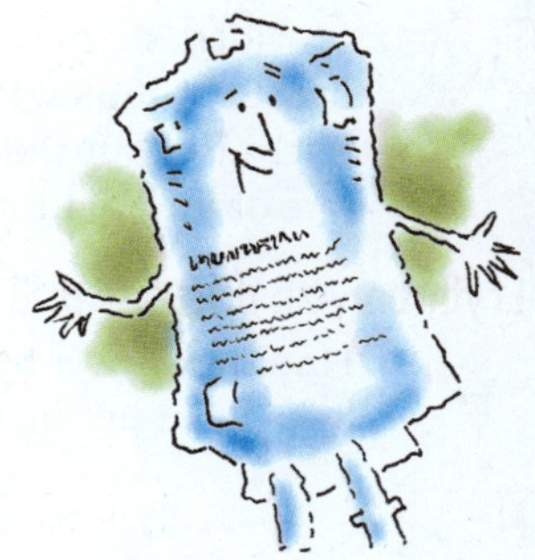

It's always good to brush up on a facility's protocol... no matter how busy the shift becomes!

Added attractions

TPN solutions contain a 10% or greater dextrose concentration. Amino acids are added to maintain or restore nitrogen balance, and vitamins, electrolytes, and trace minerals are added to meet individual patient needs.

Lipids may also be added to the solution, but they're commonly given separately to prevent their destruction by the other nutrients. Nurses also have to remember that additives increase a solution's total volume, and thus affect intake measurements.

For example, when assessing the amount of fluid remaining in the TPN solution, the nurse should anticipate an additional 20 to 50 mL more than expected.

What goes up... must come down

Initially, TPN is usually infused at a slower rate, around 40 mL/hr, then gradually increased to the full maintenance dose. Since TPN is high in dextrose, the infusion rate is gradually decreased before discontinuing TPN all together. Due to the high glucose content, patient's glucose levels are closely monitored as well when receiving TPN therapy.

For safety reasons, TPN must be administered and regulated through an IV pump. In addition, special in-line IV filters should be used to reduce the patient's exposure to particulate matter during PN therapy especially when lipids are administered.

Let the vitamins infuse!

Using the flow rate formula, determine the flow rate of a TPN solution supplied in 2,000 mL bag to be infused over a 24-hour period:

$$\text{Flow rate (mL/hr)} = \frac{\text{Total volume ordered (in mL)}}{\text{Total time (in hours)}}$$

$$X = \frac{2{,}000 \text{ mL}}{24 \text{ hours}} = 83.333 \text{ mL/hr}$$

Rounding to the nearest whole number, the infusion rate is 83 mL/hr.

More practice with IV infusion calculations

These problems are typical of the infusion calculations a nurse is likely to encounter.

Real-world problems

A patient has an order for 500 mg of erythromycin IV. The pharmacy provides 500 mg erythromycin in 50 mL of sterile water to be infused over 30 minutes. With no IV pump available, the nurse chooses a microdrip infusion set calibrated to 60 gtt/mL. Determine the drip rate of the erythromycin solution:

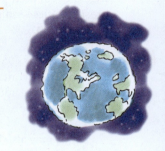

Erythromycin drip rate drill

Find the answer by using the drip rate formula:

Step 1: Set up the formula with the information provided:

$$X = \frac{50 \text{ mL}}{30 \text{ min}} \times \frac{60 \text{ gtt}}{1 \text{ mL}}$$

Step 2: Cancel units that appear in both the numerator and the denominator:

$$X = \frac{50 \cancel{\text{mL}}}{30 \text{ min}} \times \frac{60 \text{ gtt}}{1 \cancel{\text{mL}}}$$

The shortcut method could also be used to help speed up the calculation process!

Step 3: Multiply 50 by 60:

$$X = \frac{50 \times 60 \text{ gtt}}{30 \text{ min}}$$

Step 4: Solve for X. Divide 3,000 by 30:

$$X = \frac{3{,}000 \text{ gtt}}{30 \text{ min}}$$

$$X = 100 \text{ gtt/min}$$

The drip rate is 100 gtt/min.

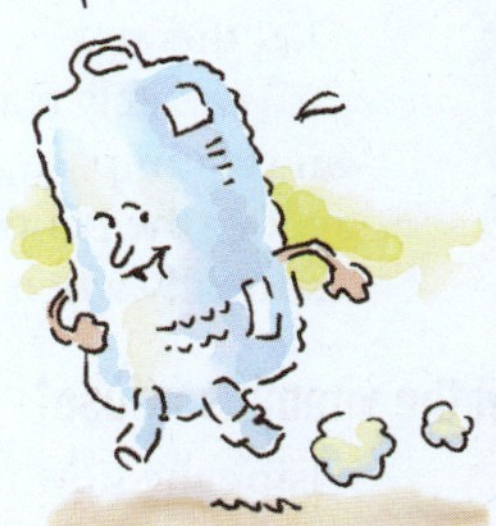

This should ring 'er bell

Recall the formula for calculating infusion time:

$$\text{Infusion Time} = \frac{\text{Total volume ordered (in mL)}}{\text{Flow rate (mL/hr)}}$$

A patient has an order for an infusion of 1,000 mL of lactated Ringer (LR) at 125 mL/hr. The nurse started the infusion at 0700 using a primary infusion set with a calibration of 10 gtt/mL.

- What's the total transfusion time?
- At what time does the nurse anticipate the infusion to be completed?

Dosage drill

Test your math skills with this drill

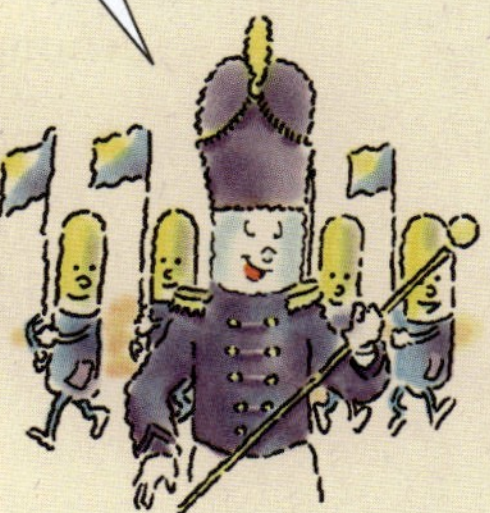
Be sure to show how you arrive at your answer.

A patient has an order for 250 mL of 0.3% sodium chloride to infuse over 4 hours. What is the flow rate for this solution?

Your answer: ______________

Step 1: Set up the formula with the information provided:

$$X = \frac{250 \text{ mL}}{4 \text{ hours}}$$

Step 2: Solve for *X*. Divide 250 by 4:

$$X = 62.5 \text{ mL/hr}$$

If necessary, round to the nearest whole number. The flow rate is 63 mL/hr.

Step 1: Set up the formula with the information provided:

$$X = \frac{1{,}000 \text{ mL}}{125 \text{ mL/hr}}$$

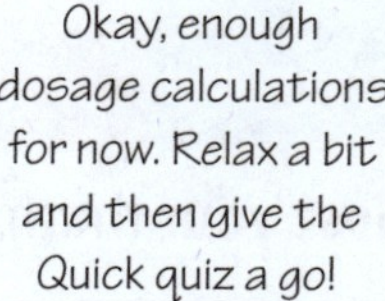
Okay, enough
dosage calculations
for now. Relax a bit
and then give the
Quick quiz a go!

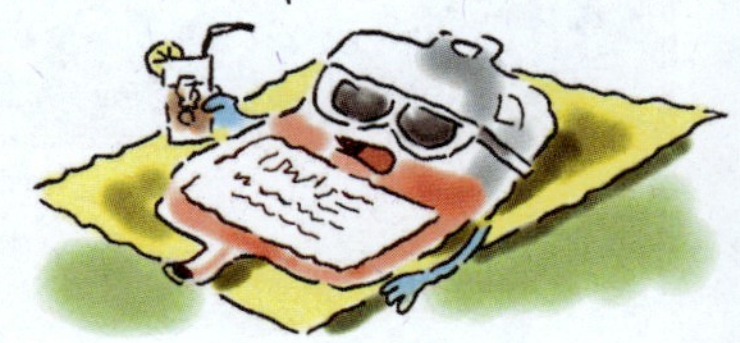

Step 2: Cancel units that appear in both the numerator and the denominator:

$$X = \frac{1{,}000 \cancel{\text{mL}}}{125 \cancel{\text{mL}}\text{/hr}}$$

Step 2: Solve for *X*. Divide 1,000 by 125:

$$X = \frac{1{,}000}{125 \text{ hr}}$$

$$X = 8 \text{ hours}$$

The total infusion time is 8 hours.

What time will the infusion be completed?

Determine by adding 8 hours to 0700. The infusion will be completed at 1500.

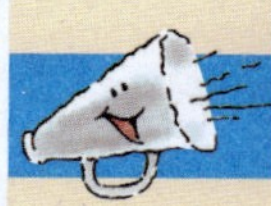

That's a wrap!

Calculating IV infusions review

Some important information about calculating IV infusions is highlighted below:

Drip rate

- Represents the number of drops infused per minute (gtt/min).
- Drop factor represents the number of drops per mL of solution that the IV tubing is designed to deliver expressed as gtt/mL.
- Drip rate formula:

$$\text{Drip rate (gtts/min)} = \frac{\text{Volume to be infused (in mL)}}{\text{Time (in minutes)}} \times \text{Drop factor (gtts/mL)}$$

Drip rate shortcut

Remember the shortcut numbers:

- 10 gtt/mL, divide the hourly flow rate by 6.
- 15 gtt/mL, divide the hourly flow rate by 4.
- 20 gtt/mL, divide the hourly flow rate by 3.
- 60 gtt/mL, divide the hourly flow rate by 1.

Flow rate

- Represents the number of mL of fluid administered over 1 hour expressed as mL/hr.
- Flow rate formula:

$$\text{Flow rate (mL/hr)} = \frac{\text{Total volume ordered (in mL)}}{\text{Total time (in hours)}}$$

Calculating IV infusions review (*continued*)

Infusion time

- The amount of time required for infusion of a specified volume of IV fluid or mediation.
- Infusion time formula:

$$\text{Infusion time} = \frac{\text{Total volume ordered (in mL)}}{\text{Flow rate (mL/hr)}}$$

Regulating IV flow by gravity

- The number of drops going into the drip chamber over 1 minute. Save time and divide the drip rate by 4, and count those drops for 15 seconds.
- Flow rate (infusion) is adjusted using the roller clamp.
- Time-tape IV bags when administering low-risk gravity drip IV infusions.

Regulating IV flow with electronic infusion pumps (IV pumps)

- Program the device based on the flow rate (mL/hr).
- Considered the safest method of regulating IV therapy infusions.

PCA pump

- Allows the patient to self-administer an analgesic or to deliver a continuous infusion rate (basal dose) of medication
- Safety measures in place to prevent overdose.
- Requires use of an access code and/or PCA key to prevent unauthorized use of the device.

PCA Summary

Frequent monitoring and documentation are required for a patient on PCA therapy. Documentation includes:

- Verification of medication being infused against the MAR or eMAR.
- Total attempts versus the number of actual administrations patient received.
- Total basal dose patient received, if applicable.
- Total dose and total volume of solution patient received.
- Patient's pain level and tolerance to therapy.

Electrolyte and nutrient infusions

- Verify that medications to be infused together are compatible.
- Perform calculations if an additive is to be added to an IVPB solution.
- Typically comes in IVPB form in 50 mL or 100 mL bags.
- Infusion using secondary tubing for IVPB is preferred.
- May need to calculate the flow rate or the drip rate.

Blood infusions

- Calculate the drip rate or flow rate according to the infusion time.
- Use special administration sets which contain filters and special tubing for blood transfusion according to a facility's policy.

PN administration

- PPN used for supplementing a patient's nutrient needs. May be infused through a peripheral IV.
- TPN used for a patient's daily caloric intake. Infused through a central venous catheter only.
- Initially infused at 40 mL/hr, then increased to maintenance dose.
- Both must be administered via an IV pump.

Quick quiz

1. A patient has an order to start IV fluids at 75 mL/hr. Based on this infusion rate, which drop factor tubing should the nurse use to deliver the fluids?

A. 15 gtt/mL
B. 10 gtt/mL
C. 20 gtt/mL
D. 60 gtt/mL

Answer: D. According to the drip guidelines, use microdrip tubing for all flow rates 80 mL/hr or less. The nurse should choose the infusion set with a drop factor of 60 gtt/mL.

2. A nurse reviews an order that states to infuse 1,000 mL of 0.9% sodium chloride over 10 hours. The available infusion set has a calibration of 15 gtt/mL. After 5 hours, 650 mL have been infused instead of 500 mL. What action would the nurse take after recalculating the drip rate for the remaining solution?

A. Change the drip rate to 18 gtt/min.
B. Change the drip rate to 35 gtt/min.
C. Change the drip rate to 17 gtt/min.
D. Change the drip rate to 25 gtt/min.

Answer: A. To solve this problem, the nurse must first determine the amount of fluid remaining by subtracting 650 mL from 1,000 mL (1,000 – 650 = 350 mL). Then, convert the time remaining to minutes (10 – 5 = 5 hr) (5 hr × 60 min = 300 min remaining). Use the drip rate formula to determine the new drip rate.

$$\text{Drip rate (gtts/min)} = \frac{\text{Volume to be infused (in mL)}}{\text{Time (in minutes)}} \times \text{Drop factor (gtts/mL)}$$

- Set up the formula with the information provided and cancel units that appear in both the numerator and the denominator:

$$X = \frac{350\ \cancel{\text{mL}}}{300\ \text{min}} \times \frac{15\ \text{gtt}}{1\ \cancel{\text{mL}}}$$

- Multiply 350 × 15:

$$X = \frac{350 \times 15\ \text{gtt}}{300\ \text{min}}$$

- Solve for *X*. Divide 5,250 by 300:

$$X = \frac{5{,}250\ \text{gtt}}{300\ \text{min}}$$

$$X = 17.5\ \text{gtt/min}$$

Since a partial drop cannot be counted, round to the nearest whole number which is 18 gtt/min.

3. Using the golden microdrip rule, what would be the drip rate for a microdrip set with a drop factor of 60 gtt/mL?

   A. half the rate of the hourly flow rate.
   B. 10 times greater than the hourly flow rate.
   C. the same rate as the hourly flow rate.
   D. 4 times greater than the hourly flow rate.

Answer: C. The drip rate is the same as the hourly flow rate because the number of minutes in an hour (60 minutes) is the same as the drop factor.

4. A PCA pump can be programmed to deliver a dose of medication on demand in addition to what other delivery method?

   A. dropped rate
   B. basal rate
   C. ratio rate
   D. lock-out rate

Answer: B. The basal rate is a continuous infusion administered by a PCA pump.

5. The nurse needs to infuse 1,500 mL of D_5W over 10 hours. What flow rate will the nurse use to program an IV pump for this infusion?

   A. 50 mL/hr
   B. 100 mL/hr
   C. 150 mL/hr
   D. 250 mL/hr

Answer: C. The nurse would program an IV pump at a flow rate of 150 mL/hr. To determine the flow rate, use the flow rate formula:

$$\text{Flow rate (mL/hr)} = \frac{\text{Total volume ordered (in mL)}}{\text{Total time (in hours)}}$$

- Set up the formula with the information provided. Solve for *X*. Divide 1,500 by 10:

$$X = \frac{1{,}500 \text{ mL}}{10 \text{ hours}} = 150 \text{ mL/hr}$$

6. A patient has an order for an infusion of D_5W at 75 mL/hr. The tubing set available is calibrated at 20 gtt/mL. What's the drip rate?

   A. 20 gtt/min
   B. 25 gtt/min
   C. 50 gtt/min
   D. 75 gtt/min

Answer: B. The nurse would set the drip rate to 25 gtt/min. Use the drip rate formula to determine the drip rate.

- Set up the formula with the information provided and cancel units that appear in both the numerator and the denominator:

$$X = \frac{75 \not{\text{mL}}}{60 \text{ min}} \times \frac{20 \text{ gtt}}{1 \not{\text{mL}}}$$

- Multiply 75×20:

$$X = \frac{75 \times 20 \text{ gtt}}{60 \text{ min}}$$

- Solve for *X*. Divide 1,500 by 60:

$$X = \frac{1{,}500 \text{ gtt}}{60 \text{ min}}$$

$$X = 25 \text{ gtt/min}$$

Scoring

☆☆☆ If you answered all eight items correctly, excellent! Enjoy every drop of success.

☆☆ If you answered five to seven items correctly, great job! Your drop factor is beyond measure. (All right, if you insist, we'll give you 15 gtt/mL.)

☆ If you answered fewer than five items correctly, no problem! Go with the flow, keep calculation, and infuse in peace and joy.

Suggested References

A compendium of transfusion practice guidelines—American Red Cross. (2021, January). https://www.redcross.org/content/dam/redcrossblood/hospital-page-documents/334401_compendium_v04jan2021_bookmarkedworking_rwv01.pdf

Epstein, E. M., & Waseem, M. (2023 Jan–). Crystalloid fluids. [Updated 2023 Jul 3]. In: *StatPearls [Internet]*. StatPearls Publishing.https://www.ncbi.nlm.nih.gov/books/NBK537326/

Hidden medication loss when using a primary administration set for small-volume intermittent infusions. Institute For Safe Medication Practices. (2020, December 3). https://www.ismp.org/resources/hidden-medication-loss-when-using-primary-administration-set-small-volume-intermittent

Open Resources for Nursing (Open RN). (2023). Chapter 1 Initiate IV therapy. In K. Ernstmeyer & E. Christman. (Eds.), *Nursing advanced skills* [Internet]. Chippewa Valley Technical College. https://www.ncbi.nlm.nih.gov/books/NBK594499/

Pastino, A., Lakra, A. (2023 Jan–). Patient-controlled analgesia. [Updated 2023 Jan 29]. In *StatPearls [Internet]*. StatPearls Publishing. https://www.ncbi.nlm.nih.gov/books/NBK551610/

Smart pumps in practice: Survey results reveal widespread use, but optimization is challenging. (2019, June 18). Institute for Safe Medication Practices. https://www.ismp.org/resources/smart-pumps-practice-survey-results-reveal-widespread-use-optimization-challenging

Worthington, P., Gura, K. M., Kraft, M. D., Nishikawa, R., Guenter, P., & Sacks, G. S. (2020). Update on the use of filters for parenteral nutrition: An aspen position paper. *Nutrition in Clinical Practice, 36*(1), 29–39. https://doi.org/10.1002/ncp.10587

Part VI

Special calculations

Chapter 14

Calculating pediatric dosages

Just the facts

In this chapter, you'll learn how to:

- prepare medications and administer them to infants and children by the four major routes
- calculate safe pediatric medication dosages according to body weight and body surface area
- recognize recommended pediatric infusion guidelines and protocols
- calculate pediatric fluid needs based on body weight, calories of metabolism, and body surface area

A look at calculating pediatric dosages

When calculating medication dosages for pediatric patients, remember that children aren't just small adults. Due to their size, metabolism, and other factors, children have special medication needs and require special care. Moreover, an incorrect dose is more likely to harm a child than an adult. For safety reasons, some medications may require two nurses to verify the calculations and ensure appropriate medication dosages.

Why is this chapter so important? Children have special dosage calculation needs.

Same routes, different needs

Although children and adults receive medications by the oral (PO), subcutaneous (subcut), intramuscular (IM), intravenous (IV), and topical routes, the similarity ends there. The pharmacokinetics, pharmacodynamics, and pharmacotherapeutics of medications differ greatly between children and adults.

For example, a child's immature body system may be unable to handle certain medications. Also, a child's total volume of body water is much greater proportionally than an adult's total water body volume, and so medication distribution is altered. Due to these differences, you must be especially careful when calculating dosages for children. (See *A trio of timesaving tips*, p. 264.)

Diversity, equity, and inclusion

Children, like adults, also bring developmental, cultural, religious, and personal backgrounds which may impact medication compliance, access to care, or understanding of medication administration. Nurses need to be aware of the unique differences of children and families when implementing safe medication administration.

Administering pediatric medications

The methods used to prepare medications and administer them to pediatric patients also differ from the methods used for adults, depending on which route is used. There are specific administration guidelines and precautions for each route as well. However, there is one step that is always the same no matter the age of the patient. Always verify the child's identity using two patient identifiers. Involve the caregiver and the patient in the identification process, when possible. (See *Giving medications to children*.)

Oral route

Infants and young children who can't swallow tablets or capsules are given oral medications in liquid form. Nurses may need to be creative so the child will take the medication completely. Infants may take liquid medications through a nipple or using a therapeutic hugging technique may assist with holding a toddler who refuses to swallow medications. Consider each child's developmental stage to adapt to

Advice from the experts

A trio of timesaving tips

When calculating safe pediatric dosages, save time and avoid errors by following these incredibly easy suggestions:

- Carry a calculator for use in solving equations.
- Consult a formulary or medication handbook to verify a medication dose. When in doubt, call the pharmacist.
- Keep your patient's weight, in kilograms, in an accessible area such as the bedside. This eliminates having to estimate it or weigh them in a rush.

Advice from the experts

Giving medications to children

When giving oral and parenteral medications to children, safety is essential. Keep these points in mind:

- Check the child's mouth to make sure they have swallowed all the oral medications.
- Carefully mix oral medications that come in suspension form.
- Give intramuscular (IM) injections in the vastus lateralis muscle, deltoid, or ventrogluteal muscle. Sites are age based.
- Inject the appropriate amount of fluid for the child's age and location.
- Rotate injection sites.
- Get assistance from caregiver or health care workers when necessary.
- Provide therapeutic interventions for painful procedures (sucking, therapeutic holding, distraction, or developmental play).

their needs. When a liquid preparation isn't available, verify if crushing a tablet and mixing it with a small amount of liquid is safe. Medications may be cut with a pill cutter to safely break the pills into the appropriate dose. Be sure to check with the pharmacist to ensure it is safe to cut or crush the medication. Don't use essential fluids, such as breast milk and infant formula, as this may lead to feeding refusal. Additionally, mix medications only with a small amount of liquid as the child won't receive the entire dose unless they take the entire liquid.

Remember: Never crush timed-release capsules or tablets or enteric-coated medications. Crushing destroys the coating that causes medications to release at the right time and prevent stomach irritation.

Measuring device advice

If a child can drink from a cup, measure and give liquid medications in a cup that's calibrated in metric and household units. If the child is very young or can't drink from a cup, use a medication dropper, syringe, or hollow-handle spoon. These devices are sold individually and come prepackaged with some medications. Reinforce proper medication amount with the caregivers who will be administering new doses at home.

Mix it up

If the liquid medication is prepared as a suspension or as an insoluble medication in a liquid base, mix it thoroughly before measuring and then administer it. This ensures that none of the medication remains settled out of the solution. Whenever an oral medication is given, check the child's mouth to make sure that the entire medication was swallowed.

Subcutaneous route

Pediatric patients also may receive childhood immunizations (such as the measles, mumps, and rubella vaccine and other virus vaccines) and medications such as insulin by the subcut route. When giving subcut injections, make sure each injection contains no more than 1 mL of solution. Any area with sufficient subcut tissue may be used—the upper arm, abdomen, and thigh are the most common.

IM route

Vaccines, such as those against diphtheria, pertussis, and tetanus, are commonly administered by the IM route. (See *IM injections for infants*, p. 266.) When giving IM injections, make sure each injection has the appropriate amount of solution for the location. Give IM injections in the vastus lateralis (outer thigh), deltoid, or the ventrogluteal muscle at a 90-degree angle.

IM injections for infants

When giving IM injections to infants, use the vastus lateralis muscle. Don't inject into the gluteus muscle until it's fully developed, which occurs when the child learns to walk. Use a 22G to 25G needle that's 5/8″ to 1″ in length. These illustrations show how to give an IM injection using one- and two-person methods. Inject at a 90-degree angle.

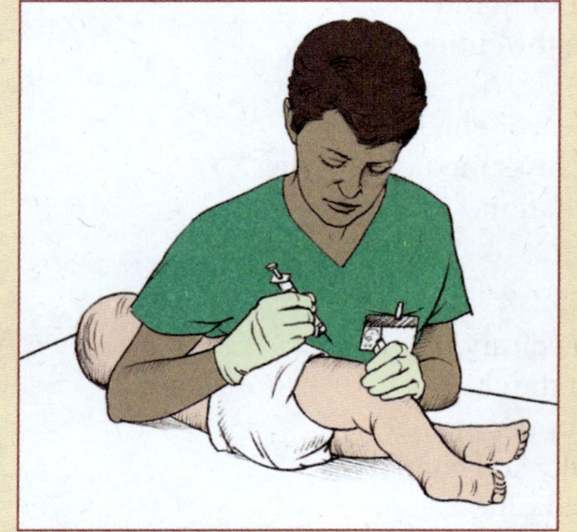

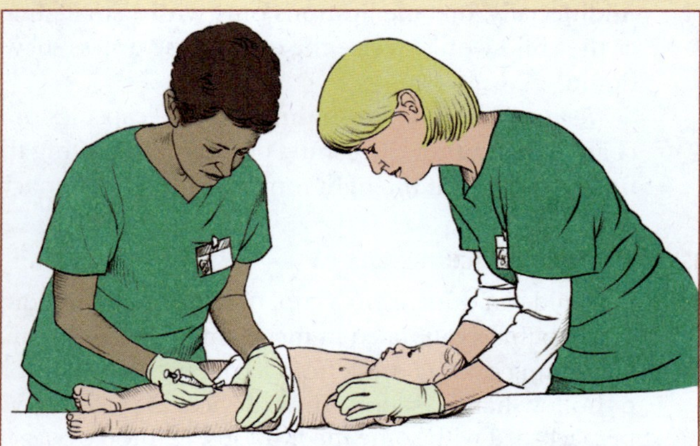

Pediatric IM Guidelines. (referenced at end of the document)

Age of child	Location	Needle length and gauge	Maximum volume of solution
Infant	Vastus lateralis	5/8–1″; 22–25 g	1 mL
Toddler	Vastus lateralis	1–1¼″; 22–25 g	1 mL
Older child[a]	Vastus lateralis, deltoid, ventrogluteal	1–1½″; 22–25 g	Up to 2 mL for vastus lateralis and ventrogluteal; 1 mL for deltoid

[a]For children ages 7–18 years of age, the CDC recommends the administration of IM vaccines in the deltoid muscle.

Finding the nerve

Be aware of the risk of nerve damage when selecting the site, needle length, and injection technique.

IV route

Fluids and medications may also be administered by the IV route. IV site placement may be in a peripheral or central vein. Since pediatric patients can tolerate only a limited amount of fluid, dilute IV medications, and administer IV fluids cautiously. Always use an infusion pump with infants and small children. Syringe pumps may be necessary to administer small amounts for IV medications at a controlled rate.

Infiltration and inflammation alert!

Inspect IV sites frequently for signs of infiltration (cool, blanched, and puffy skin) or inflammation (warm and reddened skin). Do this before, during, and after the infusion as children's vessels are immature and can be easily damaged by medications. If infiltration occurs, stop the infusion, remove the catheter, and consider placement for a new IV site. Emla cream or another numbing agent may be utilized prior to placing an IV site with the appropriate licensed practitioner's order and documentation.

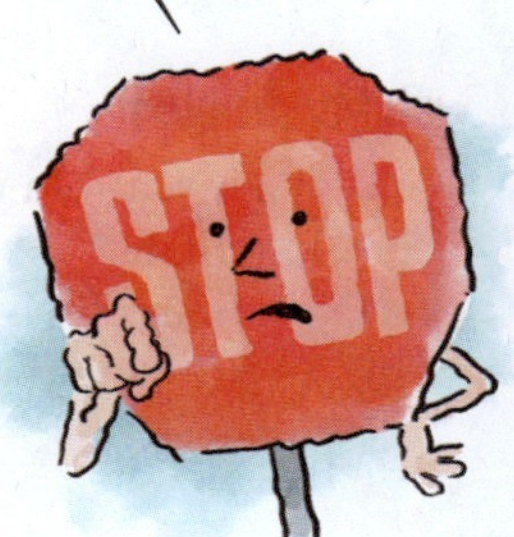
If there are signs of infiltration, stop the infusion, remove the catheter, and look for an alternate IV site. Make sure you notify the licensed practitioner.
STOP

Topical route

Medications may be administered topically in children as with adults. However, in infants and small children, the absorption of topical medications is greater because these children have:

- a thinner stratum corneum
- increased skin hydration
- a greater ratio of total body surface area (BSA) to weight.

Also, the use of disposable diapers with a plastic-coated layer can increase topical medication absorption in the diaper area due to the plastic coating can act like an occlusive dressing.

When applying topical medications on pediatric patients, clean the skin with soap and water to remove the previous application, and apply the new medication according to the licensed practitioner's order and the medication manufacturer's recommendations.

Calculation methods

To calculate and verify the safety of pediatric medication dosages, use the dosage-per-kilogram-of-body-weight method or the BSA method. Other methods, such as those based on age or the standard dosing used for adults, are less accurate and typically aren't used.

Whichever method is used, remember that nurses are professionally and legally responsible for checking the safety of a prescribed dose prior to administration. Double-check calculations with the pharmacist or another registered nurse.

Dosage per kilogram of body weight

Many pharmaceutical companies provide information about safe medication dosages for pediatric patients in milligrams per kilogram (mg/kg) of body weight. This is the most accurate and common way to calculate pediatric dosages. Pediatric dosages are usually expressed as *mg/kg/day* or *mg/kg/dose*. Based on this information, pediatric doses can be determined by multiplying the child's weight in kilograms by the required number of milligrams of medication per kilogram.

Shifting weight: From pounds to kilograms

When weight measurements are provided in pounds (lb), the nurse must convert from pounds to kilograms (kg) before calculating the dosage per kilogram of body weight. Remember that 1 kg equals 2.2 lb. (See Real-world problems below for an example.)

Real-world problems

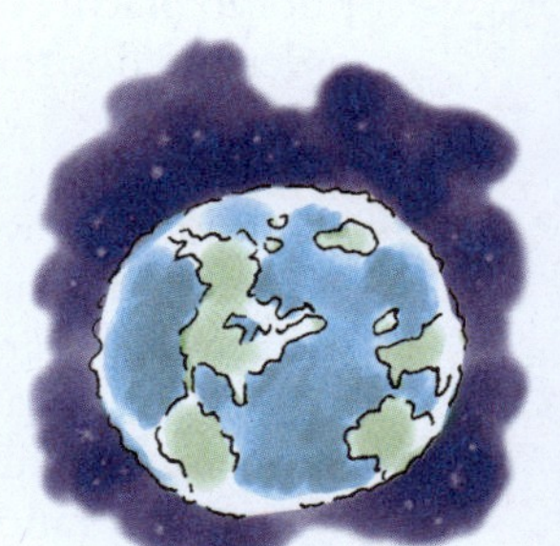

The following examples show how to use proportions to convert pounds to kilograms, how to calculate mg/kg/dose for one-time or as needed (PRN) medications, and how to calculate mg/kg/day for doses given round-the-clock to maintain a continuous medication effect.

A weighty problem

If a 6-year-old patient weighs 41.5 lb, how much do they weigh in kilograms?

Here's how to solve this problem using ratios.

Step 1: Set up the proportion, remembering that 2.2 lb equals 1 kg:

$$X\text{:}41.5\text{ lb::}1\text{ kg:}2.2\text{ lb}$$

Step 2: Multiply the extremes and the means:

$$X \times 2.2\text{ lb} = 1\text{ kg} \times 41.5\text{ lb}$$

Step 3: Solve for *X*. Divide each side of the equation by 2.2 lb and cancel units that appear in both the numerator and denominator:

$$\frac{X \times \cancel{2.2\text{ lb}}}{\cancel{2.2\text{ lb}}} = \frac{1\text{ kg} \times 41.5\ \cancel{\text{lb}}}{2.2\ \cancel{\text{lb}}}$$

$$X = \frac{41.5\text{ kg}}{2.2}$$

$$X = 18.9\text{ kg}$$

The child weighs 18.9 kg, which may be rounded off to 19 kg.

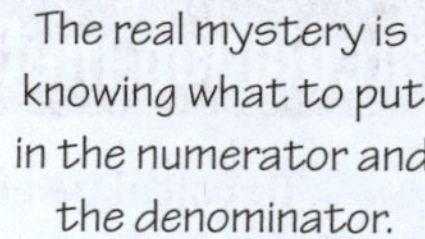

The real mystery is knowing what to put in the numerator and the denominator.

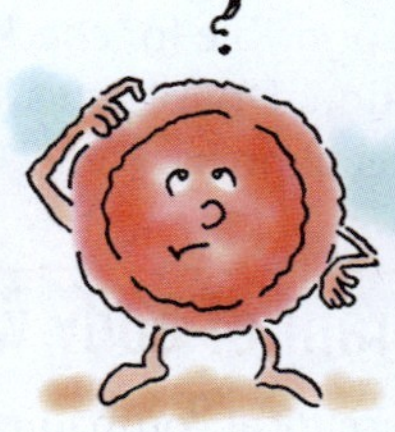

?

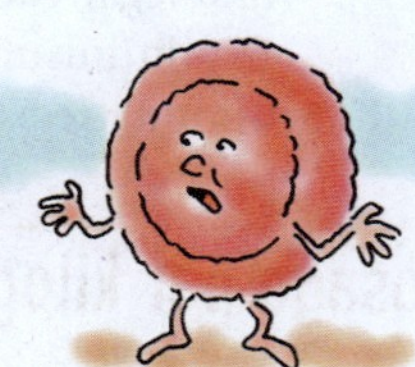

Note this: If you prefer using Dimensional Analysis to calculate dosages, feel free to do so! Refer back to Chapter 4 if you get stuck!

Milligram mystery

The licensed practitioner orders a single dose of 20 mg/kg of amoxicillin oral suspension for a toddler who weighs 20 lb (9.1 kg). What's the dose in milligrams?

Here's how to solve this problem using fractions.

Step 1: Set up the proportion with the ordered dosage in one fraction and the unknown dosage and the patient's weight in the other fraction:

$$\frac{20 \text{ mg}}{1 \text{ kg/dose}} = \frac{X}{9.1 \text{ kg/dose}}$$

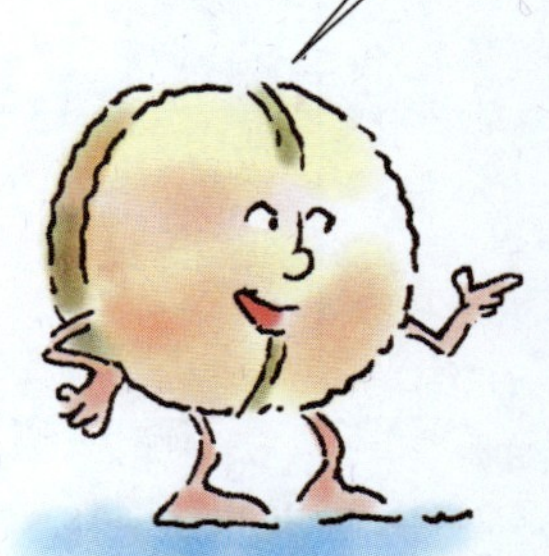
First, figure out the child's weight in kilograms; then the right dosage can be calculated.

Step 2: Cross-multiply the fractions:

$$X \times 1 \text{ kg/dose} = 20 \text{ mg} \times 9.1 \text{ kg/dose}$$

Step 3: Solve for X. Divide each side of the equation by 1 kg/dose and cancel units that appear in both the numerator and denominator:

$$\frac{X \times 1 \cancel{\text{kg/dose}}}{1 \cancel{\text{kg/dose}}} = \frac{20 \text{ mg} \times 9.1 \cancel{\text{kg/dose}}}{1 \cancel{\text{kg/dose}}}$$

$$X = 182 \text{ mg}$$

The patient needs 182 mg of amoxicillin.

A perplexing penicillin problem

The licensed practitioner orders *penicillin V potassium oral suspension 56 mg/kg/day in four divided doses* for a patient who weighs 55 lb. The suspension that's available is penicillin V potassium 125 mg/5 mL. How many mL should the nurse administer for each dose?

Solve this problem using ratios and fractions following the incredibly easy steps:

Step 1: First, convert the child's weight from pounds to kilograms by setting up the following proportion:

$$X{:}55 \text{ lb}{::}1 \text{ kg}{:}2.2 \text{ lb}$$

Step 2: Multiply the extremes and the means:

$$X \times 2.2 \text{ lb} = 1 \text{ kg} \times 55 \text{ lb}$$

Dosage drill

Test your math skills with this drill

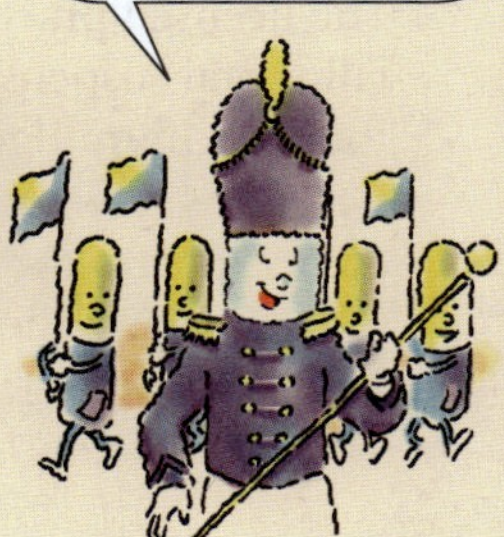
Be sure to show how you arrive at your answer.

How many milligrams (mg) of medication will a nurse give to a 32-lb child if the order calls for 25 mg/kg?

Your answer: ____________

Step 1: Find the child's weight in kilograms by setting up ratios and a proportion and solving for *X*.

$$2.2 \text{ lb}:1 \text{ kg}::32 \text{ lb}:X \text{ kg}$$

$$2.2 \text{ lb} \times X \text{ kg} = 1 \text{ kg} \times 32 \text{ lb}$$

$$\frac{\cancel{2.2 \text{ lb}} \times X \text{ kg}}{\cancel{2.2 \text{ lb}}} = \frac{1 \text{ kg} \times 32 \cancel{\text{ lb}}}{2.2 \cancel{\text{ lb}}}$$

$$X = \frac{32 \text{ kg}}{2.2}$$

$$X = 14.5454 \text{ kg}$$

Step 2: Find the total number of milligrams to give based on the child's weight.

$$1 \text{ kg}:25 \text{ mg}::14.5454 \text{ kg}:X \text{ mg}$$

$$1 \text{ kg} \times X \text{ mg} = 25 \text{ mg} \times 14.5454 \text{ kg}$$

$$\frac{\cancel{1 \text{ kg}} \times X \text{ mg}}{\cancel{1 \text{ kg}}} = \frac{25 \text{ mg} \times 14.5454 \cancel{\text{ kg}}}{1 \cancel{\text{ kg}}}$$

$$X = 25 \text{ mg} \times 14.5454$$

$$X = 363.6 \text{ mg}$$

The nurse would give 363.6 mg of medication.

Step 3: Solve for X. Divide each side of the equation by 2.2 lb and cancel units that appear in both the numerator and denominator:

$$\frac{X \times \cancel{2.2\text{ lb}}}{\cancel{2.2\text{ lb}}} = \frac{1\text{ kg} \times 55\ \cancel{\text{lb}}}{2.2\ \cancel{\text{lb}}}$$

$$X = \frac{55\text{ kg}}{2.2}$$

$$X = 25\text{ kg}$$

- The child weighs 25 kg.

Step 4: Determine the total daily dosage by setting up a proportion with the patient's weight and the unknown dosage on one side and the ordered dosage on the other side:

$$\frac{25\text{ kg}}{X} = \frac{1\text{ kg}}{56\text{ mg}}$$

Step 5: Cross-multiply the fractions:

$$X \times 1\text{ kg} = 56\text{ mg} \times 25\text{ kg}$$

Step 6: Solve for X. Divide each side of the equation by 1 kg and cancel units that appear in both the numerator and denominator:

$$\frac{X \times 1\ \cancel{\text{kg}}}{1\ \cancel{\text{kg}}} = \frac{56\text{ mg} \times 25\ \cancel{\text{kg}}}{1\ \cancel{\text{kg}}}$$

$$X = \frac{56\text{ mg} \times 25}{1}$$

$$X = 1{,}400\text{ mg}$$

- The child's daily dosage is 1,400 mg.

Step 7: Divide the daily dosage by 4 doses to determine the dose to administer every 6 hours:

$$X = \frac{1{,}400\text{ mg}}{4\text{ doses}}$$

$$X = 350\text{ mg/dose}$$

- The child should receive 350 mg every 6 hours.

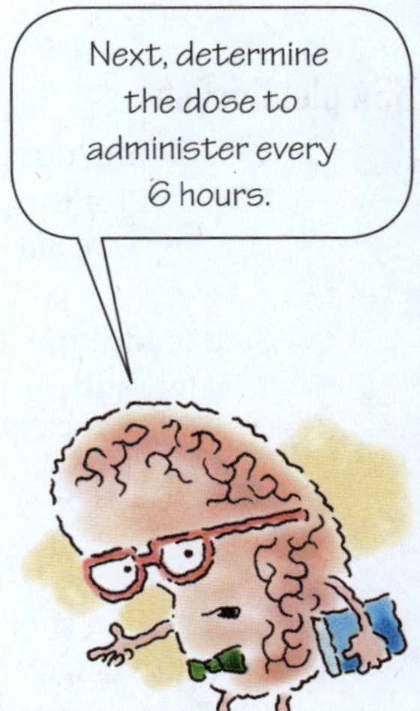
Next, determine the dose to administer every 6 hours.

Step 8: Calculate the volume to give for each dose by setting up a proportion with the unknown volume and the amount in one dose on one side and the available dose on the other side:

$$\frac{X}{350\text{ mg}} = \frac{5\text{ mL}}{125\text{ mg}}$$

Step 9: Cross-multiply the fractions:

$$X \times 125 \text{ mg} = 5 \text{ mL} \times 350 \text{ mg}$$

Step 10: Solve for X. Divide each side of the equation by 125 mg and cancel units that appear in both the numerator and denominator:

$$\frac{X \times \cancel{125 \text{ mg}}}{\cancel{125 \text{ mg}}} = \frac{5 \text{ mL} \times 350 \cancel{\text{ mg}}}{125 \cancel{\text{ mg}}}$$

$$X = \frac{5 \text{ mL} \times 350}{125}$$

$$X = \frac{1{,}750 \text{ mL}}{125}$$

$$X = 14 \text{ mL}$$

The nurse should administer 14 mL of the oral suspension at each dose.

Dosage by body surface area (BSA)

The BSA method is used to calculate safe pediatric dosages for a limited number of medications, such as antineoplastic or chemotherapeutic agents. It's also used to calculate safe dosages for adult patients receiving these extremely potent medications or medications requiring great precision.

BSA plot thickens

Calculating dosages by BSA involves two incredibly easy steps:

Step 1: Plot the patient's height and weight on a chart called a *nomogram* to determine the BSA in square meters (m^2). (See *What's in a nomogram?*, p. 274.)

Step 2: Multiply the BSA by the prescribed pediatric dose in $mg/m^2/day$. Here's the formula:

$$\text{child's dose in mg} = \text{child's BSA in m}^2 \times \frac{\text{pediatric dose in mg}}{\text{m}^2/\text{day}}$$

The BSA method can also be used to calculate a child's dose based on the average adult BSA—1.73 m^2—and an average adult dose.

The formula looks like this:

$$\text{child's dose in mg} = \frac{\text{child's BSA in m}^2}{\text{average adult BSA } (1.73 \text{ m}^2)} \times \text{average adult dose}$$

Dosage drill

Test your math skills with this drill

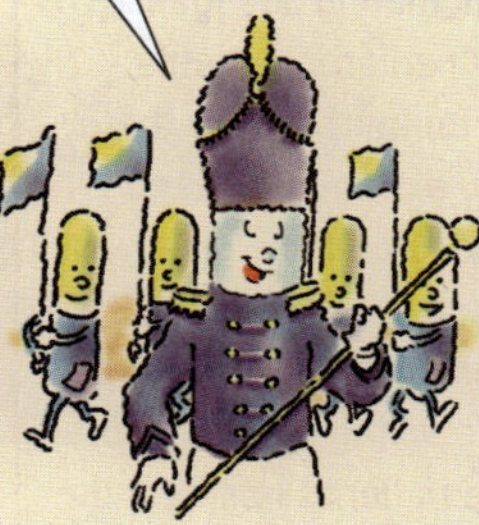
Be sure to show how you arrive at your answer.

A 52-lb (23.6-kg) child receives 5 mg/kg of phenytoin for seizure control in two divided doses. The bottle contains a concentration of 125 mg/5 mL. How many milliliters per dose should the nurse instruct the parents to administer?

Your answer: ____________

Step 1: Calculate the required milligrams.

$$1\text{ kg}:5\text{ mg}::23.6\text{ kg}:X\text{ mg}$$

$$1\text{ kg} \times X\text{ mg} = 5\text{ mg} \times 23.6\text{ kg}$$

$$\frac{\cancel{1\text{ kg}} \times X\text{ mg}}{\cancel{1\text{ kg}}} = \frac{5\text{ mg} \times 23.6\ \cancel{\text{kg}}}{1\ \cancel{\text{kg}}}$$

$$X = 118\text{ mg}$$

Step 2: Calculate the required milliliters.

$$125\text{ mg}:5\text{ mL}::118\text{ mg}:X\text{ mL}$$

$$125\text{ mg} \times X\text{ mL} = 5\text{ mL} \times 118\ \cancel{\text{mg}}$$

$$\frac{\cancel{125\text{ mg}} \times X\text{ mL}}{\cancel{125\text{ mg}}} = \frac{5\text{ mL} \times 118\ \cancel{\text{mg}}}{125\ \cancel{\text{mg}}}$$

$$X = \frac{590\text{ mL}}{125}$$

$X = 4.7\text{ mL}$ (rounded to the nearest tenth space)

Step 3: Determine the amount per dose.

$$4.7\text{ mL}:2\text{ doses}::X\text{ mL}:1\text{ dose}$$

$$4.7\text{ mL} \times 1\text{ dose} = 2\text{ doses} \times X\text{ mL}$$

$$\frac{4.7\text{ mL} \times 1\ \cancel{\text{dose}}}{2\ \cancel{\text{doses}}} = \frac{\cancel{2\text{ doses}} \times X\text{ mL}}{\cancel{2\text{ doses}}}$$

$$X = \frac{4.7}{2}$$

$$X = 2.35\text{ mL/dose}$$

The parents should give 2.35 mL of phenytoin for each dose.

What's in a nomogram?

Body surface area (BSA) is critical when calculating dosages for pediatric patients or for medications that are extremely potent and need to be given in precise amounts. The nomogram shown here allows the nurse to plot the patient's height and weight to determine the BSA. Here's how it works:

- Locate the patient's height in the left column of the nomogram and their weight in the right column.
- Use a ruler to draw a straight line connecting the two points. The point where the line intersects the surface area column indicates the patient's BSA in square meters.
- For an average-sized child, use the simplified nomogram in the box. Just find the child's weight in pounds on the left side of the scale, and then read the corresponding BSA on the right side.

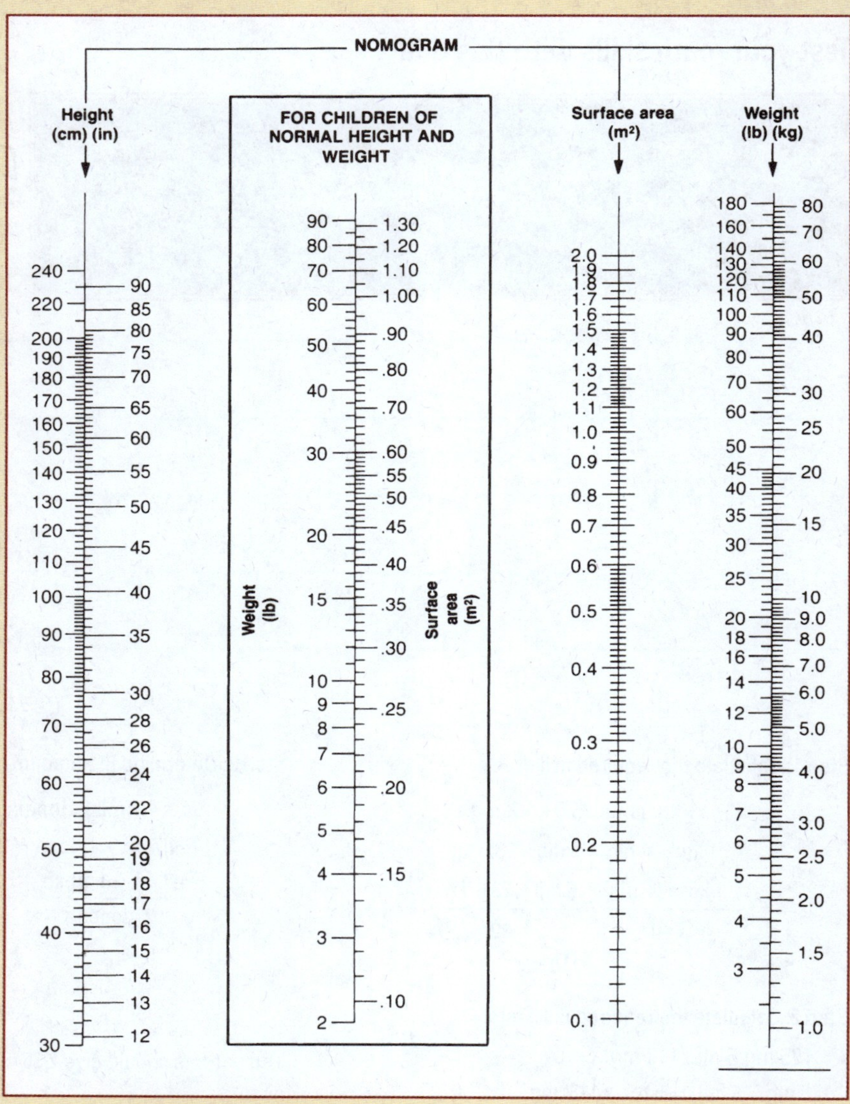

Real-world problems

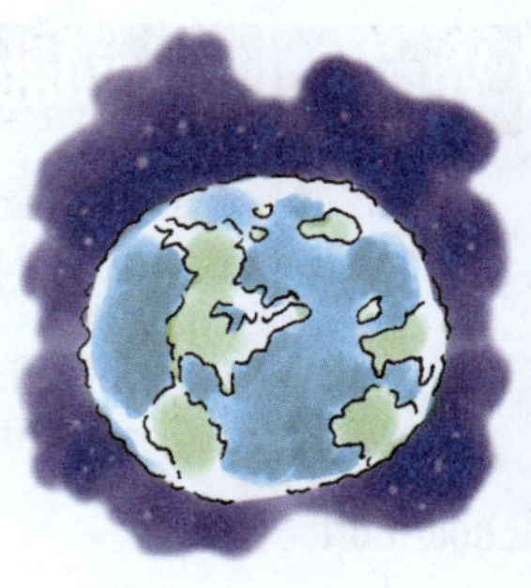

The following problems show how these two formulas are used in the BSA method of dosage calculation.

An engrossing ephedrine equation

The licensed practitioner orders *ephedrine 100 mg/m²/day* for a child who's 40″ tall and weighs 64 lb. How much ephedrine should the child receive daily?

Step 1: Use the nomogram to determine that the child's BSA is 0.96 m^2.

Step 2: Using the appropriate formula, determine the daily dosage:

$$X = 0.96\ m^2 \times \frac{100\ mg}{1\ m^2/day}$$

Step 3: Solve for X:

$$X = 0.96\ \cancel{m^2} \times \frac{100\ mg}{1\ \cancel{m^2}/day}$$

$$X = 96\ mg/day$$

The child needs 96 mg of ephedrine per day.

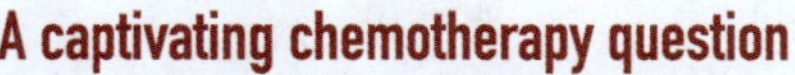

A captivating chemotherapy question

A child who needs chemotherapy is 36″ tall and weighs 40 lb. What's the safe medication dose if the average adult dose is 1,000 mg?

Step 1: Use the nomogram to determine that the child's BSA is 0.72 m^2.

Step 2: Set up an equation using the appropriate formula. Divide the child's BSA by 1.73 m^2 (the average adult BSA), and multiply by the average adult dose, 1,000 mg:

$$X = \frac{0.72\ m^2}{1.73\ m^2} \times 1{,}000\ mg$$

Step 3: Solve for X. Cancel units that appear in both the numerator and denominator.

Step 4: Multiplying the child's BSA by the average adult dose

Step 5: Divide the result by the average adult BSA:

$$X = \frac{0.72\ \cancel{m^2} \times 1{,}000\ mg}{1.73\ \cancel{m^2}}$$

$$X = 416\ mg$$

The safe dose for this child is 416 mg.

Think, think, think… When calculating a pediatric dose that's based on an adult dose, use the appropriate formula—the one including the average adult BSA.

Verifying calculations

Although the licensed practitioner determines the medication dosage, the nurse is an important "last line of defense" who verifies that the ordered dosage is safe. Depending on the facility, nurses may have access to several reliable sources of information, including online computer services, medication references, and other staff.

Look it up

Some nursing medication handbooks contain usual (recommended) pediatric dosages for commonly prescribed medications (pediatric medication references specifically developed for the special needs of infants and children are also available). The pharmacist is another excellent resource for verifying medication safety. Remember to always double-check complex calculations with another nurse.

Real-world problems

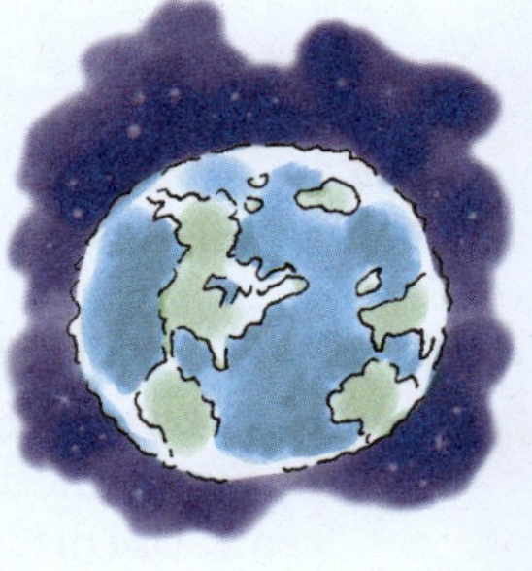

Here are some real-world examples of verifying calculations.

Clearing the way for chloral hydrate

The licensed practitioner orders *chloral hydrate 75 mg PO* to sedate a 3-kg neonate for an electroencephalogram. The medication resource states that the usual (recommended) dosage of chloral hydrate for a neonate is 25 mg/kg/dose for sedation prior to a procedure. Did the licensed practitioner order the correct dosage? Solve this problem using fractions following these incredibly easy steps:

Step 1: Set up the proportion with the usual dosage in one fraction and the unknown dosage and the patient's weight in the other fraction:

$$\frac{25\text{ mg}}{1\text{ kg/dose}} = \frac{X}{3\text{ kg/dose}}$$

Step 2: Cross-multiply the fractions:

$$X \times 1\text{ kg/dose} = 25\text{ mg} \times 3\text{ kg/dose}$$

Step 3: Solve for X. Divide each side of the equation by 1 kg/dose and cancel units that appear in both the numerator and denominator:

$$\frac{X \times 1\ \cancel{\text{kg/dose}}}{1\ \cancel{\text{kg/dose}}} = \frac{25\text{ mg} \times 3\ \cancel{\text{kg/dose}}}{1\ \cancel{\text{kg/dose}}}$$

$$X = 75\text{ mg}$$

The patient needs 75 mg of chloral hydrate.

Dosage drill

Test your math skills with this drill

The average, adult dose of codeine phosphate for pain is 60 mg PO every 4 hours. How much should a nurse administer in a single dose to a child with a body surface area of 0.55 m^2?

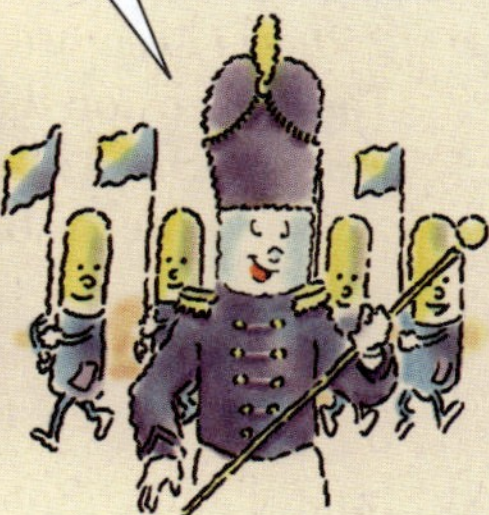
Be sure to show how you arrive at your answer.

Your answer: ____________

Set up ratios and a proportion, then solve for *X* to find the answer.

$$1.73\ m^2{:}60\ mg{::}0.55\ m^2{:}X\ mg$$

$$1.73\ m^2 \times X\ mg = 60\ mg \times 0.55\ m^2$$

$$\frac{\cancel{1.73\ m^2} \times X\ mg}{\cancel{1.73\ m^2}} = \frac{60\ mg \times 0.55\ \cancel{m^2}}{1.73\ \cancel{m^2}}$$

$$X = \frac{33\ mg}{1.73}$$

$$X = 19.1\ mg \text{ (rounded to the nearest tenth space)}$$

The nurse should administer 19.1 mg of the codeine phosphate in a single dose.

This is exactly what the licensed practitioner ordered and, therefore, the dose is safe to administer.

Penicillin puzzler

The licensed practitioner orders *penicillin V potassium oral suspension 250 mg PO every 6 hours* for a patient who weighs 55 lb. Is the dose safe? The suspension that's available is penicillin V potassium 125 mg/5 mL. How much mL should the nurse administer for each dose?

Solve the problem using ratios and fractions with these incredibly easy steps:

Step 1: Convert the child's weight from pounds to kilograms by setting up the following proportion:

$$X\text{:}55\text{ lb}::1\text{ kg}:2.2\text{ lb}$$

Step 2: Multiply the extremes and the means:

$$X \times 2.2\text{ lb} = 1\text{ kg} \times 55\text{ lb}$$

Step 3: Solve for *X*. Divide each side of the equation by 2.2 lb and cancel units that appears in both the numerator and denominator:

$$\frac{X \times 2.2\text{ \cancel{lb}}}{2.2\text{ \cancel{lb}}} = \frac{1\text{ kg} \times 55\text{ \cancel{lb}}}{2.2\text{ \cancel{lb}}}$$

$$X = \frac{55\text{ kg}}{2.2}$$

$$X = 25\text{ kg}$$

- The child weighs 25 kg.

Step 4: Verify the usual (recommended) dosage. The medication reference states to give penicillin V potassium 25 to 50 mg/kg/day orally in divided doses every 6 to 8 hours. This indicates a safe daily dosage range—a low dosage (25 mg/kg/day) and a high dosage (50 mg/kg/day). These are also the minimum (low) dosage and the maximum (high) dosage for the day.

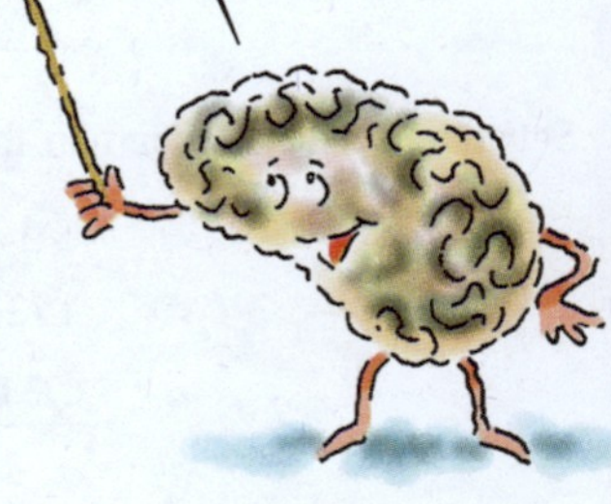

The first step is to determine whether the ordered dose is safe based on the usual or recommended dosage listed in a drug reference. The second step is to calculate what volume to give for each dose.

Step 5: Determine the usual total daily dosage range by setting up two proportions with the patient's weight on one side and the usual dosage (either the low dosage or the high dosage) on the other side.

- Let's look at the high dose first:

$$\frac{25\text{ kg}}{X} = \frac{1\text{ kg}}{50\text{ mg}}$$

Step 6: Cross-multiply the fractions:

$$X \times 1\text{ kg} = 50\text{ mg} \times 25\text{ kg}$$

Step 7: Solve for X. Divide each side of the equation by 1 kg and cancel units that appear in both the numerator and denominator:

$$\frac{X \times 1\ \cancel{kg}}{1\ \cancel{kg}} = \frac{50\ mg \times 25\ \cancel{kg}}{1\ \cancel{kg}}$$

$$X = \frac{50\ mg \times 25}{1}$$

$$X = 1{,}250\ mg$$

- The child's maximum daily dosage is 1,250 mg.

Step 8: Divide the daily dosage by 4 doses to determine the maximum safe dose to administer every 6 hours:

$$X = \frac{1{,}250\ mg}{4\ doses}$$

X = 312.5 mg/dose or 313 mg/dose

- Now repeat the same steps to determine the low or minimum dose:

$$\frac{25\ kg}{X} = \frac{1\ kg}{25\ mg}$$

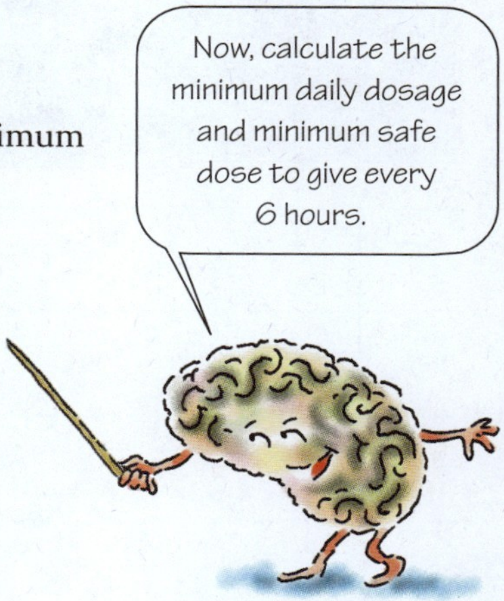

Step 9: Cross-multiply the fractions:

$$X \times 1\ kg = 25\ mg \times 25\ kg$$

Step 10: Solve for X. Divide each side of the equation by 1 kg and cancel like units:

$$\frac{X \times 1\ \cancel{kg}}{1\ \cancel{kg}} = \frac{25\ mg \times 25\ \cancel{kg}}{1\ \cancel{kg}}$$

$$X = \frac{25\ mg \times 25}{1}$$

$$X = 625\ mg$$

- The child's minimum daily dosage is 625 mg.

Step 11: Divide the daily dosage by 4 doses to determine the minimum safe dose to administer every 6 hours:

$$X = \frac{625\ mg}{4\ doses}$$

X = 156.25, or 156 mg/dose

Now, calculate the minimum daily dosage and minimum safe dose to give every 6 hours.

Dosage drill

Test your math skills with this drill

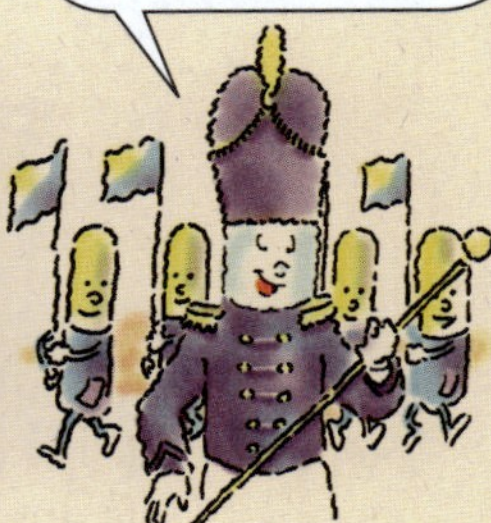
Be sure to show how you arrive at your answer.

The licensed practitioner orders furosemide (Lasix) 12 mg PO daily for a 6-kg infant diagnosed with heart failure. The medication reference on the unit states that the recommended dosage of furosemide for a child is 2 mg/kg/dose. How much should the nurse administer?

Your answer: ____________

Solving using these incredibly easy steps:

Step 1: Set up a proportion with the recommended dosage in one fraction and the unknown dosage and the patient's weight in the other fraction.

$$\frac{2 \text{ mg}}{1 \text{ kg/dose}} = \frac{X}{6 \text{ kg/dose}}$$

Step 2: Cross-multiply the fractions.

$$2 \text{ mg} \times 6 \text{ kg/dose} = X \times 1 \text{ kg/dose}$$

Step 3: Solve for X. Divide each side of the equation by 1 kg/dose and cancel units that appear in both the numerator and denominator.

$$\frac{2 \text{ mg} \times 6 \cancel{\text{ kg/dose}}}{1 \cancel{\text{ kg/dose}}} = \frac{X \times 1 \cancel{\text{ kg/dose}}}{1 \cancel{\text{ kg/dose}}}$$

$$X = 12 \text{ mg}$$

The nurse should administer 12 mg of furosemide, which is exactly the amount that was ordered. The dose is safe to administer.

- The safe daily dosage range is 625 mg to 1,250 mg per day for this child. The licensed practitioner ordered 250 mg every 6 hours (or 4 doses per day) or a total dosage of 1,000 mg (250 mg/dose × 4 doses). This falls within the safe daily range.
- The child can safely receive 250 mg every 6 hours.

Step 12: Calculate the volume to give for each dose by setting up a proportion with the unknown volume and the amount in one dose on one side and the available dose on the other side:

$$\frac{X}{250\text{ mg}} = \frac{5\text{ mL}}{125\text{ mg}}$$

$$X \times 125\text{ mg} = 5\text{ mL} \times 250\text{ mg}$$

Step 13: Solve for *X*. Divide each side of the equation by 125 mg and cancel units that appear in both the numerator and denominator:

$$\frac{X \times \cancel{125\text{ mg}}}{\cancel{125\text{ mg}}} = \frac{5\text{ mL} \times 250\ \cancel{\text{mg}}}{125\ \cancel{\text{mg}}}$$

$$X = \frac{5\text{ mL} \times 250}{125}$$

$$X = \frac{1{,}250\text{ mL}}{125}$$

$$X = 10\text{ mL}$$

The nurse should administer 10 mL of the oral suspension for each dose.

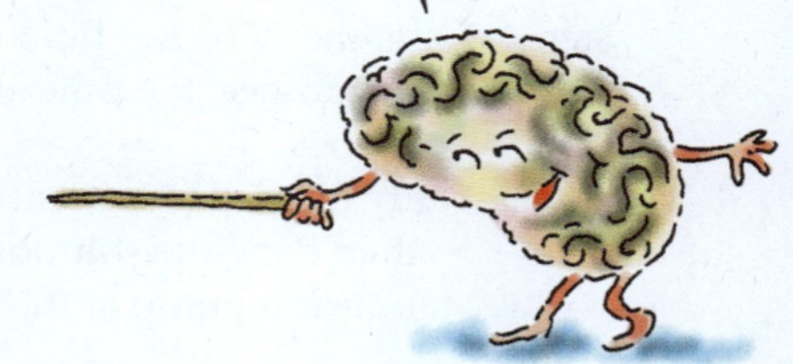
If the calculations are correct, the ordered dose is safe to give, and the patient should receive 10 mL for each dose.

IV guidelines

IV fluids and medications are administered by continuous or intermittent infusion. Since pediatric IV medication administration is so complex, be sure to follow all written guidelines and protocols about dosages, fluid volumes for dilution, and administration rates when giving the medication.

Continuous infusions

A continuous infusion is used when the pediatric patient requires around-the-clock fluids, medication therapy, or both. Fluids may be infused to maintain volume or to correct an existing fluid or electrolyte imbalance.

To prepare for a continuous medication infusion, gather the necessary supplies including a volume-control device. The pharmacy may provide a premixed medication solution, or the nurse may have to add the medication to a small-volume IV bag. Be sure to follow the manufacturer's guidelines for mixing the solution carefully. Remember that pediatric patients can tolerate only small amounts of fluid. A syringe pump may be necessary for small amounts of intermittent infusions.

Usually, a volume-control device such as the Buretrol set, which maintains flow rate by using a positive-pressure pumping mechanism, is used for continuous, as well as intermittent infusion. A small-volume bag of IV fluid with a microdrip set is another option. (See *IV infusion control.*)

IV infusion control

Accurate fluid administration is extremely important for pediatric patients. Hence, syringes, infusion pumps, and other volume-control devices are used extensively to regulate continuous and intermittent IV infusions. One typical device, the Buretrol set, is shown below.

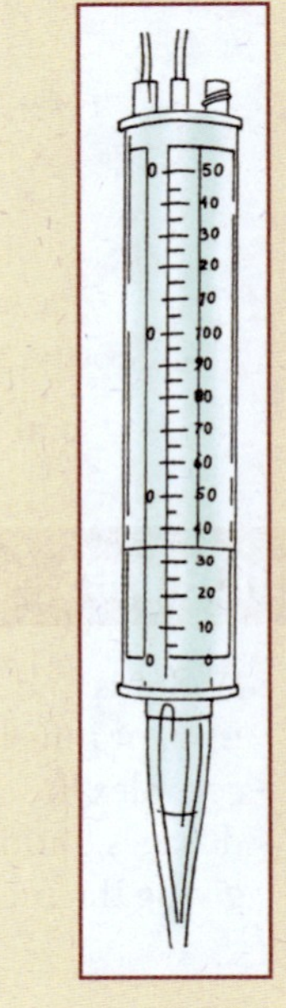

Infusion basics: 5 steps

Follow these incredibly easy steps to start a continuous infusion:

Step 1: Calculate the dosage.

Step 2: Draw up the medication in a syringe; then add the medication to the IV bag or fluid chamber through the medication additive port, using an aseptic technique.

Step 3: Mix the medication thoroughly.

Step 4: Label the IV bag or fluid chamber with the medication's name, the dosage, the time and date it was mixed, and the nurse's initials.

Step 5: Verify the patient's identity using two patient identifiers, and then hang the solution and administer the medication by infusion pump at the prescribed flow rate.

Intermittent infusions

Intermittent infusion is used commonly in acute and home care settings. If the pediatric patient is capable of normal enteral fluid intake, IV fluids or medication infusions may be necessary only at periodic intervals. A vascular access device can be kept in place, eliminating the need for continuous fluid infusion. The child can remain mobile, minimizing the potential for volume overload.

Adjusting the volume

Volume-control devices have 100- to 150-mL fluid chambers, which are calibrated in 1-mL increments to allow accurate fluid administration. Medication-filled syringes with microtubing can also be used to infuse small volumes via syringe pumps. Accuracy is especially important with pediatric patients because children can't tolerate as much fluid as adults and are more prone to fluid and electrolyte imbalances. The rate of IV infusion must be carefully controlled to ensure proper absorption and to prevent or minimize toxicity associated with rapid infusion. Use an infusion pump whenever possible. Remember to provide a flush following IV syringe medications at the same rate of the infusion. An order is required for postmedication administration flushes. Most facilities have protocols concerning IV flushes; check with the facility's policy.

Starting an infusion: 10 steps

If using a volume-control device, follow these incredibly easy steps to start an intermittent infusion:

Step 1: Carefully calculate the prescribed volume of medication. Some facilities consider the medication volume as part of the diluent volume. For example, if 100 mg of a medication is contained in 5 mL of fluid and the total fluid volume should be 50 mL, add 45 mL of diluent because 45 mL of diluent plus 5 mL of fluid medication volume equals a total of 50 mL.

Step 2: After careful calculation, draw up the prescribed volume of medication into a syringe.

Step 3: Add the medication to the fluid chamber through the medication additive port, using aseptic technique.

Step 4: Mix the medication thoroughly.

Step 5: Attach the volume-control device to an electronic infusion pump to control the infusion rate. If using a small-volume IV bag instead of a volume-control device and pump, use a microdrip set, which has a drop factor of 60 gtt/mL.

Step 6: Calculate the appropriate flow rate, verify the patient's identity using two patient identifiers, and infuse the medication.

Step 7: Label the volume-control device with the name of the medication, the dosage, the time and date it was mixed, and the nurse's initials.

Step 8: When the infusion is complete, flush the line to clear the tubing of the medication. A specific flush volume may be ordered by the licensed practitioner, or a standard volume protocol is followed based on the tubing volume, the patient's condition, or both. Administer the flush at the same rate as the medication. Label the volume-control device to indicate that the flush is infusing.

Step 9: With an intermittent infusion, disconnect the device when the flush is complete.

Step 10: During the infusion, check the IV site frequently for infiltration because children's veins are more prone to this problem.

Calculating pediatric fluid needs

Pediatric patients' needs are proportionally greater than those of adults, making children more vulnerable to changes in fluid and electrolyte balance. Since their extracellular fluid has a higher percentage of water, children's fluid exchange rates are two to three times greater than those of adults, leaving them more susceptible to dehydration.

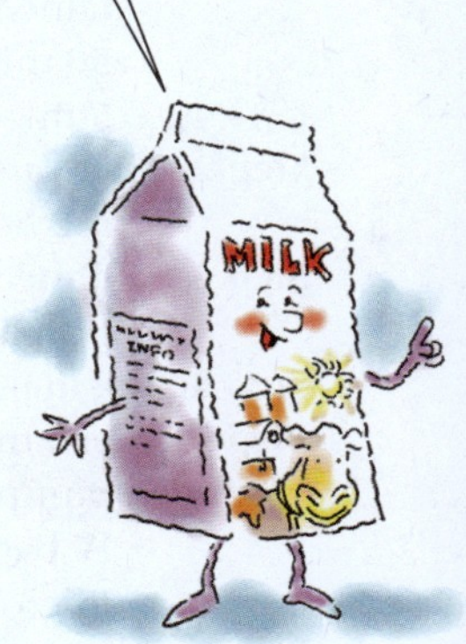

Children need two to three times more fluid intake than adults to avoid dehydration. Encourage fluids like water, apple juice, or milk—like me!!
MILK

Three ways to figure fluids

Determining and meeting the fluid needs of children are important nursing responsibilities. Calculate the number of milliliters of fluid a child needs based on:

- weight in kilograms
- metabolism (calories required)
- BSA in square meters.

Although results may vary slightly, all three methods are appropriate. Keep in mind that fluid replacement can also be affected by clinical conditions that cause fluid retention or loss. Children with these conditions should receive fluids based on their individual needs.

Fluid needs based on weight

Use three different formulas to calculate a child's fluid needs based on their weight.

Formula for Daily IV Fluid Calculations:

- 100 mL/kg for first 10 kg of body weight
- 50 mL/kg for the next 10 kg of body weight
- 20 mL/kg remaining kg of body weight

Fluid formula for tiny tots

A child who weighs less than 10 kg requires 100 mL of fluid per kilogram of body weight. To determine this child's fluid needs:

- Convert their weight from pounds to kilograms.
- Then multiply the results by 100 mL/kg/day.

Here's the formula:

$$\text{weight in kg} \times 100 \text{ mL/kg/day} = \text{fluid needs in mL/day}$$

Fluid formula for middleweights

A child weighing 10 to 20 kg requires 1,000 mL of fluid per day for the first 10 kg plus 50 mL for every kilogram over 10. To determine this child's fluid needs, follow these incredibly easy steps:

Step 1: Convert their weight from pounds to kilograms.

Step 2: Subtract 10 kg from the child's total weight.

Step 3: Multiply the result by 50 mL/kg/day to find the child's additional fluid needs.

Here's the formula:

$$(\text{total kg} - 10 \text{ kg}) \times 50 \text{ mL/kg/day} = \text{additional fluid need in mL/day}$$

Step 4: Add the additional daily fluid need to the 1,000 mL/day required for the first 10 kg. The total is the child's daily fluid requirement:

$$1{,}000 \text{ mL/day} + \text{additional fluid need} = \text{fluid needs in mL/day}$$

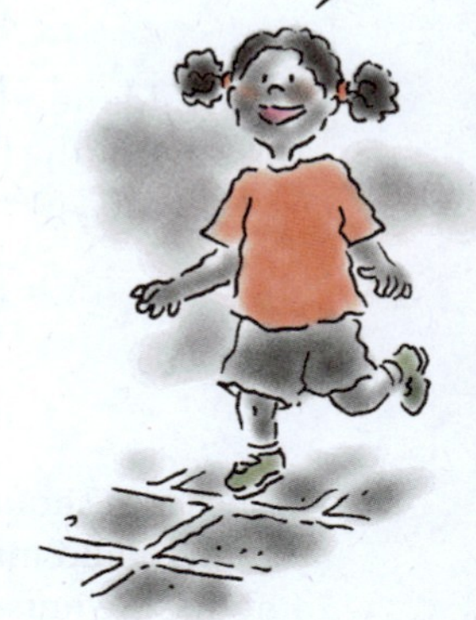

My fluid needs keep changing as I grow…think I'm due for a change now!

Fluid formula for bigger kids

A child weighing more than 20 kg requires 1,500 mL of fluid for the first 20 kg plus 20 mL for each additional kilogram. To determine this child's fluid needs, follow these incredibly easy steps:

Step 1: Convert the child's weight from pounds to kilograms.

Step 2: Subtract 20 kg from the child's total weight.

Step 3: Multiply the result by 20 mL/kg to find the child's additional fluid need.

Here's the formula:

$$(\text{total kg} - 20 \text{ kg}) \times 20 \text{ mL/kg/day} = \text{additional fluid need in mL/day}$$

Step 4: Since the child needs 1,500 mL of fluid per day for the first 20 kg, add the additional fluid need to 1,500 mL. The total is the child's daily fluid requirement:

$$1{,}500 \text{ mL/day} + \text{additional fluid need} = \text{fluid needs in mL/day}$$

Use this information to solve the following problem.

Finding a fluid solution

How much fluid should be given to a 44-lb patient over 24 hours to meet their maintenance needs?

Step 1: Convert 44 lb to kilograms by setting up a proportion with fractions. (Remember that 1 kg equals 2.2 lb.)

$$\frac{44 \text{ lb}}{X} = \frac{2.2 \text{ lb}}{1 \text{ kg}}$$

Step 2: Cross-multiply the fractions.

Step 3: Solve for X. Divide both sides of the equation by 2.2 lb and cancel units that appear in both the numerator and denominator:

$$X \times 2.2 \text{ lb} = 44 \text{ lb} \times 1 \text{ kg}$$

$$\frac{X \times \cancel{2.2 \text{ lb}}}{\cancel{2.2 \text{ lb}}} = \frac{44 \cancel{\text{ lb}} \times 1 \text{ kg}}{2.2 \cancel{\text{ lb}}}$$

$$X = \frac{44 \text{ kg}}{2.2}$$

$$X = 20 \text{ kg}$$

- The child weighs 20 kg.

Step 4: Subtract 10 kg from the child's weight.

Step 5: Multiply the result by 50 mL/kg/day to find the child's additional fluid need:

$$X = (20 \text{ kg} - 10 \text{ kg}) \times 50 \text{ mL/kg/day}$$

$$X = 10 \cancel{\text{kg}} \times 50 \text{ mL/}\cancel{\text{kg}}\text{/day}$$

$$X = 500 \text{ mL/day additional fluid need}$$

Remember to follow the guidelines for subtracting kilograms and multiplying by milliliters per kilogram outlined on the previous page.

Step 6: Add the additional fluid needed to the 1,000 mL/day required for the first 10 kg (because the child weighs between 10 and 20 kg).

$$X = 1{,}000 \text{ mL/day} + 500 \text{ mL/day}$$

$$X = 1{,}500 \text{ mL/day}$$

$$1{,}500 \text{ mL/24 hr} = 62.5 \text{ mL/hr.}$$

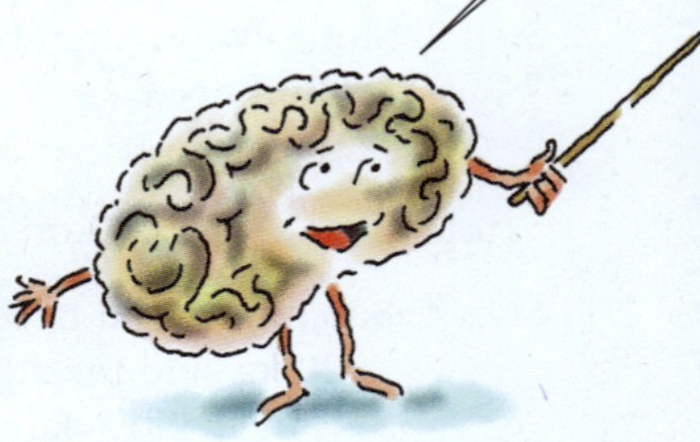

The child should receive 1,500 mL of fluid in 24 hours to meet their fluid maintenance needs. By dividing 1,500 mL by 24 hours, the nurse will set the IV pump at 62.5 mL per hour.

Fluid needs based on calories

Fluid needs can be calculated based on calories as water is necessary for metabolism. A child should receive 120 mL of fluid for every 100 kilocalories (kcal) of metabolism, also commonly called *calories*.

To find a child's calorie requirements, look at a table of recommended dietary allowances or ask the dietitian to calculate it.

Fluids help burn calories

To calculate fluid requirements based on calorie requirements, follow these incredibly easy steps:

Step 1: Find the child's calorie requirements. This information can be obtained from a table of recommended dietary allowances for children, or by having a dietitian calculate it.

Step 2: Divide the calorie requirements by 100 kcal since fluid requirements are determined for every 100 calories.

Step 3: Multiply the results by 120 mL, the amount of fluid required for every 100 kcal. Here's the formula:

$$\text{fluid requirements in mL/day} = \frac{\text{calorie requirements}}{100 \text{ kcal}} \times 120 \text{ mL}$$

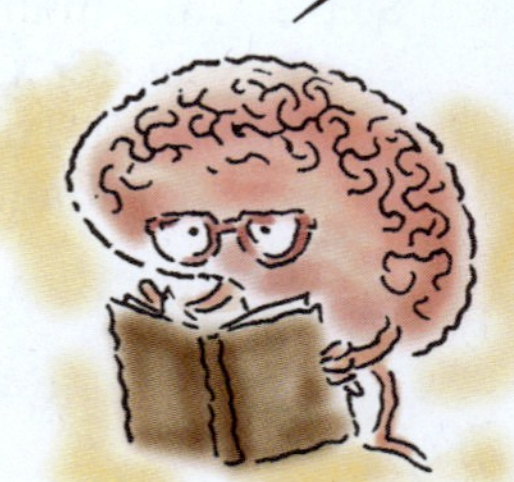

Use the information above to solve the following problem.

Calorie-conscious problem

A pediatric patient uses 900 calories/day. What are their daily fluid requirements?

- Set up the formula, inserting the appropriate numbers and substituting X for the unknown amount of fluid:

$$X = \frac{900 \cancel{\text{kcal}}}{100 \cancel{\text{kcal}}} \times 120 \text{ mL}$$

$$X = 9 \times 120 \text{ mL}$$

$$X = 1{,}080 \text{ mL}$$

The patient needs 1,080 mL of fluid per day.

Fluid needs based on BSA

Another method for determining pediatric maintenance fluid requirements is based on the child's BSA. To calculate the daily fluid needs of a child who isn't dehydrated, multiply the BSA by 1,500, as shown in this formula:

$$\text{fluid maintenance needs in mL/day} = \text{BSA in m}^2 \times 1{,}500 \text{ mL/day/m}^2$$

Use this formula to solve the following problem.

BSA-based problem

A patient is 36″ tall and weighs 40 lb (18.1 kg). If their BSA is 0.72 m^2, how much fluid do they need each day?

- Set up the equation, inserting the appropriate numbers and substituting X for the unknown amount of fluid. Then solve for X:

$$X = 0.72 \cancel{\text{m}^2} \times 1{,}500 \text{ mL/day/}\cancel{\text{m}^2}$$

$$X = 1{,}080 \text{ mL/day}$$

The child needs 1,080 mL of fluid per day.

Real-world problem

Solve the following pediatric dosage problem.

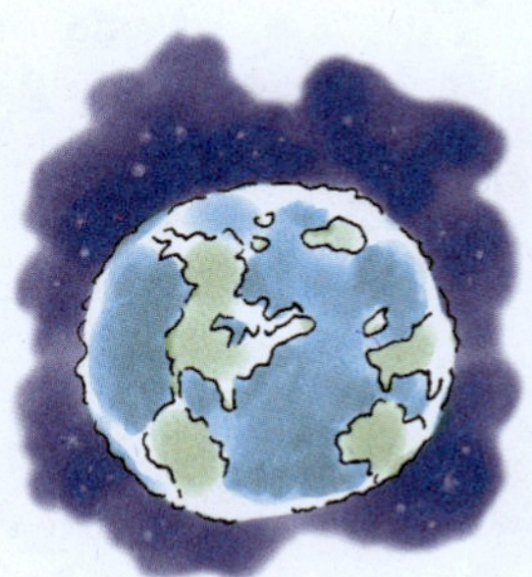

An ampicillin answer

The licensed practitioner orders a single dose of 360 mg of ampicillin for an infant who weighs 8 lb. The unit pediatric medication handbook states that the usual (recommended) ampicillin dose is 100 mg/kg/dose. After reconstituting with sterile water, the ampicillin is available in a concentration of 500 mg/5 mL. Is the dose ordered correct for the patient? What volume of ampicillin should the nurse administer to the infant?

Step 1: To determine whether the dose ordered is correct, set up the proportion to determine the child's weight in kilograms. Remember that 1 kg = 2.2 lb:

$$\frac{X}{8 \text{ lb}} = \frac{1 \text{ kg}}{2.2 \text{ lb}}$$

Step 2: Cross-multiply the fractions:

$$X \times 2.2 \text{ lb} = 8 \text{ lb} \times 1 \text{ kg}$$

Step 3: Solve for X. Divide both sides of the equation by 2.2 lb and cancel units that appear in both the numerator and denominator:

$$\frac{X \times \cancel{2.2 \text{ lb}}}{\cancel{2.2 \text{ lb}}} = \frac{8 \cancel{\text{ lb}} \times 1 \text{ kg}}{2.2 \cancel{\text{ lb}}}$$

$$X = \frac{8 \times 1 \text{ kg}}{2.2}$$

$$X = 3.63 \text{ kg}$$

- The infant weighs 3.63 kg, rounded off to 3.6 kg.

Step 4: Set up a proportion with the recommended dosage (from the pediatric medication reference) in one fraction and the unknown dosage and the patient's weight in the other fraction:

$$\frac{100 \text{ mg}}{1 \text{ kg/dose}} = \frac{X}{3.6 \text{ kg/dose}}$$

Step 5: Cross-multiply the fractions:

$$X \times 1 \text{ kg/dose} = 100 \text{ mg} \times 3.6 \text{ kg/dose}$$

Step 6: Solve for X. Divide each side of the equation by 1 kg/dose and cancel units that appear in both the numerator and denominator:

$$\frac{X \times 1 \cancel{\text{ kg/dose}}}{1 \cancel{\text{ kg/dose}}} = \frac{100 \text{ mg} \times 3.6 \cancel{\text{ kg/dose}}}{1 \cancel{\text{ kg/dose}}}$$

$$X = \frac{100 \text{ mg} \times 3.6}{1}$$

$$X = 360 \text{ mg}$$

- The correct dose was ordered: 100 mg/kg/dose for a child who weighs 8 lb (or 3.6 kg) is 360 mg.

Step 7: To determine the volume of medication that should be administered to the infant, set up a proportion with the known concentration in one fraction and the desired dose and unknown volume in the other fraction:

$$\frac{500 \text{ mg}}{5 \text{ mL}} = \frac{360 \text{ mg}}{X}$$

Step 8: Cross-multiply the fractions:

$$500 \text{ mg} \times X = 360 \text{ mg} \times 5 \text{ mL}$$

Step 9: Solve for X. Divide both sides of the equation by 500 mg and cancel units that appear in both the numerator and denominator:

$$\frac{\cancel{500 \text{ mg}} \times X}{\cancel{500 \text{ mg}}} = \frac{360 \cancel{\text{mg}} \times 5 \text{ mL}}{500 \cancel{\text{mg}}}$$

$$X = \frac{360 \times 5 \text{ mL}}{500}$$

$$X = 3.6 \text{ mL}$$

The nurse should administer 3.6 mL of reconstituted ampicillin to give the patient 360 mg.

Now that you know the dose is correct, you need to determine how much medication to administer. Just follow the steps you've been using all along.

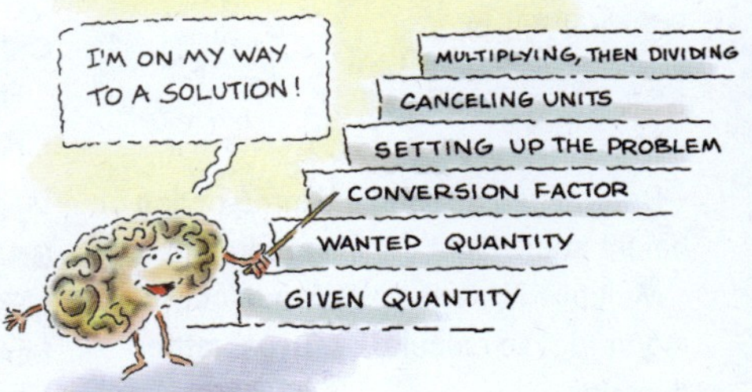

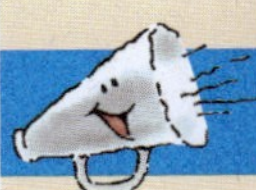

That's a wrap!

Calculating pediatric dosages review

When determining pediatric dosage calculations, be sure to keep these points in mind.

Route guidelines

- PO medications may be given as liquid suspensions.
  - Mix medication before measuring out the dose.
  - Never crush timed-release capsules or tablets or enteric-coated medications.
- Subcut route is commonly used for childhood immunizations and insulin injections.
  - Make sure the injection contains no more than 1 mL of solution.
  - Administer in any area with sufficient subcut tissue.
- IM route is commonly used for immunizations.
  - Inject the appropriate amount per location.
  - Administer in the vastus lateralis, deltoid, or ventrogluteal muscles—select on age appropriateness.
- IV medications should be diluted carefully and administered cautiously.
  - Use an infusion pump with infants and small children.
- For topical route, absorption is greater in infants and small children.

(*continued*)

Calculating pediatric dosages review (*continued*)

– Wipe off any remaining medication after application.
– Apply according to the order and medication manufacturer's recommendations.

Dosage per kilogram

- Dosages are expressed as *mg/kg/day* or *mg/kg/dose.*
- Multiply the child's weight in kilograms by the required milligrams of medication per kilogram.

BSA

- Measured in m^2
- Determined through the intersection of height and weight on a nomogram
- Multiplied by the prescribed dose in $mg/m^2/day$ to calculate safe pediatric dosages

Weight-based formulas for fluid needs

- A child weighing less than 10 kg: weight in kg × 100 mL = fluid needs in mL/day
- A child weighing 10 to 20 kg: (total kg–10 kg) × 50 mL = additional fluid need in mL/day; 1,000 mL/day + additional fluid need = fluid needs in mL/day
- A child weighing more than 20 kg: (total kg–20 kg) × 20 mL = additional fluid need in mL/day; 1,500 mL/day + additional fluid need = fluid needs in mL/day

Calorie-based formula for fluid needs

- Fluid-to-calorie ratio: 120 mL per 100 kcal
- Fluid requirements in mL/day = (calorie requirements = 100 kcal) × 120 mL

BSA-based formula for fluid needs

- For a well-dehydrated child: fluid maintenance needs in mL/day = BSA in m^2 × 1,500 $mL/day/m^2$

Quick quiz

1. The suggested pediatric dosage for a medication is 35 mg/kg/day. What amount should be administered to an infant weighing 5 kg?

A. 250 mg
B. 175 mg
C. 75 mg
D. 50 mg

Answer: B. To solve this problem, set up a proportion with the suggested dosage in one ratio and the unknown quantity in the other. Multiply the means and extremes, and then divide each side of the equation by the value that appears on the *X* side of the equation. Cancel units that appear in the numerator and denominator.

2. A child uses 1,000 calories per day. What is the child's daily fluid requirement?

A. 1,200 mL
B. 1,000 mL
C. 500 mL
D. 200 mL

Answer: A. Use the equation for calculating fluid needs based on kilocalories, inserting the appropriate numbers. Then solve for *X*.

3. A patient is 40″ tall, weighs 64 lb, and has a BSA of 0.96 m^2. How much fluid do they require per day?
   A. 140 mL
   B. 1,040 mL
   C. 1,400 mL
   D. 1,440 mL

Answer: D. Use the equation for calculating fluid needs based on BSA, inserting the appropriate numbers. Then solve for *X*.

4. What would the daily fluid need be for a child who weighs 8 kg?
   A. 1,000 mL/day
   B. 900 mL/day
   C. 800 mL/day
   D. 600 mL/day

Answer: C. Set up the equation using the formula weight in kilograms multiplied by 100 mL/kg/day. Cancel like units.

$$8 \cancel{\text{kg}} \times 100 \text{ mL}/\cancel{\text{kg}}/\text{day}$$
$$= 800 \text{ mL/day}$$

5. What chart is used to determine BSA?
   A. Monogram
   B. Nomogram
   C. Pediagram
   D. Infogram

Answer: B. A nomogram allows the nurse to plot the patient's height and weight to determine BSA.

Scoring

☆☆☆ If you answered all five items correctly, way to go! You're the pride and joy of precise pediatric dosages.

☆☆ If you answered four items correctly, we're impressed! There's nothing infantile about your abilities.

☆ If you answered fewer than four items correctly, review and try again! You'll be a specialist in special calculations before you know it.

Suggested References

Centers for Disease Control and Prevention. (2020). Intramuscular (IM) injections–vaccine administration. https://www.cdc.gov/vaccines/hcp/admin/downloads/IM-Injection-children.pdf

Hockenberry, M. J., Duffy, E. A., & Gibbs, K. (2023). *Wong's nursing care of infants and children* (12th ed.). Elsevier.

Chapter 15

Calculating obstetric medications dosages

Just the facts

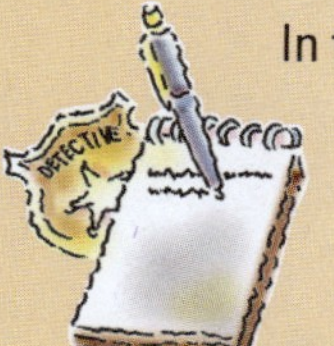

In this chapter, you'll learn how to:

- assess the mother and fetus during medication administration
- identify common obstetric medications and their adverse effects
- calculate obstetric dosages

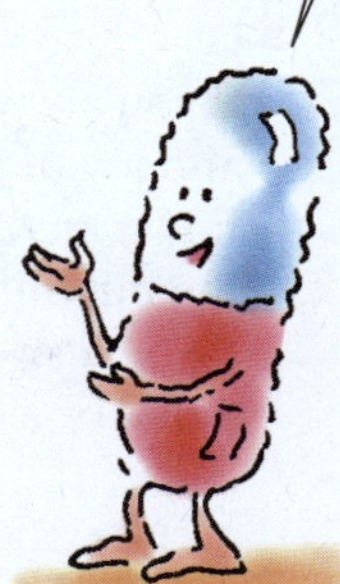

Every medication received during pregnancy can affect both mom and fetus. This special patient population needs to have extra care and precautionary measures in place when it comes to medication administration.

A look at obstetric medication administration

During pregnancy, labor and delivery, and the postpartum period, medications are commonly given to the mother for four reasons:

1. to control pregnancy-induced hypertension
2. to inhibit preterm labor
3. to induce labor or augment labor
4. to prevent postpartum hemorrhage

Because medications administered to the mother before delivery can also affect the fetus, both mother and fetus require meticulous monitoring. *Remember:* Nurses are caring for two patients at once, so there's a narrow margin for error.

Assessing the mother and fetus

When administering medications, the nurse should frequently check the mother's vital signs, urine output, uterine contractions, and deep tendon reflexes. Carefully assess fluid intake and output along with breath sounds to reduce the mother's risk of fluid overload, which can lead to acute pulmonary edema. (See *Assessing the mother's body systems*, p. 293.)

Assessing the mother's body systems

Assessment is a critical part of obstetric nursing. Here's what to assess in each of the mother's body systems.

Neurologic system

- Deep tendon reflexes when magnesium sulfate is infusing
- Pain
- Orientation (because disorientation can indicate hypoxemia or water intoxication)

Cardiovascular system

- Vital signs
- Extremities for peripheral edema with large-volume infusions
- Pulses and skin temperature in the lower extremities for evidence of deep vein thrombosis
- IV site to check for infiltration

Respiratory system

- Breath sounds
- Oxygenation
- Lungs for pulmonary edema with large-volume infusions

GI system

- Abdomen for contractions when oxytocin is infusing
- Abdomen for bowel sounds after delivery
- Ability to pass flatus or move bowels before discharge

Genitourinary system

- Urine output
- Fluid balance to check for decreased renal function

Fluid monitoring is especially critical in women with pregnancy-induced hypertension, which can cause decreased renal function. It's also important with medications given to inhibit preterm labor because of their antidiuretic effect.

The fetus is also the focus

While evaluating the mother, be sure to evaluate the fetus's response to medication therapy. Constantly assess fetal heart tones and heart rate by connecting the mother to an electronic fetal monitor. This monitor records the fetal heart rate and also provides a tracing of it.

Be alert for a sudden increase or decrease in fetal heart rate, which may signal an adverse reaction to treatment. If either occurs, discontinue the medication immediately. (See *It's got a good beat: Contractions and fetal heart rate*, p. 294.)

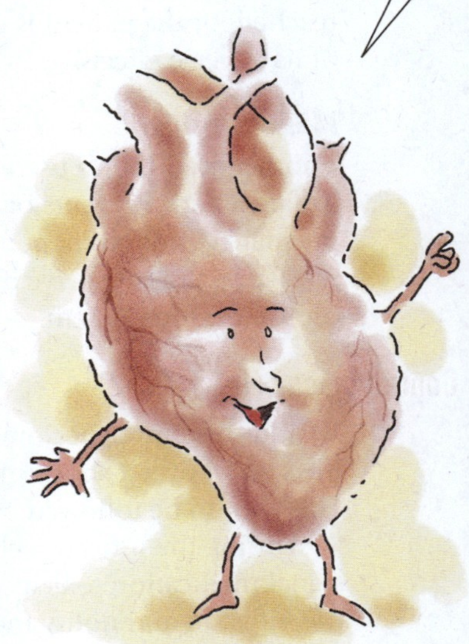

Continuous monitoring of fetal heart tones and heart rate is necessary during medication therapy.

Common obstetric medications

Medications used during pregnancy, labor, and delivery, and the postpartum period include the following:

- terbutaline
- magnesium sulfate
- dinoprostone
- oxytocin (See *The lowdown on four obstetric medications*, pp. 295–296.)

Advice from the experts

It's got a good beat: Contractions and fetal heart rate

Electronic fetal monitoring allows nurses to assess the mother's contractions as well as the fetal heart rate. Follow these incredibly easy steps:

1. Evaluate the mother's contraction pattern.
2. Note the characteristics of the contractions.
   - What's the frequency?
   - What's the duration?
   - What's the intensity?
3. Evaluate the fetal heart rate after establishing a baseline.
   - Is the rate within normal range?
   - Is tachycardia present?
   - Is bradycardia present?
4. What is the fetal heart rate variability: minimal, moderate, or marked.
5. Assess for changes in fetal heart rate characteristics.
   - Is acceleration or increased heart rate present with contractions?
   - Is deceleration or decreased heart rate present with contractions?
   - Is the deceleration early, late, or variable?

Terbutaline

Terbutaline is used to inhibit preterm labor. It stimulates the beta$_2$-adrenergic receptors in the uterine smooth muscle and inhibits contractility.

A preterm proposition

To administer terbutaline, mix it in a compatible IV solution and administer it through an infusion pump. Then titrate the dose every 10 minutes until the contractions subside, the maximum dose is reached, or the patient is unable to tolerate the medication because of its adverse effects.

Magnesium sulfate

Another medication used during labor and delivery is magnesium sulfate, which prevents or controls seizures that may be caused by pregnancy-induced hypertension. This medication acetylcholine released by motor nerve impulses which results in depressing the central nervous system.

Control those seizures

To administer magnesium sulfate, first give a loading dose (a high dose given over a short time to rapidly reach a therapeutic drug level). This should be followed by an infusion at a lower dose, as prescribed.

During the infusion, closely assess patellar reflexes loss of these signal medication toxicity. If toxicity is suspected, immediately stop the infusion and notify the licensed practitioner. Calcium gluconate may be ordered as an antidote.

Before you give that medication!

The lowdown on four obstetric medications

This table lists some common medications used in the obstetric setting along with their actions, adverse reactions, and nursing considerations.

Medication	Action	Adverse reactions	Nursing considerations
Terbutaline	Relaxes uterine muscle by acting on beta$_2$-adrenergic receptors; inhibits uterine contractions	**Maternal** • *Blood:* increased liver enzymes • *Central nervous system (CNS):* seizures, nervousness, tremor, headache, drowsiness, flushing, sweating • *Cardiovascular (CV):* increased heart rate, changes in blood pressure, palpitations, chest discomfort • *Eye, ear, nose, and throat (EENT):* tinnitus • *GI:* nausea, vomiting, altered taste • *Respiratory:* dyspnea, wheezing	• Use cautiously in patients with diabetes, hypertension, hyperthyroidism, severe cardiac disease, seizure disorder, and arrhythmias. • Protect from light. *Don't use if discolored.* • Explain the need for the medication to the patient and family. • Give subQ injection in lateral deltoid area. • Inform the patient about the possibility of paradoxical bronchospasm. • Although not approved by the Food and Drug Administration for treatment of preterm labor, this medication is considered very effective and is used in many hospitals. • Monitor the patient's blood glucose level. • Monitor the neonate for hypoglycemia.
Magnesium sulfate	Decreases acetylcholine released by nerve impulse; prevents seizures by blocking neuromuscular transmission	**Maternal** • *CNS:* sweating, drowsiness, depressed reflexes, flaccid paralysis, hypothermia, flushing, blurred vision • *CV:* hypotension, circulatory collapse, depressed cardiac function, heart block • *GI:* diarrhea • *Other:* fatal respiratory paralysis, hypocalcemia with tetany	• Use cautiously in labor and in those with impaired renal function, myocardial damage, or heart block. • This medication may be used as a tocolytic agent to inhibit premature labor; it can decrease the frequency and force of uterine contractions. • Keep calcium gluconate available to reverse magnesium sulfate intoxication. • Watch for respiratory depression. • Monitor intake and output. • Monitor deep tendon reflexes. • Maximum infusion is 150 mg/min. • Signs of hypermagnesemia begin to appear at blood levels of 4 mEq/L. • This medication should be stopped at least 2 hours before delivery to avoid fetal respiratory depression. • Monitor the neonate for magnesium sulfate toxicity.

(*continued*)

The lowdown on four obstetric medications (*continued*)

Medication	Action	Adverse reactions	Nursing considerations
Dinoprostone	A prostaglandin that produces strong, prompt contractions of uterine smooth muscle; facilitates cervical dilations by directly softening the cervix	**Maternal** • *CNS:* fever, headache, dizziness, anxiety, paresthesia, weakness, syncope • *CV:* chest pain, arrhythmias, hypotension • *EENT:* blurred vision, eye pain • *GI:* nausea, vomiting, diarrhea • *Genitourinary:* vaginal pain, vaginitis, endometritis **Fetal** • *CNS:* hypotonia, hyperstimulation • *Respiratory:* respiratory depression • *CV:* bradycardia • *Other:* intrauterine fetal sepsis	• Use only with the patient in or near a delivery suite. Critical care facilities should be available. • After administration of the gel form of the medication the patient should remain supine for 15–30 minutes. May be repeated in 6 hours if no cervical response. • Have the patient remain supine for 2 hours after insertion of the vaginal insert form of the medication. • Remove the vaginal insert with onset of active labor or 12 hours after insertion. • Monitor the fetus accordingly. • If hyperstimulation of the uterus occurs, gently flush the vagina with sterile saline solution. • Treat dinoprostone-induced fever (usually self-limiting and transient) with water sponging and increased fluid intake, not with aspirin.
Oxytocin	Causes potent and selective stimulation of uterine and mammary gland, smooth muscle and antidiuretic effect	**Maternal** • *Blood:* afibrinogenemia (may be from postpartum bleeding) • *CNS:* subarachnoid hemorrhage resulting from hypertension; seizures or coma resulting from water intoxication • *CV:* hypotension, increased heart rate, systemic venous return, increased cardiac output, arrhythmias • *Other:* hypersensitivity, tetanic uterine contractions, abruptio placentae, impaired uterine blood flow, increased uterine motility, uterine rupture **Fetal** • *Blood:* hyperbilirubinemia, hypercapnia • *CV:* bradycardia, tachycardia, premature ventricular contractions, variable deceleration of heart rate • *Respiratory:* hypoxia, asphyxia, death • *CNS:* brain damage, seizures • *EENT:* retinal hemorrhage • *GI:* hepatic necrosis	• Oxytocin is contraindicated in cephalopelvic disproportion; where delivery requires conversion, as in transverse lie; in fetal distress; when delivery isn't imminent; and in other obstetric emergencies. • Administer by piggyback infusion so the medication can be discontinued without interrupting the IV line. *Don't give by IV bolus injection.* • Don't infuse in more than one site. • Monitor and record uterine contractions, heart rate, blood pressure, intrauterine pressure, fetal heart rate, and character of blood loss every 15 minutes. • Have magnesium sulfate (20% solution) available for relaxation of myometrium. • Monitor fluid intake and output. Antidiuretic effect may lead to fluid overload, seizures, and coma.

Dinoprostone

Dinoprostone, a medication used to induce labor, is used to dilate the cervix in pregnant patients at or near term.

Scope it out

Dinoprostone is available as an endocervical gel, a vaginal insert, or a vaginal suppository. In some states in the United States, administration of this medication doesn't fall within a nurse's scope of practice, and it must be administered by a licensed practitioner.

Warm and... gel-like

For administration of dinoprostone, have the patient lie on their back; the cervix will then be examined using a speculum. Then assist with insertion of the gel, using aseptic technique. A catheter provided with the medication is used to administer the gel into the cervical canal just below the level of the internal os. Warm the gel to room temperature before using. It isn't necessary to warm the vaginal inserts before giving; however, a minimal amount of water-soluble jelly may be used to aid insertion.

Oxytocin

Oxytocin—the medication most commonly used to induce labor or to augment labor—selectively stimulates uterine smooth muscle.

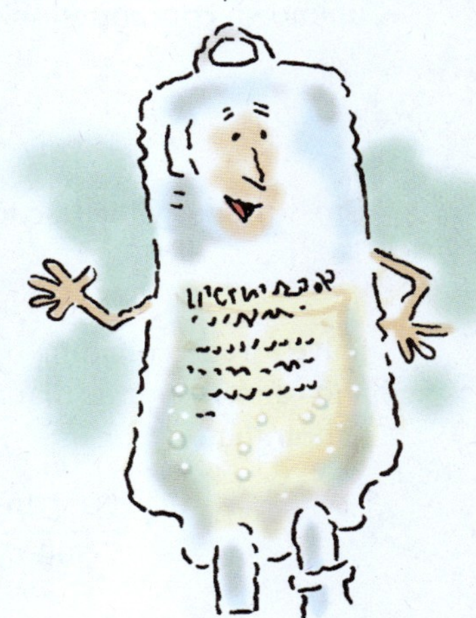

Oxytocin is given to help induce labor or augment labor contractions!

Compelling contractions

After mixing oxytocin with a compatible solution, administer it by piggyback infusion with an IV infusion pump and titrate until a normal contraction pattern occurs. When labor is firmly established, a licensed practitioner may prescribe a decrease in the infusion rate. Carefully monitor contraction strength because the medication can cause tachysystole contractions that can lead to uterine rupture as well as fetal and maternal death. Do not exceed 20 milliunits/min.

Bleeding blockade

Oxytocin may also be used to control bleeding after delivery of the placenta. To control bleeding, add the medication to 1 L of IV fluid, and then infuse it at a rate that controls bleeding. Never administer oxytocin by IV push.

Dosage calculations

In the labor and delivery unit, nurses must be especially careful to calculate and administer medications accurately. For instance, when dealing with life-threatening problems, such as hemorrhage and seizures caused by pregnancy-induced hypertension.

Administering accurate dosages to the mother helps avoid fetal complications. Be sure to examine medication labels closely. They contain valuable information for calculating dosages.

Real-world problems

These examples show how to calculate obstetric medications using proportions.

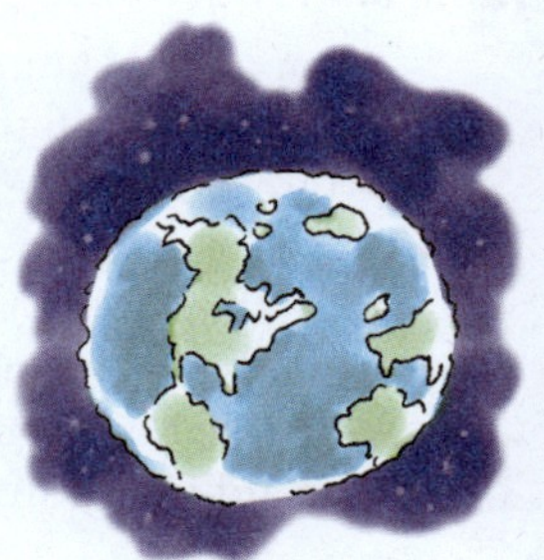

Overdue? Order oxytocin

A patient is 10 days overdue, so the licensed practitioner prescribes oxytocin to stimulate labor. The order reads: *add 30 units of oxytocin to 500 mL Lactated Ringer's and infuse via pump at 2 milliunits/min for 20 minutes and then increase flow rate of 1 to 2 milliunits/minute every 30 to 60 minutes as needed.* What's the solution's concentration? What's the flow rate needed to deliver 2 milliunits/min for 20 minutes? What's the flow rate needed to deliver 1 milliunits/min?

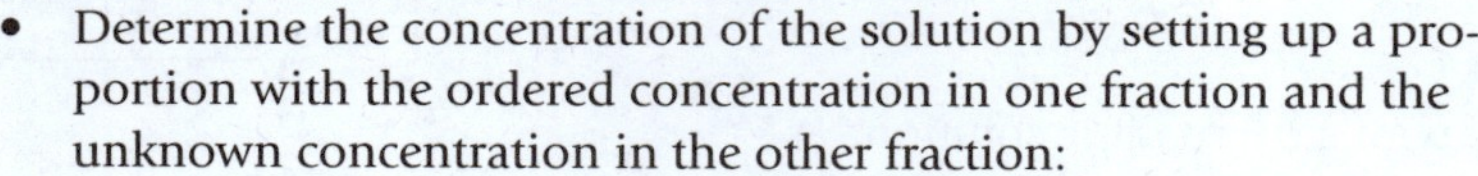

- Determine the concentration of the solution by setting up a proportion with the ordered concentration in one fraction and the unknown concentration in the other fraction:

$$\frac{30 \text{ units}}{500 \text{ mL}} = \frac{X}{1 \text{ mL}}$$

- Cross-multiply the fractions:

$$X \times 500 \text{ mL} = 30 \text{ units} \times 1 \text{ mL}$$

- Solve for *X* by dividing both sides of the equation by 500 mL and canceling units that appear in both the numerator and denominator:

$$\frac{X \times \cancel{500 \text{ mL}}}{\cancel{500 \text{ mL}}} = \frac{30 \text{ units} \times 1 \cancel{\text{ mL}}}{500 \cancel{\text{ mL}}}$$

$$X = \frac{30 \text{ units}}{500}$$

$$X = 0.06 \text{ units}$$

- The amount 0.06 units can be written in milliunits: 1 milliunit is 1/1,000 of a unit; 1,000 milliunits is 1 unit. Therefore, 0.06 units times 1,000 equals 60 milliunits. So, the concentration is 60 milliunits/mL.
- Next, determine the flow rate. If the prescribed dosage of oxytocin is 2 milliunits/min for 20 minutes, the patient receives a total of 40 milliunits. To calculate the rate needed to provide that dose, set up a proportion with the known concentration in one fraction and the total oxytocin dose and unknown flow rate in the other:

$$\frac{60 \text{ milliunits}}{1 \text{ mL}} = \frac{40 \text{ milliunits}}{X}$$

- Cross-multiply the fractions:

$$X \times 60 \text{ milliunits} = 1 \text{ mL} \times 40 \text{ milliunits}$$

- Solve for X by dividing both sides of the equation by 60 milliunits and canceling units that appear in both the numerator and denominator:

$$\frac{X \times \cancel{60 \text{ milliunits}}}{\cancel{60 \text{ milliunits}}} = \frac{1 \text{ mL} \times 40 \cancel{\text{ milliunits}}}{60 \cancel{\text{ milliunits}}}$$

$$X = \frac{40 \text{ mL}}{60}$$

$$X = 0.67 \text{ mL}$$

- The flow rate is 0.67 mL/20 minutes. Because this medication must be delivered by infusion pump, compute the hourly flow rate by multiplying the 20-minute rate by three:

$$0.67 \text{ mL/20 min} \times 3 = 2 \text{ mL/hr}$$

- The hourly flow rate is 2 mL/hr. Finally, calculate the flow rate to be used after the first 20 minutes, resulting in 1 milliunits/min (60 milliunits/hr). Having calculated the solution's concentration as 60 milliunits/mL, set up a proportion with the known concentration in one fraction and the increased oxytocin dose and the unknown flow rate in the other fraction:

$$\frac{60 \text{ milliunits}}{1 \text{ mL}} = \frac{40 \text{ milliunits}}{X}$$

Some medications infuse over a shorter period of time than 1 hour or 60 minutes. For this example, the initial infusion must run over 20 minutes. Therefore, 60 minutes divided by 20 minutes = 3. Multiply 20 × 3 to obtain the hourly rate!

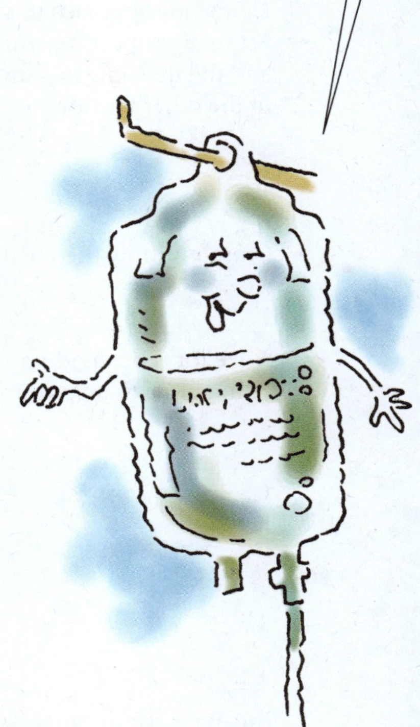

- Cross-multiply the fractions:

$$X \times 60 \text{ milliunits} = 1 \text{ mL} \times 60 \text{ milliunits}$$

- Solve for X by dividing both sides of the equation by 60 milliunits and canceling units that appear in both the numerator and denominator:

$$\frac{X \times \cancel{60 \text{ milliunits}}}{\cancel{60 \text{ milliunits}}} = \frac{1 \text{ mL} \times 60 \cancel{\text{ milliunits}}}{60 \cancel{\text{ milliunits}}}$$

$$X = 1 \text{ mL}$$

- After 20 minutes, reset the pump to deliver 1 mL/hr.
  That's 1 mL/60 minutes, or 0.017 mL/min. Because there are 60 milliunits/mL, multiply 60 by 0.017 mL/min to verify that this flow rate does provide 1 milliunits/minute.

Seizure? Stop it with magnesium sulfate

A patient is at risk for a seizure due to pregnancy-induced hypertension. The licensed practitioner orders *4 g (4,000 mg) magnesium sulfate in 250 mL D_5W to be infused at 2 g/hr.* What's the flow rate in mL/hr?

Here's one approach to solving this problem:

- Set up a proportion with the known concentration in one fraction and the flow rate in grams and the unknown flow rate in milliliters in the other fraction:

$$\frac{4 \text{ g}}{250 \text{ mL}} = \frac{2 \text{ g}}{X}$$

- Cross-multiply the fractions:

$$X \times 4 \text{ g} = 250 \text{ mL} \times 2 \text{ g}$$

- Solve for X by dividing each side of the equation by 4 g and canceling units that appear in both the numerator and denominator:

$$\frac{X \times \cancel{4 \text{ g}}}{\cancel{4 \text{ g}}} = \frac{250 \text{ mL} \times 2 \cancel{\text{g}}}{4 \cancel{\text{g}}}$$

$$X = \frac{250 \text{ mL} \times 2}{4}$$

$$X = \frac{500 \text{ mL}}{4}$$

$$X = 125 \text{ mL}$$

The magnesium sulfate solution should be infused at 125 mL/hr.

Let's seize that problem again

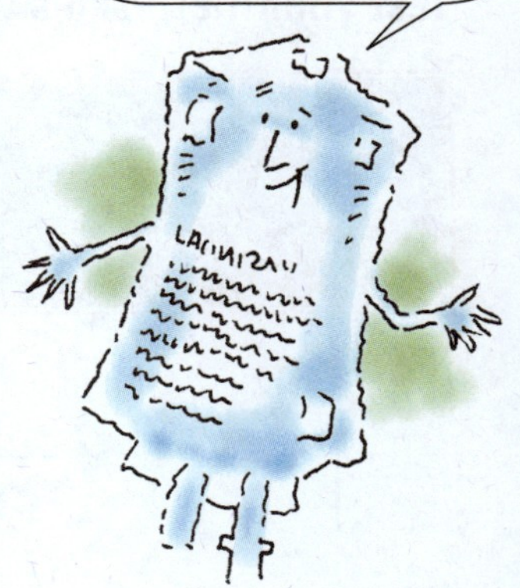

Let's try to solve
the same problem
using another method.

Here's another approach to solving the same problem.

- First, calculate the strength of the solution by setting up a proportion with the known strength in one fraction and the unknown strength in the other fraction:

$$\frac{4\text{ g}}{250\text{ mL}} = \frac{X}{1\text{ mL}}$$

- Cross-multiply the fractions:

$$X \times 250\text{ mL} = 4\text{ g} \times 1\text{ mL}$$

- Solve for X by dividing each side of the equation by 250 mL and canceling units that appear in both the numerator and denominator:

$$\frac{X \times \cancel{250\text{ mL}}}{\cancel{250\text{ mL}}} = \frac{4\text{ g} \times 1\cancel{\text{mL}}}{250\cancel{\text{mL}}}$$

$$X = \frac{4\text{ g}}{250}$$

$$X = 0.016\text{ g}$$

- The solution's strength is 0.016 g/mL. Next, calculate the flow rate by setting up another proportion with the solution concentration in one fraction and the unknown flow rate in the other fraction:

$$\frac{1\text{ mL}}{0.016\text{ g}} = \frac{X}{2\text{ g}}$$

- Cross-multiply the fractions:

$$X \times 0.016\text{ g} = 1\text{ mL} \times 2\text{ g}$$

- Solve for X by dividing each side of the equation by 0.016 g and canceling units that appear in both the numerator and denominator:

$$\frac{X \times \cancel{0.016\text{ g}}}{\cancel{0.016\text{ g}}} = \frac{1\text{ mL} \times 2\cancel{\text{g}}}{0.016\cancel{\text{g}}}$$

$$X = \frac{2\text{ mL}}{0.016}$$

$$X = 125\text{ mL}$$

The same flow rate of 125 mL/hr is obtained using this method.

Dosage drill

Test your math skills with this drill

A patient with gestational hypertension is receiving 8 g of magnesium sulfate in 1 L of dextrose 5% in water at 125 mL/hr. How many grams per hour is the patient receiving?

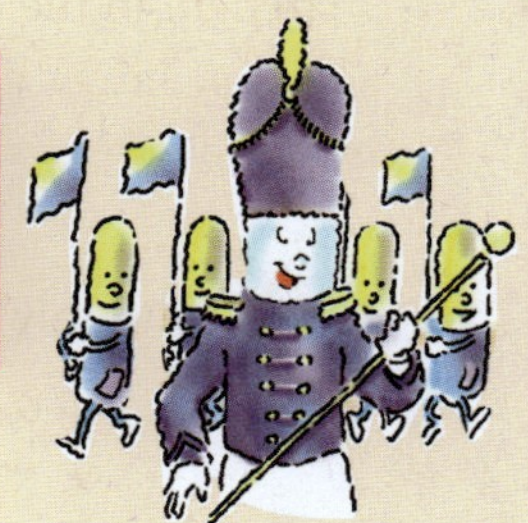

Your answer: ______________

To find the answer, set up ratios and a proportion and solve for X. Remember that 1 L = 1,000 mL.

$$1{,}000\text{ mL}:8\text{ g}::125\text{ mL}:X\text{ g}$$

$$1{,}000\text{ mL} \times X\text{ g} = 125\text{ mL} \times 8\text{ g}$$

$$\frac{\cancel{1{,}000\text{ mL}} \times X\text{ g}}{\cancel{1{,}000\text{ mL}}} = \frac{125\ \cancel{\text{mL}} \times 8\text{ g}}{1{,}000\ \cancel{\text{mL}}}$$

$$X = \frac{1{,}000}{1{,}000}$$

$$X = 1\text{ g/hr}$$

The patient is receiving 1 g of magnesium sulfate per hour.

Preterm labor? Try terbutaline

A patient is in preterm labor. An order for *10 mg terbutaline sulfate in 250 mL D_5W to infuse at 5 mcg/min has been prescribed.* What's the flow rate for this solution?

- First, find the solution's strength. Set up a proportion with the known strength in one fraction and the unknown strength in the other fraction:

$$\frac{10 \text{ mg}}{250 \text{ mL}} = \frac{X}{1 \text{ mL}}$$

- Cross-multiply the fractions:

$$X \times 250 \text{ mL} = 10 \text{ mg} \times 1 \text{ mL}$$

- Solve for X by dividing each side of the equation by 250 mL and canceling units that appear in both the numerator and denominator:

$$\frac{X \times \cancel{250 \text{ mL}}}{\cancel{250 \text{ mL}}} = \frac{10 \text{ mg} \times 1 \cancel{\text{ mL}}}{250 \cancel{\text{ mL}}}$$

$$X = \frac{10 \text{ mg}}{250}$$

$$X = 0.04 \text{ mg}$$

- The strength of the solution is 0.04 mg/mL. Next, convert to micrograms (mcg) by multiplying by 1,000 (0.04 mg × 1,000 = 40 mcg/mL). Then calculate the flow rate needed to deliver the prescribed dose of 5 mcg/min. To do this, set up a proportion with the known solution strength in one fraction and the unknown flow rate in the other:

$$\frac{1 \text{ mL}}{40 \text{ mcg}} = \frac{X}{5 \text{ mcg}}$$

- Cross-multiply the fractions:

$$X \times 40 \text{ mcg} = 1 \text{ mL} \times 5 \text{ mcg}$$

- Solve for X by dividing each side of the equation by 40 mcg and canceling units that appear in both the numerator and denominator:

$$\frac{X \times \cancel{40 \text{ mcg}}}{\cancel{40 \text{ mcg}}} = \frac{1 \text{ mL} \times 5 \cancel{\text{ mcg}}}{40 \cancel{\text{ mcg}}}$$

$$X = \frac{5 \text{ mcg}}{40}$$

$$X = 0.125 \text{ mL}$$

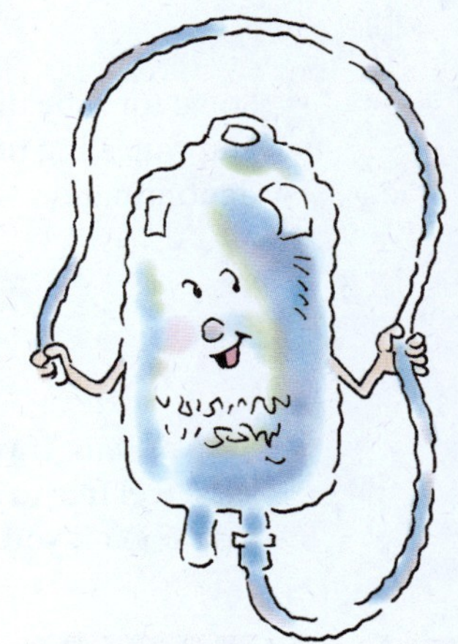

Nothing feels better than getting the right answer twice!

- The flow rate is 0.125 mL/min. Because the infusion must be administered with a pump, compute the hourly flow rate by setting up a proportion with the known flow rate per minute in one fraction and the unknown flow rate per hour in the other fraction:

$$\frac{0.125 \text{ mL}}{1 \text{ min}} = \frac{X}{60 \text{ min}}$$

- Cross-multiply the fractions:

$$X \times 1 \text{ min} = 0.125 \text{ mL} \times 60 \text{ min}$$

- Solve for X by dividing each side of the equation by 1 minute and canceling units that appear in both the numerator and denominator:

$$\frac{X \times \cancel{1 \text{ min}}}{\cancel{1 \text{ min}}} = \frac{0.125 \text{ mL} \times 60 \cancel{\text{min}}}{1 \cancel{\text{min}}}$$

$$X = 7.5 \text{ mL}$$

Note this: If you prefer Dimensional Analysis to calculate dosages, feel free to do so! Refer back to Chapter 4 of this incredibly easy book if you get stuck!

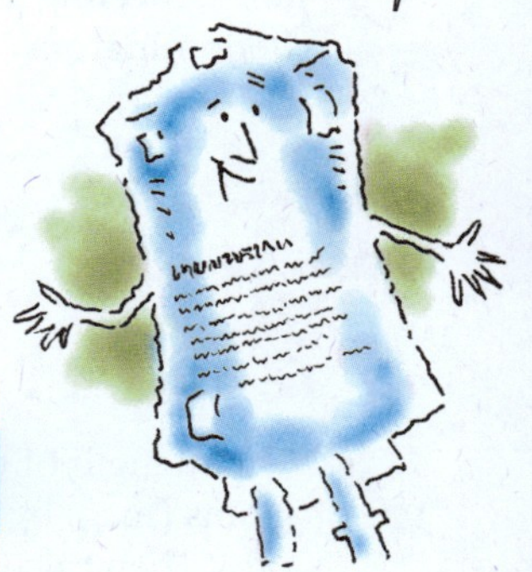

Most IV pumps allow inputting the mL/hr to the tenth decimal place. If your calculation contains a 10th decimal, then you should input it for a more accurate measurement.

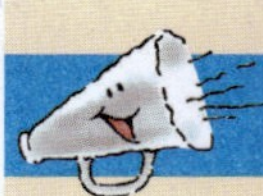

That's a wrap!

Calculating obstetric medication dosages review

Here are some important facts about obstetric medication dosages to keep in mind.

Assessing the mother during medication administration

- Frequently check vital signs, urine output, uterine contractions, and deep tendon reflexes.
- Monitor and record fluid intake and output.
- Assess breath sounds.

Evaluating fetal response to medication therapy

- Monitor fetal heart rate during mother's medication therapy.
- If sudden increase or decrease occurs, immediately discontinue the medication.

Common obstetric medication

Terbutaline

- Inhibits preterm labor.
- Administered via an infusion pump and titrated every 10 minutes as needed.

Magnesium sulfate

- Prevents or controls seizures caused by pregnancy-induced hypertension.
- Given as a loading dose first, then followed with infusion at a lower dose.
- Suspected toxicity requires stopping infusion immediately and notifying the licensed practitioner.

Calculating obstetric medication dosages review (*continued*)

Oxytocin

- Selectively stimulates uterine smooth muscle to induce labor or augment labor.
- May also be used to control bleeding after delivery of the placenta.
- Administered IV piggyback with an infusion pump and titrated until normal contraction pattern occurs.
- Requires careful monitoring of contraction strength because medication can cause tachysystole contractions and even death.

Dinoprostone

- Ripens the cervix (to induce labor) in pregnant patients at or near term.
- Available as endocervical gel, vaginal inserts, or vaginal suppositories.

Dosage calculations

- Accurate dosages of medications given to the mother help avoid fetal complications.
- Proportions can be used to solve obstetric dosage calculations.

Quick quiz

1. The order reads to give 20 units oxytocin in 1,000 mL of lactated Ringer's solution. What is the solution's concentration?

A. 20 units/mL
B. 2 units/mL
C. 0.2 unit/mL
D. 0.02 unit/mL

Answer: D. To solve this problem, set up a proportion with the known concentration in one fraction and the unknown concentration in the other fraction. Then solve for *X*.

2. The nurse is aware that a sudden increase or decrease in the fetal heart rate after medication treatment is a result of which outcome?

A. A sign that the infant is about to be delivered
B. A change due to an adverse reaction to the medication
C. A temporary reaction to many obstetric medications
D. An indication that the medication has reached its peak level

Answer: B. Changes in the fetal heart rate may signal an adverse reaction to the medication; therefore, discontinue the medication immediately.

3. Which medication should be kept readily available to reverse magnesium sulfate intoxication?

A. Potassium chloride
B. Atropine
C. Calcium gluconate
D. Sodium chloride

Answer: C. During magnesium sulfate infusion, calcium gluconate should be readily available to reverse magnesium intoxication should it occur.

4. The order states infuse *20 mg terbutaline sulfate in 1,000 mL D_5W at 0.01 mg/min for 20 minutes.* What is the flow rate?
   A. 1 mL
   B. 10 mL
   C. 100 mL
   D. 200 mL

Answer: B. First, calculate the concentration, which is 0.02 mg/mL. Then determine the amount of medication provided in 20 minutes by multiplying 0.01 by 20 minutes to get 0.2 mg. Finally, set up a proportion with the concentration in one fraction and the total amount of medication and the unknown flow rate in the other fraction. Solve for *X*.

5. If 5 g of magnesium sulfate are added to 1 L of normal saline solution, what is the concentration of magnesium sulfate?
   A. 0.05 mg/mL
   B. 0.5 mg/mL
   C. 5 mg/mL
   D. 50 mg/mL

Answer: C. First, convert 5 g to 5,000 mg and 1 L to 1,000 mL. Then divide the 1,000 into 5,000 to obtain the concentration: 5 mg/mL.

6. The licensed provider orders *20 g magnesium sulfate in 1,000 mL D_5W to be infused at 2 g/hr.* What is the flow rate in milliliters per hour?
   A. 1 mL/hour
   B. 10 mL/hour
   C. 100 mL/hour
   D. 300 mL/hour

Answer: C. To solve this problem, set up a proportion with the ordered concentration in one fraction and the flow rate in grams and the unknown flow rate in milliliters in the other. Solve for *X*.

7. What is the best way to administer oxytocin?
   A. IV piggyback infusion
   B. IV bolus injection
   C. Direct IV infusion
   D. IM injection

Answer: A. Administer oxytocin by IV piggyback infusion using an infusion pump so that the medication can be discontinued without interrupting the IV line.

Scoring

☆☆☆ If you answered all seven items correctly, fantastic! Your labors have helped you become a confident calculator.

☆☆ If you answered five or six items correctly, keep at it! You'll soon be able to deftly deliver medications in any delivery unit.

☆ If you answered fewer than five items correctly, chin up! You still have one chapter left to conquer the Quick quiz.

Suggested References

American College of Nurse-Midwives; Carlson, N. S., Dunn Amore, A., Ellis J. A., Page, K., & Schafer, R. (2022). American College of Nurse-Midwives clinical bulletin no.18. Induction of labor. *Journal of Midwifery and Women's Health, 67*(1), 140–149.

American College of Obstetricians and Gynecologists. (2009). ACOG Practice Bulletin No. 106: Intrapartum fetal heart rate monitoring: nomenclature, interpretation, and general management principles. *Obstetrics & Gynecology, 114*(1), 192–202.

American College of Obstetricians and Gynecologists. (2020). Gestational hypertension and preeclampsia. ACOG Practice Bulletin No. 222. *Obstetrics & Gynecology, 135*(6), e237–e260. Retrieved September 30, 2023, from https://www.preeclampsia.org/frontend/assets/img/advocacy_resource/Gestational_Hypertension_and_Preeclampsia_ACOG_Practice_Bulletin,_Number_222_1605448006.pdf

Erickson, E. N., & Carlson, N. S. (2020). Predicting postpartum hemorrhage after low-risk vaginal birth by labor characteristics and oxytocin administration. *Journal of Obstetrics, Gynecology, and Neonatal Nursing, 49*(6), 549–563.

Xi, M., & Gerriets, V. (2022). Prostaglandin E2 (Dinoprostone). National Library of Medicine. Retrieved September 30, 2023, from https://www.ncbi.nlm.nih.gov/books/NBK545279/

Chapter 16

Calculating critical care infusions

Just the facts

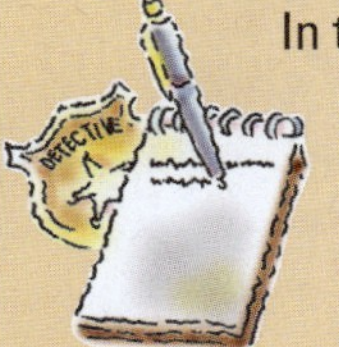

In this chapter, you'll learn how to:

- distinguish points to consider when giving critical care medications
- calculate dosages for IV push medications
- calculate IV flow rates for critical care medications
- calculate medications not ordered at a specific flow rate or dosage

A look at critical care dosages

Critically ill patients being cared for in acute care settings often receive special medications that are not only potent but also have potential serious adverse effects if not infused and maintained properly. Nurses who care for these types of patients usually work in areas where advanced training is necessary to be able to assess, monitor, and evaluate patients' conditions. It is extremely important to accurately calculate, titrate, and monitor the flow of critical care medications.

Medications used in critical care areas must be regulated carefully. As these IV medications are potent, they may be supplied in smaller units of measure such as micrograms (mcg) versus milligrams (mg). Furthermore, the dosage of these medications may be ordered based on a patient's body weight in kilograms (kg). All critical care medications that require continuous infusions must be administered using an IV pump device and never infused using gravity regulation. Examples of critical care medications include lidocaine, epinephrine, nitroglycerin, norepinephrine, phenylephrine, dobutamine, dopamine, and nitroprusside which are all mixed with IV fluids.

Administering IV injections

When needing medications to take an immediate effect (onset time), the licensed practitioner will order a medication to be administered as an IV push (IVP). Since IV medications enter directly into the blood stream, the onset time is quicker. This is especially important when administering medications in emergency situations. These potent, fast-acting medications rapidly control heart rate, respiration, blood pressure, cardiac output, or kidney function. Although these medications act fast, they usually have a short duration of action and may require a continuous IV infusion to achieve the desired effects.

Nurses working with critically ill patients must be SUPER quick and accurate with dosage calculations.

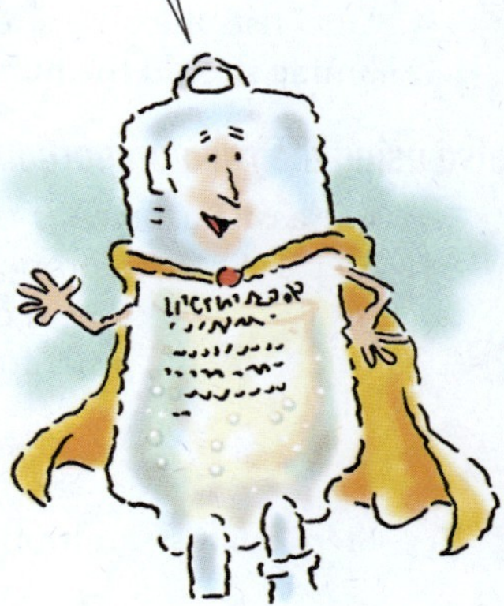

One critical difference

Generally, IVP medications are ordered by dosage, which can sometimes include the specific unit of measure to administer over a short time (such as mg/min or mcg/kg/min). The nurse calculates critical care dosages the same way as with other non-critical medications. The nurse, however, must take extra precaution because medications used on critical care units are extremely potent and may have serious adverse effects including death.

Although dosage calculations of IVP medications are very similar to those for intramuscular (IM) medications, the actual administration is very different. Administration rates vary with each IVP; therefore, nurses must know how slowly or quickly to deliver—or "push"—a medication. This information can be found in medication resources such as drug books, an online library, or a pharmacist. It's better to be safe than sorry with rapid-acting medications.

Emergency medications, such as atropine and lidocaine, are usually supplied in prefilled syringes to be administered via IVP. (See *Preparing emergency closed-system medications*.) Prefilled syringes are not only easier to prepare and administer, but they eliminate the need to perform calculations during stressful situations.

Be prepared to be under stress

Nurses are responsible for calculating and administering dosages accurately. Many medications used in critical care areas are supplied in small vials; therefore, it's important for nurses to double-check the label to make sure they're giving the right dose or concentration. For example, epinephrine comes in two concentrations (1:1,000 [1 mg/mL] and 1:10,000 [1 mg:10 mL]). Giving the wrong concentration could be fatal.

Performing calculations during an emergency is stressful, which can increase the chances of making an error. Nurses must be extra aware and cautious in stressful situations. (See *Stress busters*, p. 310.)

Preparing emergency closed-system medications

To prepare a closed-system device, follow these incredibly easy steps:

- Hold the medication chamber in one hand.
- Hold the syringe section in the other hand.
- Flip the protective caps off both ends.
- Insert the medication chamber into the syringe section.
- Finally, remove the needle or needleless cap and expel air and any extra medication.

Calculating dosages

The following examples demonstrate how to calculate IVP medications.

Are you label able?

A patient is admitted with frequent ventricular dysrhythmias. The licensed practitioner orders procainamide hydrochloride 100 mg IVP every 5 minutes prn until dysrhythmias disappear. If the medication label lists the dose strength as 50 mg/mL, how many mL of procainamide should the nurse administer to the patient every 5 minutes?

Solve using the *ratio proportion method*

For assistance, refer to Chapter 3.

Step 1: Set up a proportion with the ordered dose and the unknown volume in one fraction and the dose strength in mg/mL in the other fraction:

$$\frac{100 \text{ mg}}{X} = \frac{50 \text{ g}}{1 \text{ mL}}$$

Step 2: Cross-multiply the fractions:

$$X \times 50 \text{ mg} = 1 \text{ mL} \times 100 \text{ mg}$$

Step 3: Solve for *X*. Divide each side of the equation by 100 mg and cancel the units that appear in both the numerator and denominator:

$$\frac{X \times \cancel{50 \text{ mg}}}{\cancel{50 \text{ mg}}} = \frac{1 \text{ mL} \times 100 \cancel{\text{ mg}}}{50 \cancel{\text{ mg}}}$$

$$X = \frac{100 \text{ mL}}{50}$$

$$X = 2 \text{ mL}$$

The nurse should administer 2 mL of procainamide IVP.

Solve using the *formula method*

For assistance, refer to Chapter 10.

Recall the formula:

$$X = \frac{\text{Desired dose (D)}}{\text{Have on hand (H)}} \times \text{Quantity (Q) (aka volume)}$$

Step 1: Set up the formula with the information provided:

- Desired dose: 100 mg
- Have on hand: 50 mg
- Quantity: 1 mL

$$X = \frac{100 \text{ mg}}{50 \text{ mg}} \times 1 \text{ mL}$$

Advice from the experts

Stress busters

Here are four hot tips to help prepare and thus reduce stress levels when performing dosage calculations during an emergency:

- Memorize the calculation formulas or have them available at all times.
- Have a calculator available for quick use.
- Have the patient's weight available in kilograms (kg). The nurse may need to covert from pounds (lb) to kilograms (kg).
- Be familiar with the different critical care medications, as well as a facility's medication policy and protocols.

Step 2: Cancel the units that appear in both the numerator and the denominator:

$$X = \frac{100 \cancel{mg}}{50 \cancel{mg}} \times 1 \text{ mL}$$

Step 3: Multiply the desired dose by quantity (100 × 1):

$$X = \frac{100 \text{ mL}}{50}$$

Step 4: Solve for *X*. Divide the numerator by the denominator (100 ÷ 50):

$$X = 2 \text{ mL}$$

The nurse should administer 2 mL of procainamide IVP.

Rapid heartbeat riddle

A patient suddenly develops supraventricular tachycardia (SVT). The licensed practitioner orders *6 mg adenosine IVP stat*. If the only vial available contains 3 mg/mL of adenosine, how many mL should the nurse give?

Solve using the *ratio proportion method*

Step 1: Set up a proportion with the available solution in one ratio and the ordered dose and the unknown volume in the other ratio:

$$3 \text{ mg} : 1 \text{ mL} :: 6 \text{ mg} : X$$

Step 2: Multiply the means and the extremes:

$$X \times 3 \text{ mg} = 1 \text{ mL} \times 6 \text{ mg}$$

Step 3: Solve for *X*. Divide both sides of the equation by 3 mg and cancel units that appear in both the numerator and denominator:

$$\frac{X \times \cancel{3 \text{ mg}}}{\cancel{3 \text{ mg}}} = \frac{1 \text{ mL} \times 6 \cancel{mg}}{3 \cancel{mg}}$$

$$X = \frac{6 \text{ mL}}{3}$$

$$X = 2 \text{ mL}$$

The nurse should administer 2 mL of adenosine by IVP.

Solve using the *formula method*

Step 1: Set up the formula with the information provided:

- Desired dose: 6 mg
- Have on hand: 3 mg
- Quantity: 1 mL

$$X = \frac{6 \text{ mg}}{3 \text{ mg}} \times 1 \text{ mL}$$

Step 2: Cancel the units that appear in both the numerator and the denominator:

$$X = \frac{6\ \cancel{mg}}{3\ \cancel{mg}} \times 1\ mL$$

Step 3: Multiply the desired dose by quantity (6 × 1):

$$X = \frac{6\ mL}{3}$$

Step 4: Solve for *X*. Divide the numerator by the denominator (6 ÷ 3):

$$X = 2\ mL$$

The nurse should administer 2 mL of adenosine by IVP.

Digoxin difficulty

A patient with a history of atrial fibrillation takes digoxin tablets at home but currently has an order to be NPO. The licensed practitioner prescribes 0.125 mg of digoxin IV once for an elevated heart rate. The available digoxin vial contains 0.25 mg/mL. How many mL will the nurse administer?

Solve using the *formula method*

Step 1: Set up the formula with the information provided:

- Desired dose: 0.125 mg
- Have on hand: 0.25 mg
- Quantity: 1 mL

$$X = \frac{0.125\ mg}{0.25\ mg} \times 1\ mL$$

Step 2: Cancel the units that appear in both the numerator and the denominator:

$$X = \frac{0.125\ \cancel{mg}}{0.25\ \cancel{mg}} \times 1\ mL$$

Step 3: Multiply the desired dose by quantity (0.125 × 1):

$$X = \frac{0.125\ mL}{0.25}$$

Step 4: Solve for *X*. Divide the numerator by the denominator (0.125 ÷ 0.25):

$$X = 0.5\ mL$$

The nurse should administer 0.5 mL of digoxin.

Dosage drill

Test your math skills with this drill

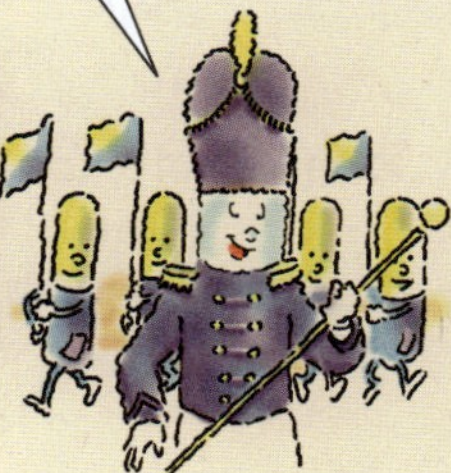
Be sure to show how you arrive at your answer.

The licensed practitioner orders amiodarone 150 mg IVP stat for a patient experiencing ventricular tachycardia (V-Tach). If the vial available contains 50 mg/mL, how many mL will the nurse administer?

Your answer: ____________

Find the answer using the ***formula method.***

Step 1: Set up the formula with the information provided:

- Desired dose: 150 mg
- Have on hand: 50 mg
- Quantity: 1 mL

$$X = \frac{150 \text{ mg}}{50 \text{ mg}} \times 1 \text{ mL}$$

Step 2: Cancel the units that appear in both the numerator and the denominator:

$$X = \frac{150 \cancel{\text{mg}}}{50 \cancel{\text{mg}}} \times 1 \text{ mL}$$

Step 3: Multiply the desired dose by quantity (150×1):

$$X = \frac{150 \text{ mL}}{50}$$

Step 4: Solve for *X*. Divide the numerator by the denominator ($150 \div 50$):

$$X = 3 \text{ mL}$$

The nurse should administer 3 mL of amiodarone IVP.

Find the answer using the ***ratio proportion method.***

Step 1: Set up the proportion using the information provided:

$$50 \text{ mg}:1 \text{ mL}::150 \text{ mg}:X$$

Step 2: Set up the equation, multiplying the means and extremes:

$$50 \text{ mg} \times X = 150 \text{ mg} \times 1 \text{ mL}$$

Step 3: Solve for *X*. Divide both sides of the equation by 50 mg and cancel units that appear in both the numerator and denominator:

$$\frac{\cancel{50 \text{ mg}} \times X}{\cancel{50 \text{ mg}}} = \frac{150 \cancel{\text{mg}} \times 1 \text{ mL}}{50 \cancel{\text{mg}}}$$

$$X = \frac{150 \text{ mL}}{50}$$

$$X = 3 \text{ mL}$$

The nurse should administer 3 mL of amiodarone IVP.

Solve using the *ratio proportion method*

Step 1: Set up the proportion using the information provided:

$$0.25 \text{ mg}:1 \text{ mL}::0.125 \text{ mg}:X$$

Step 2: Set up the equation, multiplying the means and extremes:

$$X \times 0.25 \text{ mg} = 1 \text{ mL} \times 0.125 \text{ mg}$$

Step 3: Solve for X. Divide both sides of the equation by 50 mg and cancel units that appear in both the numerator and denominator:

$$\frac{X \times 0.25 \cancel{\text{mg}}}{0.25 \cancel{\text{mg}}} = \frac{1 \text{ mL} \times 0.125 \cancel{\text{mg}}}{0.25 \cancel{\text{mg}}}$$

$$X = \frac{0.125 \text{ mL}}{0.25}$$

$$X = 0.5 \text{ mL}$$

The nurse should administer 0.5 mL of digoxin.

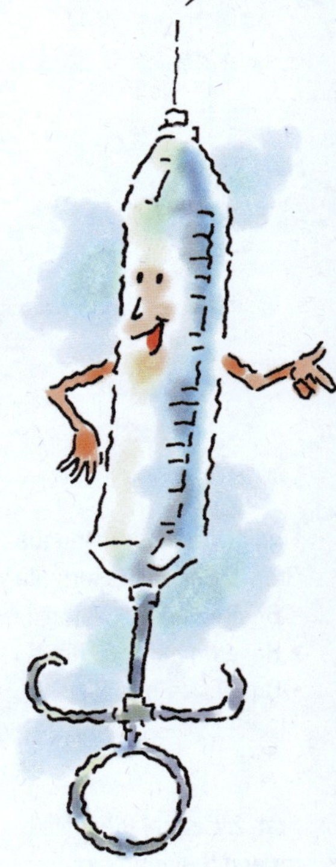

When giving an IVP injection, it's very important to note how long to push the medication... too fast or too slow can have serious consequences.

Calculating IV flow rates

Patients who are critically ill often require medications that treat life-threatening problems. Nurses must work swiftly to perform dosage calculations, prepare and administer medications, and then observe the patient closely to evaluate the effectiveness of the medication.

Critical care medications can be prescribed by a patient's weight. These weight-based medications are ordered by the amount of medication per kilogram (kg) of body weight per minute (min). Others may be ordered by the dose per minute. This section reviews how to perform dosage calculations of critical care medications to determine the IV flow rates in:

- micrograms per kilogram per min (mcg/kg/min)
- micrograms per min (mcg/min)
- milligrams per min (mg/min).

Three critical components

Nurses may need to perform calculations of critical care medications before administering. Depending on how a medication is ordered, the nurse will need certain information to perform dosage calculations. These components may include:

- the patient's weight in kilograms (kg)
- the concentration of the medication (mg/mL or mcg/mL)
- the desired dosage (mg/min, mcg/min, mcg/kg/minute).

The low down on concentration

Performing calculations for critical care medications can be complex. To help with calculations, find the lowest available concentration of a medication by reducing to how much medication is in 1 mL of fluid. To calculate the concentration, use this formula:

$$X = \frac{\text{Amount of medication (mg or mcg)}}{\text{Amount of fluid (mL)}}$$

Here's an example:

A patient has an infusion of 2 g (2,000 mg) lidocaine in 500 mL D_5W. Using the formula, find the lowest concentration of this medication.

Step 1: Set up the formula with the information provided:

$$X = \frac{2{,}000 \text{ mg}}{500 \text{ mL}}$$

Step 2: Solve for X. Divide the numerator by the denominator (2,000 ÷ 500):

$$X = 4 \text{ mg/mL}$$

The lowest concentration is 4 mg of lidocaine in 1 mL of D_5W.

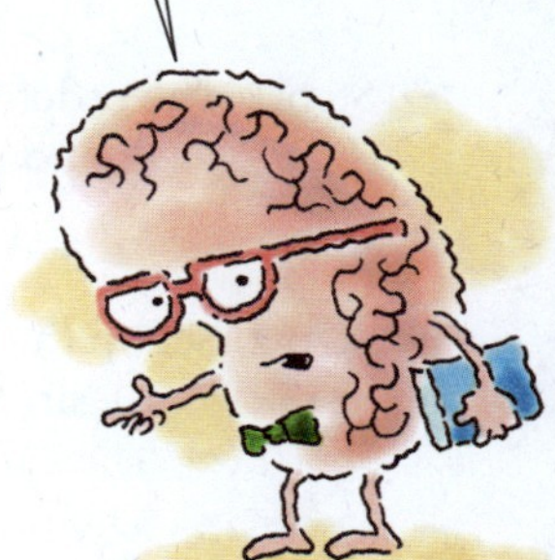
Convert, convert, convert! When performing dosage calculations, don't forget that the numerator and the denominator must be of the same unit of measure!

Figure the flow rate

Since continuous critical care medications must be infused through an IV pump, the nurse will need to determine the flow rate to program the pump. The nurse will need to complete several steps to calculate the hourly flow rate. Let's look at several different formulas to use.

Orders for Mg or Mcg/Minute

Use this formula for medications ordered to infuse with an amount of medication per minute:

$$X = \frac{\text{Ordered amount in mg or mcg/ min}}{\text{Medication Concentration (mg or mcg/mL)}} \times 60 \text{ min/hr}$$

Here's an example: A patient's order reads:

Give 2 g (2,000 mg) lidocaine in 500 mL D_5W at 2 mg/min

Determine the flow rate (mL/hr):

Step 1: Find the lowest concentration of this medication. Use the provided formula. Divide the numerator by the denominator (2,000 ÷ 500):

$$X = \frac{2{,}000 \text{ mg}}{500 \text{ mL}}$$

$$X = 4 \text{ mg/mL}$$

Step 2: Set up the formula with the information provided:

$$X = \frac{2 \text{ mg/min}}{4 \text{ mg/mL}} \times 60 \text{ min/hr}$$

Step 3: Cancel the units that appear in both the numerator and the denominator:

$$X = \frac{2 \cancel{\text{mg}}/\cancel{\text{min}}}{4 \cancel{\text{mg}}/\text{mL}} \times 60 \cancel{\text{min}}/\text{hr}$$

Step 4: Multiply the ordered amount by 60 (2×60):

$$X = \frac{120 \text{ hr}}{4 \text{ mL}}$$

Step 5: Solve for *X*. Divide the numerator by the denominator ($120 \div 4$):

$$X = 30 \text{ mL/hr}$$

The flow rate of lidocaine would be 30 mL/hr.

Solve using the *formula method*

- Nurses may also use the formula method to determine the flow rate. Recall the formula:

$$X = \frac{\text{Desired dose (D)}}{\text{Have on hand (H)}} \times \text{Quantity (Q) (aka volume)}$$

Step 1: The ordered dose is in mg/min. Multiply by 60 to determine the hourly dose (2×60):

$$X = 2 \text{ mg/min} = 120 \text{ mg/hr}$$

Step 2: Set up the formula with the information provided:

- Desired dose: 120 mg/hr
- Have on hand: 4 mg (lowest concentration)
- Quantity: 1 mL

$$X = \frac{120 \text{ mg/hr}}{4 \text{ mg}} \times 1 \text{ mL}$$

Step 3: Cancel the units that appear in both the numerator and the denominator:

$$X = \frac{120 \cancel{\text{mg}}/\text{hr}}{4 \cancel{\text{mg}}} \times 1 \text{ mL}$$

Step 4: Multiply the desired dose by quantity (120×1):

$$X = \frac{120 \text{ mL/hr}}{4}$$

Step 5: Solve for X. Divide the numerator by the denominator ($120 \div 4$):

$$X = 30 \text{ mL/hr}$$

The nurse would program an IV pump to deliver 30 mL/hr.

Solve using the *ratio proportion method*

Find the flow rate using the *ratio proportion method:*

Step 1: Find the solution's concentration by setting up a proportion with the unknown concentration in one fraction and the ordered dose in the other fraction:

$$\frac{X}{1 \text{ mL}} = \frac{2{,}000 \text{ mg}}{500 \text{ mL}}$$

Step 2: Cross-multiply the fractions:

$$X \times 500 \text{ mL} = 2{,}000 \text{ mg} \times 1 \text{ mL}$$

Step 3: Solve for X. Divide each side of the equation by 500 mL and cancel units that appear in both the numerator and denominator:

$$\frac{X \times \cancel{500 \text{ mL}}}{\cancel{500 \text{ mL}}} = \frac{2{,}000 \text{ mg} \times 1 \cancel{\text{ mL}}}{500 \cancel{\text{ mL}}}$$

$$X = \frac{2{,}000 \text{ mg}}{500}$$

$$X = 4 \text{ mg}$$

The solution's lowest concentration is 4 mg/mL.

Step 4: Calculate the flow rate per minute needed to deliver the ordered dose of 2 mg/minute. Set up a proportion with the unknown flow rate per minute in one fraction and the solution's concentration in the other fraction:

$$\frac{2 \text{ mg}}{X} = \frac{4 \text{ mg}}{1 \text{ mL}}$$

Step 5: Cross-multiply the fractions:

$$X \times 4 \text{ mg} = 1 \text{ mL} \times 2 \text{ mg}$$

Step 6: Solve for X. Divide each side of the equation by 4 mg and cancel units that appear in both the numerator and denominator:

$$\frac{X \times \cancel{4 \text{ mg}}}{\cancel{4 \text{ mg}}} = \frac{1 \text{ mL} \times 2 \cancel{\text{ mg}}}{4 \cancel{\text{ mg}}}$$

$$X = \frac{2 \text{ mL}}{4}$$

$$X = 0.5 \text{ mL}$$

The patient should receive 0.5 mL/min of lidocaine.

Step 7: Find the hourly flow rate. Set up a proportion with the unknown flow rate per hour in one fraction and the flow rate per minute in the other fraction:

$$\frac{X}{60\text{ min}} = \frac{0.5\text{ mL}}{1\text{ min}}$$

Step 8: Cross-multiply the fractions:

$$X \times 1\text{ min} = 0.5\text{ mL} \times 60\text{ min}$$

Step 9: Solve for X. Divide each side of the equation by 1 minute and cancel units that appear in both the numerator and denominator:

$$\frac{X \times \cancel{1\text{ min}}}{\cancel{1\text{ min}}} = \frac{0.5\text{ mL} \times 60\ \cancel{\text{min}}}{1\ \cancel{\text{min}}}$$

$$X = 30\text{ mL}$$

The nurse would program an IV pump to deliver 30 mL/hr.

Real-world problems

The following examples show how to calculate an IV flow rate using the different formulas.

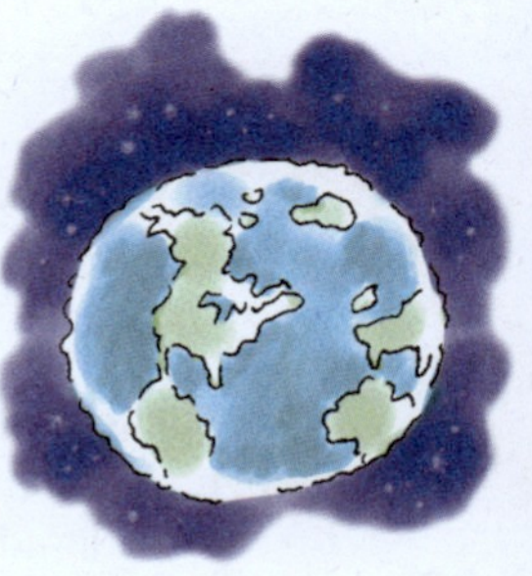

Nitro relief

A patient experiencing chest pain has an order for a nitroglycerin continuous infusion. The order reads *Start nitroglycerin 5 mcg/min, titrate to control chest pain.* Available is 50 mg of nitroglycerin added to 500 mL 0.9% NS. How will the nurse program the IV pump to start the infusion?

Recall the formula:

$$X = \frac{\text{Ordered amount in mg or mcg/ min}}{\text{Medication Concentration (mg or mcg/mL)}} \times 60\text{ min /hr}$$

Step 1: Find the lowest concentration of nitroglycerin:

$$X = \frac{50\text{ mg}}{500\text{ mL}} = 0.1\text{ mg/mL}$$

Step 2: Set up the formula with the information provided. Since nitroglycerin is ordered in mcg, convert 0.1 mg to mcg (0.1 × 1,000) = 100 mcg/mL:

$$X = \frac{5\text{ mcg/ min}}{100\text{ mcg/mL}} \times 60\text{ min/hr}$$

Step 3: Cancel the units that appear in both the numerator and the denominator:

$$X = \frac{5 \cancel{mcg}/\cancel{min}}{100 \cancel{mcg}/mL} \times 60 \cancel{min}/hr$$

Step 4: Multiply the ordered amount by 60 (5 × 60):

$$X = \frac{300 \text{ hr}}{100 \text{ mL}}$$

Step 5: Solve for *X*. Divide the numerator by the denominator (300 ÷ 100):

$$X = 3 \text{ mL/hr}$$

The nurse would program the IV pump to deliver 3 mL/hr of nitroglycerin.

Solve using the *formula method*

Find the flow rate using the *formula method:* Recall the formula:

$$X = \frac{\text{Desired dose (D)}}{\text{Have on hand (H)}} \times \text{Quantity (Q) (aka volume)}$$

Step 1: The ordered dose is in mcg/min. Multiply by 60 to determine the hourly dose:

$$X = 5 \text{ mcg/min} = 300 \text{ mcg/hr}$$

Step 2: Set up the formula with the information provided:

- Desired dose: 300 mcg/hr
- Have on hand: 0.1 mg (convert to mcg = 100 mcg)
- Quantity: 1 mL

$$X = \frac{300 \text{ mcg/hr}}{100 \text{ mcg}} \times 1 \text{ mL}$$

Step 3: Cancel the units that appear in both the numerator and the denominator:

$$X = \frac{300 \cancel{mcg}/hr}{100 \cancel{mcg}} \times 1 \text{ mL}$$

Step 4: Multiply the desired dose by quantity (300 × 1):

$$X = \frac{300 \text{ mL/hr}}{100}$$

Step 5: Solve for X. Divide the numerator by the denominator (300 ÷ 100):

$$X = 3 \text{ mL/hr}$$

The nurse would program the IV pump to deliver 3 mL/hr of nitroglycerin.

Solve using the *ratio proportion method*

Find the flow rate using the *ratio proportion method:*

Step 1: Find the solution's concentration by setting up a proportion with the unknown concentration in one fraction and the ordered dose in the other fraction:

Convert total mg to mcg:

$$1 \text{ mg}:1{,}000 \text{ mcg}::50 \text{ mg}:X \text{ mcg}$$

$$X = 50{,}000 \text{ mcg}$$

Calculate the lowest concentration:

$$\frac{50{,}000 \text{ mcg}}{500 \text{ mL}} = 100 \text{ mcg/mL}$$

Step 2: Calculate the flow rate per minute. Set up a proportion with the unknown flow rate per minute in one fraction and the solution's concentration in the other fraction:

$$\frac{5 \text{ mcg}}{X} = \frac{100 \text{ mcg}}{1 \text{ mL}}$$

Step 3: Cross-multiply the fractions:

$$X \times 100 \text{ mcg} = 1 \text{ mL} \times 5 \text{ mcg}$$

Step 4: Solve for X. Divide each side of the equation by 4 mg and cancel units that appear in both the numerator and denominator:

$$\frac{X \times \cancel{100} \cancel{\text{mcg}}}{\cancel{100} \cancel{\text{mcg}}} = \frac{1 \text{ mL} \times 5 \cancel{\text{mcg}}}{100 \cancel{\text{mcg}}}$$

$$X = \frac{5 \text{ mL}}{100}$$

$$X = 0.05 \text{ mL}$$

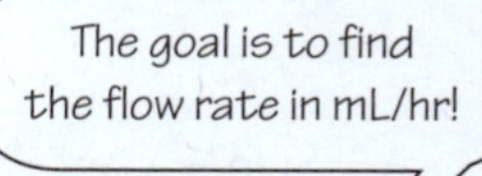

The goal is to find the flow rate in mL/hr!

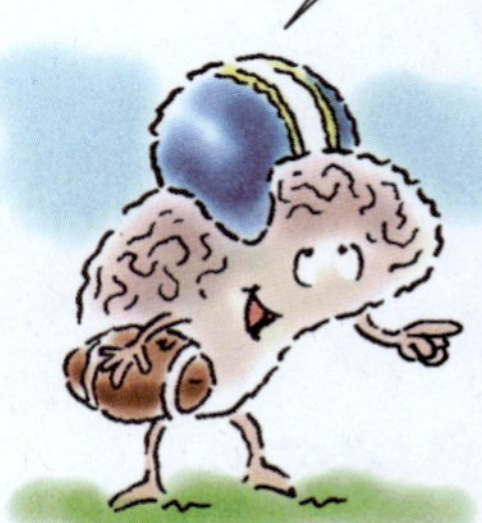

The patient should receive 0.05 mL/min of nitroglycerine.

Step 5: Find the hourly flow rate. Set up a proportion with the unknown flow rate per hour in one fraction and the flow rate per minute in the other fraction:

$$\frac{X}{60 \text{ min}} = \frac{0.05 \text{ mL}}{1 \text{ min}}$$

Dosage drill

Test your math skills with this drill

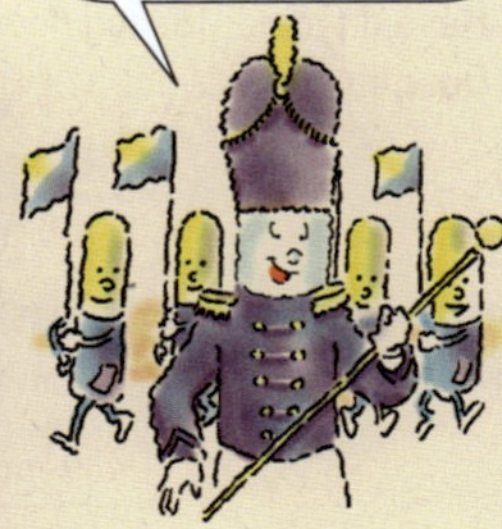
Be sure to show how you arrive at your answer.

A patient is receiving norepinephrine (Levophed) infusing at 30 mL/hr. The IV solution contains 4 mg of norepinephrine in 250 mL of D_5W. To verify that the medication is infusing at the correct rate per the order (8 mcg/min), the nurse must determine how many mcg/min of norepinephrine are infusing.

The nurse chooses to find the flow rate in mL/min to perform the calculation:

Your answer: ____________

Find the answer using the ***ratio proportion method:***

Step 1: Determine the lowest concentration of norepinephrine:

$$X = \frac{4 \text{ mg}}{250 \text{ mL}}$$

$$X = 0.016 \text{ mg/mL}$$

The lowest concentration is 0.016 mg/mL.

Step 2: Find the flow rate in mL/min. Convert 1 hour to 60 minutes:

$$X = \frac{30 \text{ mL}}{60 \text{ min}} = 0.5 \text{ mL/min}$$

Step 3: Find how many mcg/min the patient will receive:

- Multiply 0.5 mL/min by 16 mcg/mL

$$X = 8 \text{ mcg/min}$$

The nurse determines that the IV pump is programmed to the correct dose rate ordered.

Let's try a different method to verify the correct rate is infusing:

Find the flow rate using the ***formula method:***

Step 1: The ordered dose is in mcg/min. Multiply by 60 to determine the hourly dose:

$$X = 8 \text{ mcg/min} = 480 \text{ mcg/hr}$$

(*continued*)

Test your math skills with this drill (*continued*)

Step 2: Set up the formula with the information provided:

- Desired dose: 480 mcg/hr
- Have on hand: 16 mcg (lowest concentration dose)
- Quantity: 1 mL

$$X = \frac{480\text{ mcg/hr}}{16\text{ mcg}} \times 1\text{ mL}$$

Step 3: Cancel the units that appear in both the numerator and the denominator:

$$X = \frac{480\ \cancel{\text{mcg}}\text{/hr}}{16\ \cancel{\text{mcg}}} \times 1\text{ mL}$$

Step 4: Multiply the desired dose by quantity (480 × 1):

$$X = \frac{480\text{ mL/hr}}{16}$$

Step 5: Solve for *X*. Divide the numerator by the denominator (480 ÷ 16):

$$X = 30\text{ mL/hr}$$

The flow rate of 30 mL/hr for the concentration of nitroglycerin hanging is the correct rate for delivering the ordered dose of 8 mcg/min.

Let's try yet another method to verify the correct rate is infusing:

Step 1: Set up ratios and a proportion to determine the solution's concentration:

$$4\text{ mg:}250\text{ mL::}X\text{ mL:}1\text{ min}$$

$$X\text{ mg} \times 250\text{ mL} = 1\text{ mL} \times 4\text{ mg}$$

$$\frac{X\text{ mg} \times \cancel{250\text{ mL}}}{\cancel{250\text{ mL}}} = \frac{1\ \cancel{\text{mL}} \times 4\text{ mg}}{250\ \cancel{\text{mL}}}$$

$$X = \frac{4\text{ mg}}{250}$$

$$X = 0.016\text{ mg/mL, or }16\text{ mcg/mL}$$

Step 2: Determine the flow rate in mL/minute:

$$30\text{ mL:}60\text{ min::}X\text{ mL:}1\text{ min}$$

$$30\text{ mL} \times 1\text{ min} = 60\text{ min} \times X\text{ mL}$$

$$\frac{30\text{ mL} \times 1\ \cancel{\text{min}}}{60\ \cancel{\text{min}}} = \frac{\cancel{60\text{ min}} \times X\text{ mL}}{\cancel{60\text{ min}}}$$

$$X = \frac{30}{60}$$

$$X = 0.5\text{ mL/min}$$

Step 3: Determine how many mcg of the medication the patient will receive per minute:

$$X = 0.5\text{ mL/min} \times 16\text{ mcg/mL}$$

$$X = 8\text{ mcg/min}$$

There are 8 mcg of norepinephrine infusing each minute.

Step 6: Cross-multiply the fractions:

$$X \times 1\text{ min} = 100\text{ mL} \times 60\text{ min}$$

Step 7: Solve for *X*. Divide each side of the equation by 1 minute and cancel units that appear in both the numerator and denominator:

$$\frac{X \times \cancel{1}\ \cancel{\text{min}}}{\cancel{1}\ \cancel{\text{min}}} = \frac{0.05\text{ mL} \times 60\ \cancel{\text{min}}}{1\ \cancel{\text{min}}}$$

$$X = 3\text{ mL/hr}$$

The nurse would program the IV pump to deliver 3 mL/hr of nitroglycerin.

Weighing out the dobutamine

The licensed practitioner orders dobutamine to infuse at 10 mcg/kg/min for a patient who weighs 165 lb. The available concentration is 500 mg of dobutamine hydrochloride in 250 mL of D_5W. Find the flow rate to program an IV pump.

Recall this formula:

$$X = \frac{\text{Ordered amount in mg or mcg/min}}{\text{Medication Concentration (mg or mcg/mL)}} \times 60 \text{ min/hr}$$

Step 1: Convert the patient's weight into kilograms (kg):

$$X = \frac{165 \text{ lb}}{2.2 \text{ kg}} = 75 \text{ kg}$$

Step 2: Determine the dose per minute:

$$X = 10 \text{ mcg/kg/min}$$
$$X = 10 \text{ mcg} \times 75 \text{ kg/ min}$$
$$X = 750 \text{ mcg/min}$$

Step 3: Determine the lowest concentration of dobutamine:

$$X = \frac{500 \text{ mg}}{250 \text{ mL}} = 2 \text{ mg/mL}$$

Step 4: Set up the formula with the information provided. Since dobutamine is ordered in mcg, convert 2 mg to mcg (2 × 1,000) = 2,000 mcg/mL:

$$X = \frac{750 \text{ mcg/min}}{2{,}000 \text{ mcg/mL}} \times 60 \text{ min/hr}$$

Step 5: Cancel the units that appear in both the numerator and the denominator:

$$X = \frac{750 \cancel{\text{mcg}} / \cancel{\text{min}}}{2{,}000 \cancel{\text{mcg}} /\text{mL}} \times 60 \cancel{\text{min}} /\text{hr}$$

Step 6: Multiply the ordered amount by 60 (750 × 60):

$$X = \frac{45{,}000 \text{ hr}}{2{,}000 \text{ mL}}$$

Step 7: Solve for X. Divide the numerator by the denominator (45,000 ÷ 2,000):

$$X = 22.5 \text{ mL/hr}$$

The IV pump should be set to deliver 22.5 mL/hr of dobutamine.

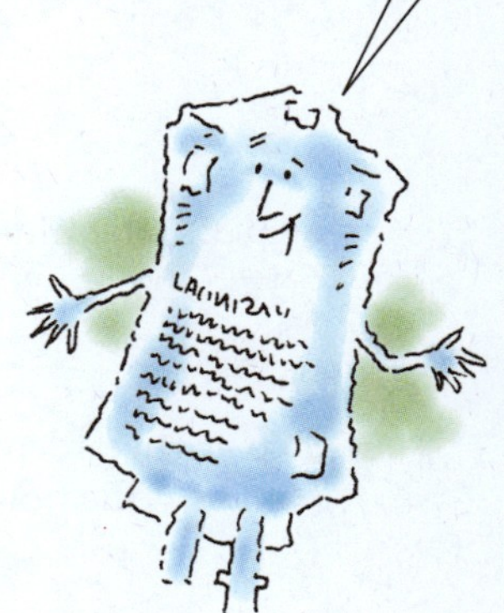

Most smart pumps used for delivering medication in critical areas are programmable to the tenth space!

Advice from the experts

Weighing in!

Some medications are prescribed to deliver a certain amount based on a patient's body weight, often referred to as weight-based dosing. A large portion of critical care medications are dosed according to weight as a patient's weight or body composition could affect their absorption, distribution, metabolism, or elimination. Therefore, it is imperative that a patient's weight be accurate and reliable.

Unstable patients ordered for bed rest will require weight measurements to be obtained from the bed scale. The reliability and accuracy of bed scales can be prone to error due to variables such as items and/or equipment being left in a patient's bed. In addition, inaccurate weight measurements or omission of weight documentation could potentially contribute to medication dosing errors (Pan et al., 2016).

Kilograms versus pounds

Weight-based medications are ordered by a patient's weight in kilograms (kg). Most medical grade scales have an option to measure a patient's weight in kilograms (kg). However, if this option is not available, the nurse will have to perform a conversion from pounds (lb) to kilograms (kg). This requires memorization of 1 kg is equal to 2.2 lb.

- If a patient's weight is provided in lb, divide by 2.2 to obtain the weight in kg.
- If a patient's weight is provided in kg, multiply by 2.2 to obtain the weight in lb.

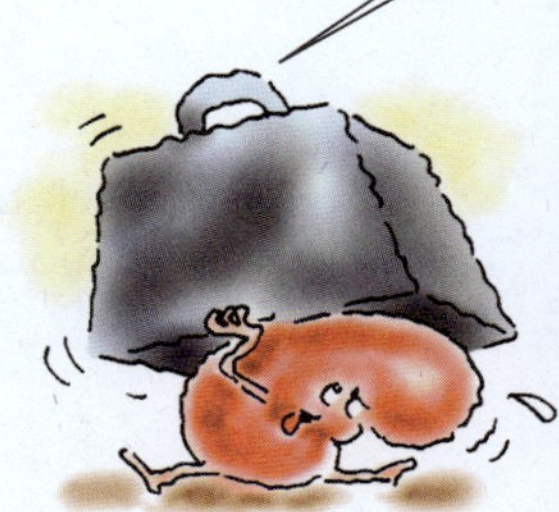

This must weigh 50 lb—not 50 kg!

Solve using the *formula method*

Find the flow rate using the *formula method:*

Step 1: Convert the patient's weight into kilograms (kg):

$$X = \frac{165 \text{ lb}}{2.2 \text{ kg}} = 75 \text{ kg}$$

Step 2: Determine the dose per minute:

$$X = 10 \text{ mcg/kg/min}$$
$$X = 10 \text{ mcg} \times 75 \text{ kg/min}$$
$$X = 750 \text{ mcg/min}$$

Step 3: Determine the lowest concentration of dobutamine:

$$X = \frac{500 \text{ mg}}{250 \text{ mL}} = 2 \text{ mg/mL}$$

Step 4: The ordered dose is in mcg/min. Multiply by 60 to determine the hourly dose:

$$750 \text{ mcg} \times 60 \text{ min} = 45{,}000 \text{ mcg/hr}$$

Step 5: Set up the formula with the information provided:

- Desired dose: 750 mcg/hr
- Have on hand: 2 mg (covert to mcg: $2 \times 1{,}000 = 2{,}000$ mcg)
- Quantity: 1 mL

$$X = \frac{45{,}000 \text{ mcg/hr}}{2{,}000 \text{ mcg}} \times 1 \text{ mL}$$

Step 6: Cancel the units that appear in both the numerator and the denominator:

$$X = \frac{45{,}000 \cancel{\text{mcg}}\text{/hr}}{2{,}000 \cancel{\text{mcg}}} \times 1 \text{ mL}$$

Step 7: Multiply the desired dose by quantity ($45{,}000 \times 1$):

$$X = \frac{45{,}000 \text{ mL/hr}}{2{,}000}$$

Step 8: Solve for X. Divide the numerator by the denominator ($45{,}000 \div 2{,}000$):

$$X = 22.5 \text{ mL/hr}$$

The IV pump should be set to deliver 22.5 mL/hr of dobutamine.

Solve using the *ratio proportion method*

Find the flow rate using the *ratio proportion method:*

Step 1: Convert the patient's weight into kilograms (kg). Set up a proportion with the weight in pounds and the unknown weight in kilograms in one fraction and the number of pounds per kilogram in the other fraction:

$$\frac{165 \text{ lb}}{X} = \frac{2.2 \text{ lb}}{1 \text{ kg}}$$

Step 2: Cross-multiply the fractions:

$$X \times 2.2 \text{ lb} = 1 \text{ kg} \times 165 \text{ lb}$$

Step 3: Solve for X. Divide each side of the equation by 2.2 lb and cancel units that appear in both the numerator and denominator:

$$\frac{X \times \cancel{2.2 \text{ lb}}}{\cancel{2.2 \text{ lb}}} = \frac{1 \text{ kg} \times 165 \cancel{\text{lb}}}{\cancel{2.2 \text{ lb}}}$$

$$X = \frac{165 \text{ kg}}{2.2}$$

$$X = 75 \text{ kg}$$

The patient weighs 75 kg.

Step 4: Determine the dose in mL/min by setting up a proportion with the patient's weight in kg and the unknown dose in mcg/min in one fraction and the known dose in mcg/kg/min in the other fraction:

$$\frac{75 \text{ kg}}{X} = \frac{1 \text{ kg}}{10 \text{ mcg/min}}$$

Step 5: Cross-multiply the fractions:

$$X \times 1 \text{ kg} = 10 \text{ mcg/min} \times 75 \text{ kg}$$

Step 6: Solve for X. Divide each side of the equation by 1 kg and cancel units that appear in both the numerator and denominator:

$$\frac{X \times \cancel{1 \text{ kg}}}{\cancel{1 \text{ kg}}} = \frac{10 \text{ mcg/min} \times 75 \cancel{\text{ kg}}}{\cancel{1 \text{ kg}}}$$

$$X = 750 \text{ mcg/min}$$

The patient should receive 750 mcg/min of dobutamine or 0.75 mg/min (Divide 750 by 1,000).

Step 7: Determine the flow rate in mL/min. Set up a proportion using the solution's concentration and solve for X:

$$\frac{0.75 \text{ mg}}{X} = \frac{500 \text{ mg}}{250 \text{ mL}}$$

$$\frac{\cancel{500 \text{ mg}} \times X}{\cancel{500 \text{ mg}}} = \frac{0.75 \cancel{\text{ mg}}\text{/min} \times 250 \text{ mL}}{500 \cancel{\text{ mg}}}$$

$$X = \frac{187.5 \text{ mL/min}}{500}$$

$$X = 0.375 \text{ mL/min}$$

Step 8: Find the flow rate in mL/hr. Multiply by 60 (60 min in hour):

$$X = 0.375 \text{ mL/min} \times 60 \text{ min/hr} = 22.5 \text{ mL/hr}$$

The patient should receive dobutamine at a rate of 22.5 mL/hr.

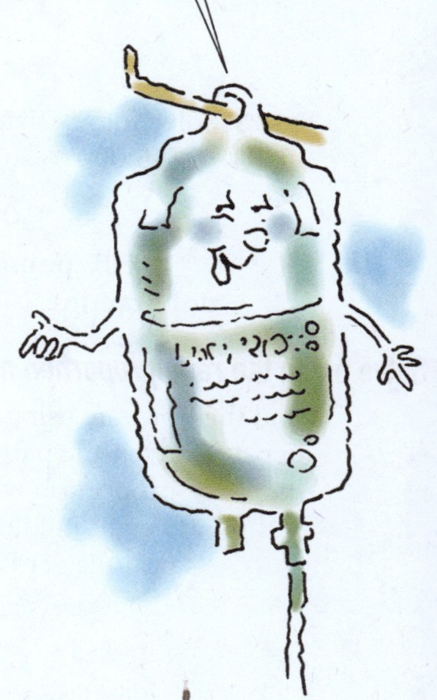

It can be confusing switching from one calculation method to another. Be consistent with using the same calculation method, and use the appropriate formulas to find the right answers.

Special cases

Critical care medications aren't always ordered at a specific flow rate or dosage. Sometimes, they're prescribed according to the patient's heart rate, blood pressure, or other parameters.

Dosage drill

Test your math skills with this drill

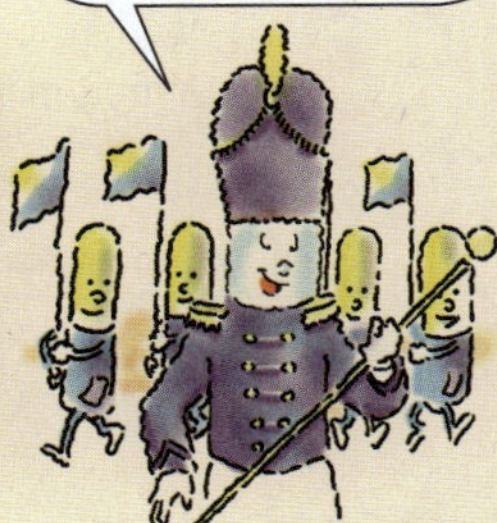
Be sure to show how you arrive at your answer.

A patient has been ordered to receive a continuous infusion of esmolol hydrochloride (Brevibloc) at 50 mcg/kg/min for a patient who weighs 73 kg. The solution contains 2.5 g esmolol in 250 mL of D_5W. How should the nurse set the pump to deliver the correct mL/hr?

Your answer: ______________

Find the flow rate using the ***formula method:***

Step 1: Determine the dose in mcg/min:

$$X = 50 \text{ mcg/kg/min}$$
$$X = 50 \text{ mcg} \times 73 \text{ kg/min}$$
$$X = 3{,}650 \text{ mcg/min}$$

Step 2: The ordered dose is in mcg/min. Multiply by 60 to determine the hourly dose:

$$3{,}650 \text{ mcg} \times 60 \text{ min} = 219{,}000 \text{ mcg/hr}$$

Step 3: Determine the lowest concentration of esmolol:

$$X = \frac{2.5 \text{ g}}{250 \text{ mL}} = 0.01 \text{ g/mL}$$

Step 4: Set up the formula with the information provided. Since esmolol is ordered in mcg, convert 0.01 g to mcg (multiply 0.01 by 1,000 by 1,000) = 10,000 mcg/mL:

- Desired dose: 219,000 mcg/hr
- Have on hand: 10,000 mcg
- Quantity: 1 mL

$$X = \frac{219{,}000 \text{ mcg/hr}}{10{,}000 \text{ mcg}} \times 1 \text{ mL}$$

Step 5: Cancel the units that appear in both the numerator and the denominator:

$$X = \frac{219{,}000 \cancel{\text{mcg}}\text{/hr}}{10{,}000 \cancel{\text{mcg}}} \times 1 \text{ mL}$$

Step 6: Multiply the desired dose by quantity (219,000 × 1):

$$X = \frac{219{,}000 \cancel{\text{mcg}}\text{/hr}}{10{,}000 \cancel{\text{mcg}}} \times 1 \text{ mL}$$

Step 7: Solve for *X*. Divide the numerator by the denominator (45,000 ÷ 2,000):

$$X = 21.9 \text{ mL/hr}$$

The IV pump should be set to deliver 21.9 mL/hr of dobutamine.

(*continued*)

Test your math skills with this drill (*continued*)

Find the answer using the ***ratio proportion method:***
Step 1: Determine the dose in mcg/min:

$$73 \text{ kg}:X \text{ mcg/min}::1 \text{ kg}:50 \text{ mcg/min}$$

$$73 \text{ kg} \times 50 \text{ mcg/min} = 1 \text{ kg} \times X \text{ mcg/min}$$

$$\frac{73 \cancel{\text{kg}} \times 50 \text{ mcg/min}}{1 \cancel{\text{kg}}} = \frac{\cancel{1 \text{kg}} \times X \text{ mcg/min}}{\cancel{1 \text{kg}}}$$

$$X = 3{,}650 \text{ mcg/min}$$

Step 2: Set up an equation to determine the volume infused per minute:

$$3.65 \text{ mg}:X \text{ mL}::2{,}500 \text{ mg}:250 \text{ mL}$$

$$3.650 \text{ mg} \times 250 \text{ mL} = X \text{ mL} \times 2{,}500 \text{ mg}$$

$$\frac{3.650 \cancel{\text{mg}} \times 250 \text{ mL}}{2{,}500 \cancel{\text{mg}}} = \frac{X \text{ mL} \times \cancel{2{,}500 \text{ mg}}}{\cancel{2{,}500 \text{ mg}}}$$

$$X = \frac{912.5}{2{,}500}$$

$$X = 0.365 \text{ mL/min}$$

Step 3: Multiply by 60 min/hr to determine the correct flow rate in mL/hr:

$$0.365 \text{ mL/min} \times 60 \text{ min/hr} = 21.9 \text{ mL/hour}$$

The nurse should set the pump to deliver 21.9 mL/hr of esmolol.

Most hospitals have policies in place which determines the starting dose and the maximum dose for titratable medications. The nurse must be familiar with these titratable medications and their limits as well. In addition, the nurse will need to perform calculations to double-check the correct dose amounts.

Here are some examples of medication calculations that may be used in special cases.

Note this: If using Dimensional Analysis to calculate dosages, feel free to refer back to Chapter 4 of this incredibly easy book if you get stuck!

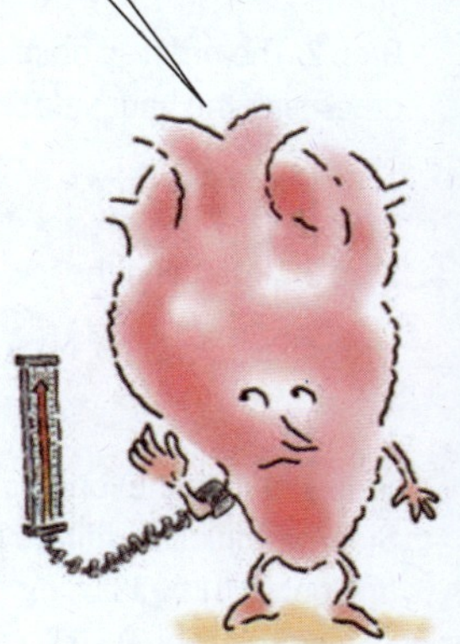

Certain medications are ordered to be titrated according to a patient's heart rate (HR), systolic blood pressure (SBP), or mean arterial pressure (MAP) parameters!

Nitroprusside number cruncher

A licensed practitioner orders a nitroprusside infusion for a patient experiencing severe hypertension. The order reads *Start nitroprusside 0.5 mcg/kg/min. Titrate to keep SBP less than 170 mm Hg. Max dose is 10 mcg/kg/min.* The patient weighs 85 kg and available is nitroprusside 50 mg added to 250 mL D_5W. At what flow rate should the nurse start the infusion?

Solve using the *formula method*

Find the flow rate using the *formula method:*
Step 1: Determine the dose per mcg/min:

$$X = 0.5 \text{ mcg/kg/min}$$
$$X = 0.5 \text{ mcg} \times 85 \text{ kg/min}$$
$$X = 42.5 \text{ mcg/min}$$

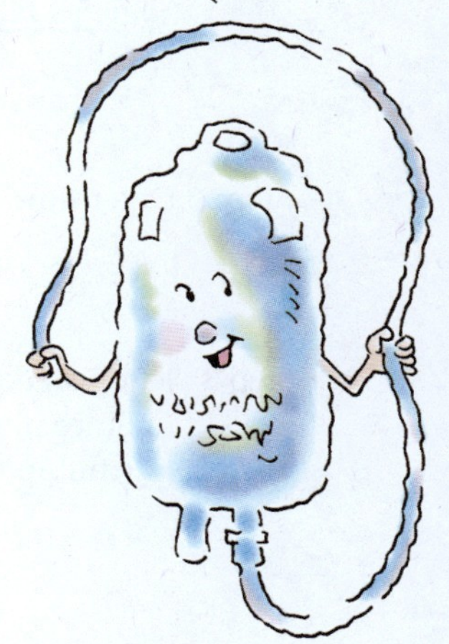

That skipped a step! The patient's weight is already provided in kg.

Step 2: The ordered dose is in mcg/min. Multiply by 60 to determine the hourly dose:

$$42.5 \text{ mcg/min} \times 60 \text{ min/hr} = 2{,}550 \text{ mcg/hr}$$

Step 3: Determine the lowest concentration of nitroprusside:

$$X = \frac{50 \text{ mg}}{250 \text{ mL}} = 0.2 \text{ mg/mL}$$

Step 4: Set up the formula with the information provided. Since nitroprusside is ordered in mcg, convert 0.2 mg to mcg (multiply 0.2 by 1,000) = 200 mcg/mL:

- Desired dose: 2,550 mcg/hr
- Have on hand: 200 mcg
- Quantity: 1 mL

$$X = \frac{2{,}550 \text{ mcg/hr}}{200 \text{ mcg}} \times 1 \text{ mL}$$

Step 5: Cancel the units that appear in both the numerator and the denominator:

$$X = \frac{2{,}550 \cancel{\text{mcg}} \text{/hr}}{200 \cancel{\text{mcg}}} \times 1 \text{ mL}$$

Step 6: Multiply the desired dose by quantity (2,550 × 1):

$$X = \frac{2{,}550 \text{ mL/hr}}{200}$$

Step 7: Solve for *X*. Divide the numerator by the denominator (2,550 ÷ 200):

$$X = 12.75 \text{ mL/hr}$$

Rounded to the nearest tenth space, the nurse should set the pump to deliver 12.8 mL/hr.

Solve using the *ratio proportion method*

Find the flow rate using the *ratio proportion method:*

Step 1: Determine the dose in mcg/min:

$$85 \text{ kg}:X \text{ mcg/min}::1 \text{ kg}:0.5 \text{ mcg/min}$$

$$85 \text{ kg} \times 0.5 \text{ mcg/min} = 1 \text{ kg} \times X \text{ mcg/min}$$

$$\frac{85 \cancel{\text{kg}} \times 0.5 \text{ mcg/min}}{1 \cancel{\text{kg}}} = \frac{1 \cancel{\text{kg}} \times X \text{ mcg/min}}{1 \cancel{\text{kg}}}$$

$$X = 42.5 \text{ mcg/min}$$

Step 2: Determine the lowest concentration of nitroprusside:

$$X = \frac{50 \text{ mg}}{250 \text{ mL}} = 0.2 \text{ mg/mL}$$

Step 3: Set up an equation to determine the volume infused per minute. Since nitroprusside is ordered in mcg, convert 0.2 mg to mcg (multiply 0.2 by 1,000) = 200 mcg/mL:

$$42.5 \text{ mcg}:X \text{ mL}::200 \text{ mcg}:1 \text{ mL}$$

$$42.5 \text{ mcg} \times 1 \text{ mL} = X \text{ mL} \times 200 \text{ mcg}$$

$$\frac{42.5 \cancel{\text{mcg}} \times 1 \text{ mL}}{200 \cancel{\text{mcg}}} = \frac{X \text{ mL} \times \cancel{200 \text{ mcg}}}{\cancel{200 \text{ mcg}}}$$

$$X = \frac{42.5 \times 1 \text{ mL}}{200}$$

$$X = 0.2125 \text{ mL/min}$$

Step 4: Multiply by 60 min/hr to determine the correct flow rate in mL/hr:

$$0.2125 \text{ mL/min} \times 60 \text{ min/hr} = 12.75 \text{ mL/hr}$$

Rounded to the nearest tenth space, the nurse should set the pump to deliver 12.8 mL/hr.

Keep the phenylephrine flowing

A patient with sustained hypotension has been ordered a vasopressor infusion. The order reads *Start phenylephrine (NEO-SYNEPHRINE) at 0.5 mcg/kg/min. Titrate to keep SBP above 90 mm Hg or MAP greater than 65*. The patient weighs 41 kg and phenylephrine is provided in a solution of 10 mg in 500 mL of NS. How will the nurse program an IV pump to start the infusion?

Recall the formula:

$$X = \frac{\text{Ordered amount in mg or mcg/min}}{\text{Medication Concentration (mg or mcg/mL)}} \times 60 \text{ min/hr}$$

Step 1: Determine the dose per minute:

$$X = 0.5 \text{ mcg/kg/min}$$
$$X = 0.5 \text{ mcg} \times 41 \text{ kg/min}$$
$$X = 20.5 \text{ mcg/min}$$

Step 2: Determine the lowest concentration of phenylephrine:

$$X = \frac{10 \text{ mg}}{500 \text{ mL}} = 0.02 \text{ mg/mL}$$

Step 3: Set up the formula with the information provided. Since phenylephrine is ordered in mcg, convert 0.02 mg to mcg (0.02 × 1,000) = 20 mcg/mL:

$$X = \frac{20.5 \text{ mcg/min}}{20 \text{ mcg/mL}} \times 60 \text{ min/hr}$$

Step 4: Cancel the units that appear in both the numerator and the denominator:

$$X = \frac{20.5 \cancel{\text{mcg}} / \cancel{\text{min}}}{20 \cancel{\text{mcg}} / \text{mL}} \times 60 \cancel{\text{min}} / \text{hr}$$

Step 5: Multiply the ordered amount by 60 (20.5 × 60):

$$X = \frac{1{,}230 \text{ hr}}{20 \text{ mL}}$$

Step 6: Solve for *X*. Divide the numerator by the denominator (1,230 ÷ 20):

$$X = 61.5 \text{ mL/hr}$$

The nurse should set the pump to deliver 61.5 mL/hr of phenylephrine.

Solve using the *formula method*

Find the flow rate using the *formula method:*
Step 1: Determine the dose per mcg/min:

$$X = 0.5 \text{ mcg/kg/min}$$
$$X = 0.5 \text{ mcg} \times 41 \text{ kg/min}$$
$$X = 20.5 \text{ mcg/min}$$

Step 2: The ordered dose is in mcg/min. Multiply by 60 to determine the hourly dose:

$$20.5 \text{ mcg/min} \times 60 \text{ min/hr} = 1{,}230 \text{ mcg/hr}$$

Step 3: Determine the lowest concentration of phenylephrine:

$$X = \frac{10 \text{ mg}}{500 \text{ mL}} = 0.02 \text{ mg/mL}$$

Step 4: Set up the formula with the information provided. Since phenylephrine is ordered in mcg, convert 0.02 mg to mcg (0.02 × 1,000) = 20 mcg/mL:

- Desired dose: 1,230 mcg/hr
- Have on hand: 20 mcg
- Quantity: 1 mL

$$X = \frac{1{,}230 \text{ mcg/hr}}{20 \text{ mcg}} \times 1 \text{ mL}$$

Step 5: Cancel the units that appear in both the numerator and the denominator:

$$X = \frac{1{,}230 \cancel{\text{mcg}} \text{/hr}}{20 \cancel{\text{mcg}}} \times 1 \text{ mL}$$

Step 6: Multiply the desired dose by quantity (1,230 × 1):

$$X = \frac{1{,}230 \text{ mL/hr}}{20}$$

Step 7: Solve for *X*. Divide the numerator by the denominator (1,230 ÷ 20):

$$X = 61.5 \text{ mL/hr}$$

The nurse should set the pump to deliver 61.5 mL/hr.

Solve using the *ratio proportion method*

Find the flow rate using the *ratio proportion method:*

Step 1: Determine the dose in mcg/min:

$$41 \text{ kg}:X \text{ mcg/min}::1 \text{ kg}:0.5 \text{ mcg/min}$$

$$41 \text{ kg} \times 0.5 \text{ mcg/min} = 1 \text{ kg} \times X \text{ mcg/min}$$

$$\frac{41 \cancel{\text{kg}} \times 0.5 \text{ mcg/min}}{1 \cancel{\text{kg}}} = \frac{1 \cancel{\text{kg}} \times X \text{ mcg/min}}{1 \cancel{\text{kg}}}$$

$$X = 20.5 \text{ mcg/min}$$

Dosage drill

Test your math skills with this drill

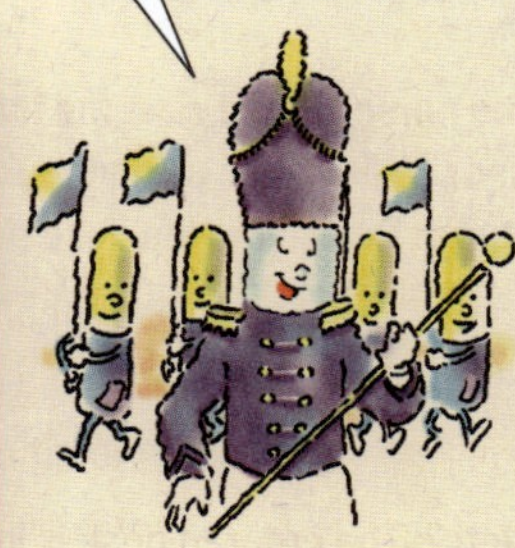
Be sure to show how you arrive at your answer.

An 80 kg patient is admitted with a severe infection. The licensed practitioner orders a dopamine infusion starting at 5 mcg/kg/min to titrate to maintain an SBP greater than 90 mm Hg or a MAP greater than 65. The pharmacy provides dopamine 800 mg in 500 mL of dextrose 5% in water. The nurse notes that the maximum dose is 15 mcg/kg/min. At what flow rate should the nurse start the infusion?

Your answer: ________________

Recall the formula:

$$X = \frac{\text{Ordered amount in mg or mcg/min}}{\text{Medication concentration (mg or mcg/mL)}} \times 60 \text{ min/hr}$$

Step 1: Determine the dose per minute:

$$X = 5 \text{ mcg/kg/min}$$
$$X = 5 \text{ mcg} \times 80 \text{ kg/min}$$
$$X = 400 \text{ mcg/min}$$

Step 2: Determine the lowest concentration of dopamine:

$$X = \frac{800 \text{ mg}}{500 \text{ mL}} = 1.6 \text{ mg/mL}$$

Step 3: Set up the formula with the information provided. Since dopamine is ordered in mcg, convert 1.6 mg to mcg $(1.6 \times 1{,}000) = 1{,}600$ mcg/mL:

$$X = \frac{400 \text{ mcg/min}}{1{,}600 \text{ mcg/mL}} \times 60 \text{ min/hr}$$

Step 4: Cancel the units that appear in both the numerator and the denominator:

$$X = \frac{400 \cancel{\text{mcg}}\text{/min}}{1{,}600 \cancel{\text{mcg}}\text{/mL}} \times 60 \cancel{\text{min}}\text{/hr}$$

Step 5: Multiply the ordered amount by 60 (400×60):

$$X = \frac{24{,}000 \text{ hr}}{1{,}600 \text{ mL}}$$

(*continued*)

Test your math skills with this drill (*continued*)

Step 6: Solve for X. Divide the numerator by the denominator (24,000 ÷ 1,600):

$$X = 15 \text{ mL/hr}$$

The nurse should start the infusion at 15 mL/hr.

Find the flow rate using the ***formula method:***

Step 1: Determine the dose per mcg/min:

$$X = 5 \text{ mcg/kg/min}$$
$$X = 5 \text{ mcg} \times 80 \text{ kg/min}$$
$$X = 400 \text{ mcg/min}$$

Step 2: The ordered dose is in mcg/min. Multiply by 60 to determine the hourly dose:

$$400 \text{ mcg/min} \times 60 \text{ min/hr} = 24{,}000 \text{ mcg/hr}$$

Step 3: Determine the lowest concentration of dopamine:

$$X = \frac{800 \text{ mg}}{500 \text{ mL}} = 1.6 \text{ mg/mL}$$

Step 4: Set up the formula with the information provided. Since dopamine is ordered in mcg, convert 1.6 mg to mcg (1.6 × 1,000) = 1,600 mcg/mL:

- Desired dose: 24,000 mcg/hr
- Have on hand: 1,600 mg
- Quantity: 1 mL

$$X = \frac{24{,}000 \text{ mcg/hr}}{1{,}600 \text{ mcg}} \times 1 \text{ mL}$$

Step 5: Cancel the units that appear in both the numerator and the denominator:

$$X = \frac{24{,}000 \cancel{\text{mcg}}\text{/hr}}{1{,}600 \cancel{\text{mcg}}} \times 1 \text{ mL}$$

Step 6: Multiply the desired dose by quantity (24,000 × 1):

$$X = \frac{24{,}000 \text{ hr}}{1{,}600 \text{ mL}}$$

Step 7: Solve for X. Divide the numerator by the denominator (24,000 ÷ 1,600):

$$X = 15 \text{ mL/hr}$$

The nurse should start the infusion at 15 mL/hr.

Find the flow rate using the ***ratio proportion method:***

Step 1: Determine the dose in mcg/min:

$$80 \text{ kg}:X \text{ mcg/min}::1 \text{ kg}:5 \text{ mcg/min}$$
$$80 \text{ kg} \times 5 \text{ mcg/min} = 1 \text{ kg} \times X \text{ mcg/min}$$
$$\frac{80 \cancel{\text{kg}} \times 5 \text{ mcg/min}}{1 \cancel{\text{kg}}} = \frac{1 \cancel{\text{kg}} \times X \text{ mcg/min}}{1 \cancel{\text{kg}}}$$
$$X = 400 \text{ mcg/min}$$

Step 2: Determine the lowest concentration of dopamine:

$$X = \frac{800 \text{ mg}}{500 \text{ mL}} = 1.6 \text{ mg/mL}$$

Step 3: Set up an equation to determine the volume infused per minute. Since dopamine is ordered in mcg, convert 1.6 mg to mcg (1.6 × 1,000) = 1,600 mcg/mL:

$$400 \text{ mcg}:X \text{ mL}::1{,}600 \text{ mcg}:1 \text{ mL}$$
$$400 \text{ mcg} \times 1 \text{ mL} = X \text{ mL} \times 1{,}600 \text{ mcg}$$

Step 4: Solve for X. Divide each side of the equation by 1 kg and cancel units that appear in both the numerator and denominator:

$$\frac{400 \cancel{\text{mcg}} \times 1 \text{ mL}}{1{,}600 \cancel{\text{mcg}}} = \frac{X \text{ mL} \times \cancel{1{,}600 \text{ mcg}}}{\cancel{1{,}600 \text{ mcg}}}$$
$$X = \frac{400 \times 1 \text{ mL}}{1{,}600}$$
$$X = 0.25 \text{ mL/min}$$

Step 5: Multiply by 60 min/hr to determine the correct flow rate in mL/hr:

$$0.25 \text{ mL/min} \times 60 \text{ min/hr} = 15 \text{ mL/hr}$$

The nurse should start the infusion at 15 mL/hr.

Step 2: Determine the lowest concentration of phenylephrine:

$$X = \frac{10 \text{ mg}}{500 \text{ mL}} = 0.02 \text{ mg/mL}$$

Step 3: Set up an equation to determine the volume infused per minute. Since phenylephrine is ordered in mcg, convert 0.02 mg to mcg (0.02 × 1,000) = 20 mcg/mL:

$$20.5 \text{ mcg}:X \text{ mL}::20 \text{ mcg}:1 \text{ mL}$$

$$20.5 \text{ mcg} \times 1 \text{ mL} = X \text{ mL} \times 20 \text{ mcg}$$

$$\frac{20.5 \cancel{\text{mcg}} \times 1 \text{ mL}}{20 \cancel{\text{mcg}}} = \frac{X \text{ mL} \times \cancel{20 \text{ mcg}}}{\cancel{20 \text{ mcg}}}$$

$$X = \frac{20.5 \times 1 \text{ mL}}{20}$$

$$X = 1.025 \text{ mL/min}$$

Step 4: Multiply by 60 min/hr to determine the correct flow rate in mL/hr:

$$1.025 \text{ mL/min} \times 60 \text{ min/hr} = 61.5 \text{ mL/hr}$$

The nurse should set the pump to deliver 61.5 mL/hr.

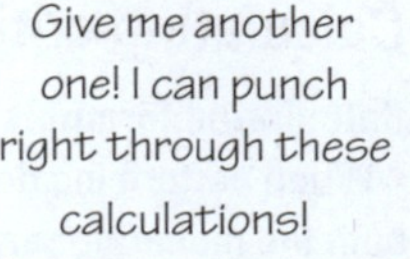

Give me another one! I can punch right through these calculations!

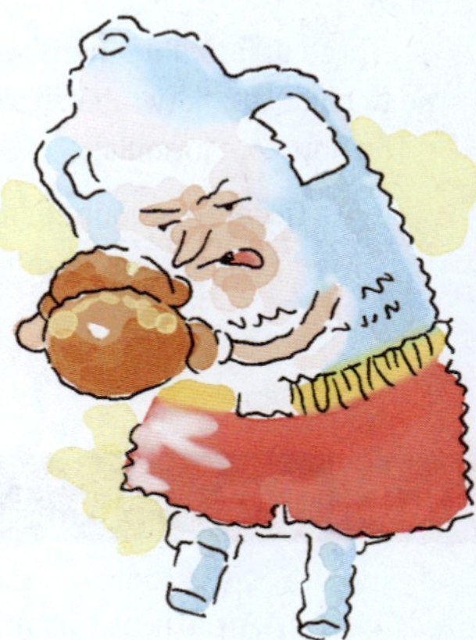

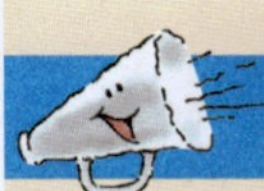

That's a wrap!

Calculating critical care infusion review

When working with critical care infusions, keep in mind these important facts.

Calculating IV push dosages

- IVP medications are usually ordered by dosages.
- Emergency medications are usually supplied in prefilled syringes.
- Some medications come in different concentrations. Double-check the label for safety!
- Know the administration times of each IVP medication before given.

Calculating a medication's concentration

$$X = \frac{\text{Amount of medication (mg or mcg)}}{\text{Amount of fluid (mL)}}$$

- Working with the lowest concentration of a solution helps with solving calculations.

Calculating the flow rate

- Most critical care medications requiring continuous infusions must be administered using an IV pump device.
- IV pumps are typically programmed by a flow rate which is mL/hr.
- Critical care medications are potent and supplied in smaller units of measure such as mcg or mg.
- Continuous IV infusions of critical care medications are ordered by:
  - micrograms per min (mcg/min).
  - milligrams per min (mg/min).

Calculating dosages by weight

- Some medications are ordered by a patient's weight in kg:
  - micrograms per kilogram per min (mcg or mg/kg/min).
- Convert lb to kg using the conversion factor: 1 kg is equal to 2.2 lb.

(*continued*)

Calculating critical care infusion review (*continued*)

Calculation formulas

- When performing dosage calculations, both the numerator and the denominator must be of the same unit of measure!
- If performing weight-based calculations, make sure the patient's weight is in kg.

Three different methods were provided to calculate flow rates in this chapter:

- The flow rate formula:

$$X = \frac{\text{Ordered amount in mg or mcg/min}}{\text{Medication Concentration (mg or mcg/mL)}} \times 60 \text{ min/hr}$$

- The formula method:

$$X = \frac{\text{Desired dose (D)}}{\text{Have on hand (H)}} \times \text{Quantity (Q) (aka volume)}$$

- The ratio proportion method:
  - Requires setting up ratios and proportions to calculate:
  - Dose per minute
  - Volume infused per minute
  - Converting minutes to hourly rates

Quick quiz

1. A patient has an infusion of dopamine with a solution containing 800 mg in 500 mL D_5W. What is the lowest concentration of this solution?
   A. 0.16 mg/mL
   B. 1.6 mg/mL
   C. 16 mg/mL
   D. 160 mg/mL

Answer: B. To determine the lowest concentration, divide the amount of medication by the amount of fluid:

$$X = \frac{\text{Amount of medication (mg or mcg)}}{\text{Amount of fluid (mL)}}$$

2. How would a nurse convert mg to mcg?
   A. Multiply mg by 10.
   B. Multiply mg by 60.
   C. Multiply mg by 100.
   D. Multiply mg by 1,000.

Answer: D. When converting a number from mg to mcg, multiply the number by 1,000 or simply move the decimal three spaces to the right.

3. How many kg does a 250 lb man weigh?
   A. 11.4 kg
   B. 114 kg
   C. 550 kg
   D. 125 kg

Answer: B. To convert lb to kg, divide by 2.2 and round to the nearest whole number. Remember to only round at the end of a problem—not within the problem itself.

4. A patient has an order for furosemide (Lasix) 80 mg IV as a one-time dose. The available vial contains 100 mg in 10 mL of normal saline solution. How many mL will the nurse give to administer this dose?
   A. 0.08 mL
   B. 0.8 mL
   C. 1.8 mL
   D. 8 mL

Answer: D. Using the ratio proportion method, set up a proportion with the available solution in one ratio and the ordered dose and the unknown volume in the other ratio. Solve for *X*. Using the formula method, set up the formula with the information provided:

$$X = \frac{\text{Desired dose (D)}}{\text{Have on hand (H)}} \times \text{Quantity (Q) (aka volume)}$$

5. A patient weighing 50 kg asks the nurse how much that is in lb. How would the nurse respond?
   A. "You weigh 28 lb."
   B. "You weigh 100 lb."
   C. "You weigh 110 lb."
   D. "You weigh 200 lb."

Answer: C. To convert kg to lb, multiply 50 kg by 2.2. Remember that lb will always be a higher number than kg!

Scoring

☆☆☆ If you answered all seven items correctly, fantastic! You can calculate confidently in critical cases.

☆☆ If you answered five or six items correctly, that isn't bad! You're a cool, calm, and collected calculator.

☆ If you answered fewer than five items correctly, keep at it! You have the best dosage calc. book ever. Keep it with you always and refer to it frequently.

Suggested Reference

Pan, S., Zhu, L., Chen, M., Xia, P., & Zhou, Q. (2016). Weight-based dosing in medication use: what should we know? *Patient Prefer Adherence, 10*, 549–560. https://doi.org/10.2147/PPA.S103156

Chapter 17

Calculating heparin and insulin dosages

Just the facts

In this chapter, you'll learn how to:

- apply basic insulin and heparin principles
- interpret insulin and heparin orders
- calculate, monitor, and regulate insulin and heparin infusions

Unit-based medications

Medications such as insulin and heparin are measured in units. The unit system is based on an international standard of medication potency, not on weight. The number of units appears on the medication label. (See *Look for the unit label*.)

Look for the unit label

The label of a parenteral medication that's measured in units includes the information shown here on this simulated label.

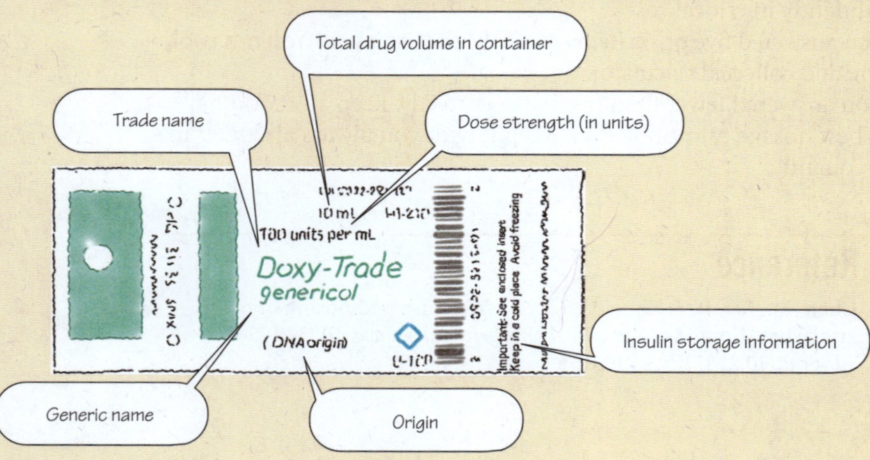

Insisting on insulin

The body needs insulin, a potent hormone produced by the pancreas, to regulate carbohydrate metabolism. The effect of insulin's impact is reflected in blood glucose levels. A lack of insulin, or having insulin resistance, leads to diabetes mellitus. (See *Differentiating diabetes*.)

According to the Centers for Disease Control and Prevention (CDC), in 2019 approximately 11.6% of the population had diabetes (2023). Moreover, the American Diabetes Association (ADA) estimates that each year in the United States an additional 1.4 million people are diagnosed with diabetes. With these alarming statistics, nurses will continue to provide diabetic care and education well into the future.

Care and management of a patient with diabetes can be quite complex, which is why the role of the educator is instrumental in teaching patients self-care and wellness. Although the goal of diabetic care is to control and maintain normal blood glucose levels, the treatment can vary from type 1 to type 2.

Complications from diabetes can range from minor to life-threatening. Depending on the severity of signs and symptoms, patients may seek medical care at an outpatient clinic or a hospital. Nurses must know how to care for and educate patients, including controlling blood glucose levels with insulin management.

Insulin may be given subcutaneously or by continuous IV infusion. The route in which insulin is ordered is usually dependent on how elevated a patient's blood sugar is and how symptomatic the patient may be. Either route, the nurse is responsible for the safe administration of insulin because errors can lead to adverse patient outcomes.

Differentiating diabetes

Diabetes is classified according to two major types: type 1 and type 2.

Type 1
In type 1 diabetes, the pancreas no longer makes insulin and blood glucose can't enter the cells to be used for energy. Patients with type 1 diabetes are insulin dependent.

Type 2
In type 2 diabetes, either the pancreas does not make enough insulin, or it can't use the insulin it does produce effectively. Type 2 diabetes can sometimes be controlled by diet and oral antidiabetic agents; however, insulin may be needed to stabilize blood glucose levels.

Types of insulin

Several different types of insulin are available to help control and regulate blood glucose levels. Insulin is classified according to its three phases of action time: onset, peak, and duration. The three phases of action times refer to the following:

- Onset: how long it takes for the insulin to start lowering glucose levels.
- Peak: the time when the insulin is at its maximum strength at lowering glucose levels.
- Duration: how long it continues to work on glucose levels.

The five major classifications include rapid acting, short acting, intermediate acting, long acting, and ultra long acting.

Before the administration of insulin, nurses must know the insulin classification and the three different phases of time for that insulin.

Insulin action times

Insulin preparations are modified through combination with larger insoluble protein molecules to slow absorption and prolong activity. An insulin preparation may be rapid acting, short acting, intermediate acting, or long acting, as shown in the table below.

Medication	Onset	Peak	Duration
Rapid acting			
Insulin lispro (Admelog, Humalog, Lyumjev) Insulin aspart (Fiasp, NovoLog) Insulin glulisine (Apidra)	Less than 15 min	1 to 2 hr	2 to 4 hr
Short acting			
Regular insulin (Novolin R, Velosulin R, Humulin-R)	30 min to 1 hr	2 to 3 hr	3 to 6 hr
Intermediate acting			
Neutral protamine hagedorn (NPH) (Humulin N, Novolin N, ReliOn)	1 to 2 hr	4 to 12 hr	18 to 24 hr
Long acting			
degludec (Tresiba) detemir (Levemir) glargine (Basaglar, Lantus)	1 to 2 hr	None	Up to 24 hr
Ultra long acting			
glargine U-300 (Toujeo)	6 hours	None	36+ hr

Source: American Diabetes Association. (n.d.). *Insulin basics.* https://diabetes.org/health-wellness/medication/insulin-basics

(See *Insulin action times.*) Patients may be ordered one or more different types of insulin in their treatment plan to help control their blood glucose levels.

Insulin alert

Insulin is considered a "high-alert" or high-risk medication, meaning that it has been associated with a high rate of errors, adverse events, and admissions to the hospital. Poor management and insulin errors can lead to significant patient harm including hypo or hyperglycemia. Contributing factors in insulin administration errors are due to name similarity, name confusion, or labeling and packaging similarities such as look-alike insulin products. Using automated dispensing systems and barcoding scanning systems has decreased some of the errors, but errors still can occur. Thus, it is imperative that nurses continue to use the "rights" of medications and the three safety checks before administration of any medication.

Selecting an insulin syringe

These syringes are examples of the different dose-specific insulin syringes that are available.

- The 1-mL U-100 syringe delivers up to 100 units of insulin.
- The low-dose 3/10- and 1/2-mL syringes deliver up to 30 or 50 units of U-100 insulin.

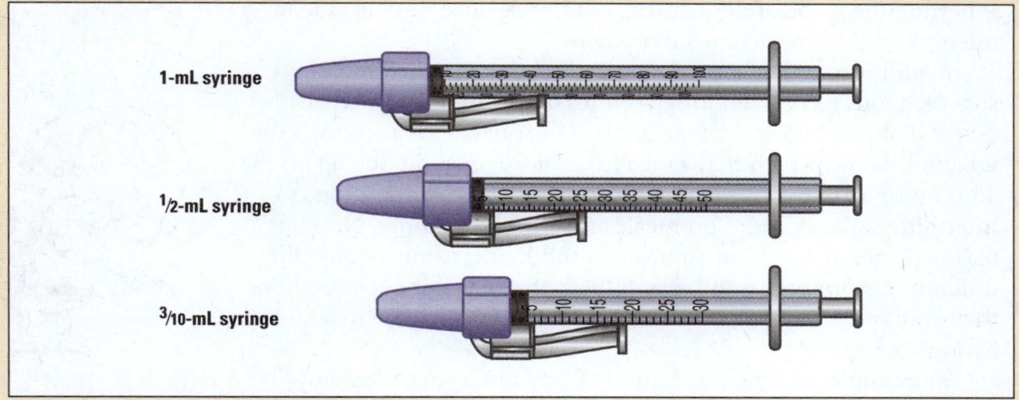

What dose do you want?

Insulin doses, expressed in units, are available in two concentrations. The most traditional insulin concentration is available in 100 units/mL (U-100) and a higher dose, which is not as common, is available in 500 units/mL (U-500).

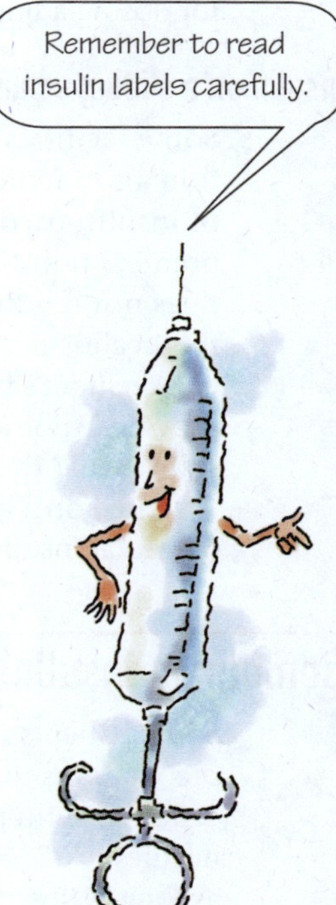

Insulin syringes

Since insulin is ordered and measured in units, nurses must only use syringes calibrated for insulin. For accuracy, these syringes are available in different sizes to accommodate smaller to larger unit doses of insulin. A U-100 syringe, the only type of insulin syringe available in the United States, is calibrated so that 1 mL holds 100 units of insulin. A low-dose U-100 syringe, holding 50 units of insulin or less, is also used for some patients. Another low-dose U-100 syringe holds 30 units of insulin or less. (See *Selecting an insulin syringe*.)

No syringes were made for the specific administration of U-500 insulin. Therefore, this insulin must be administered with a U-100 syringe as well. Nurses must exercise caution when administering this medication.

Insulin therapy

The medical management of diabetes at home may differ from when requiring an in-patient hospitalization. In fact, a new diabetes diagnosis is often made when a patient is admitted into a hospital setting. Treatment plans for managing diabetes can range from oral antidiabetics to insulin therapy. Nurses must be familiar with the treatments and evaluate their effectiveness.

Management of diabetes is complex and may be further complicated due to various medical conditions. This complex management is beyond the scope of this context, but nurses must be able to read, interpret, and implement insulin orders.

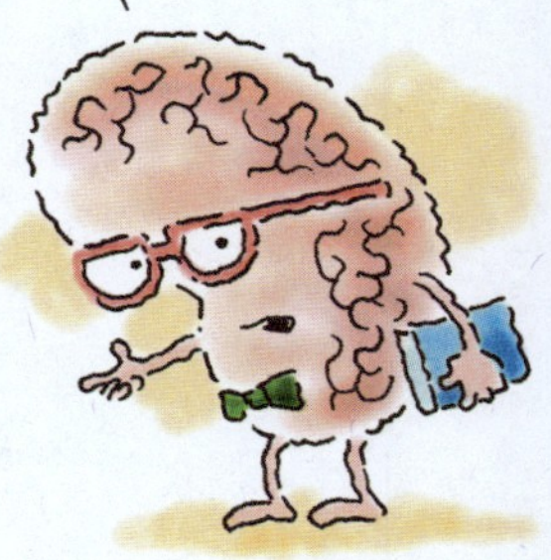

Many facilities require an independent witness check with insulin administrations!

In addition to diet control, insulin therapy may be ordered in subcutaneous or IV form for glycemic control for all patients with type 1 diabetes and some type 2. Most hospitals have protocols for insulin therapy, which may range from basing insulin dosing on the amount of carbohydrate grams consumed (aka carb counting) to intermittent doses based on meals and glucose readings. No matter the protocol or administration method, nurses must know the different insulin preparations and their pharmacokinetic properties to ensure proper timing in relation to meals and activity to avoid hypoglycemia.

For example, a licensed practitioner may order small doses of rapid-acting insulin to be given to a patient at set times, such as every 4 hours or before meals and at bedtime. If needed, intermediate-acting insulin and/or long-acting insulin (for basal coverage) may be added for dosing adjustments.

Insulin on a sliding scale

Some facilities may use a sliding scale protocol for glucose correction and management. Sliding scale uses a predetermined amount of insulin used for correction or to supplement insulin based on premeal point-of-care (POC) glucometer readings. Note that this does not require performing dosage calculations with the use of this scale.

A patient's blood glucose level results at 384 mg/dL. Based on the provided sliding scale (see *Insulin sliding scale,* p. 343), how much insulin would the nurse give the patient?

Based on a blood glucose of 384, the nurse would administer 8 units of regular insulin.

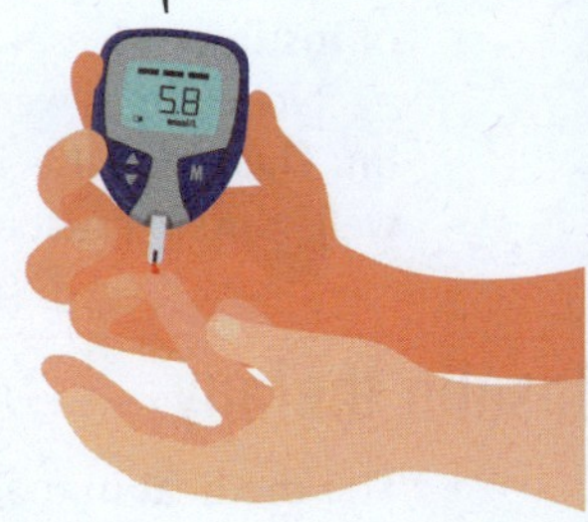

Many patients with diabetes monitor their blood glucose levels at home with a glucometer and self-administer their insulin according to set times or surrounding mealtimes.

Combining insulins

Some patients may have orders for two different types of insulin preparations to be administered at the same time. Nurses can mix certain insulin preparations together to save time and the patient a needlestick. However, not all insulins can be mixed with another such as long-acting insulins. The most common mixture consists of mixing

Insulin sliding scale

Insulin doses may be based on blood glucose levels, as shown in this table.

Blood glucose level	Insulin dose
Less than 200 mg/dL	No insulin
201–250 mg/dL	2 units regular insulin
251–300 mg/dL	4 units regular insulin
301–350 mg/dL	6 units regular insulin
351–400 mg/dL	8 units regular insulin
Greater than 400 mg/dL	Call prescriber for insulin order.

regular insulin with NPH insulin. This mixture can then be injected together in one syringe at the same site. To avoid potential errors, premixed insulin may be ordered for patients as well.

If a patient has an order for two insulin preparations that can be mixed, draw them into the same syringe following this incredibly easy procedure:

- Read the insulin order carefully.
- Read the vial labels carefully, noting the type, concentration, source, and expiration date of the medications.
- Roll the NPH vial between your palms to mix it thoroughly.
- Choose the appropriate syringe.
- Clean the tops of both vials of insulin with an antiseptic swab.
- Inject air into the NPH vial equal to the amount of insulin you need to give. Withdraw the needle and syringe, but don't withdraw any NPH insulin.
- Inject into the regular insulin vial an amount of air equal to the dose of the regular insulin. Then invert or tilt the vial and withdraw the prescribed amount of regular insulin into the syringe. Draw the clear, regular insulin first to avoid contamination by the cloudy, longer-acting insulin.
- Clean the top of the NPH vial again with an antiseptic swab. Then insert the needle of the syringe containing the regular insulin into the vial and withdraw the prescribed amount of NPH insulin.
- Mix the insulins in the syringe by pulling back slightly on the plunger and tilting the syringe back and forth.
- Recheck the medication order.
- Have a second nurse verify the withdrawn dose and cosign the medication administration record (per the facility's policies).
- Verify the patient's identity using two patient identifiers.
- Administer the insulin immediately.

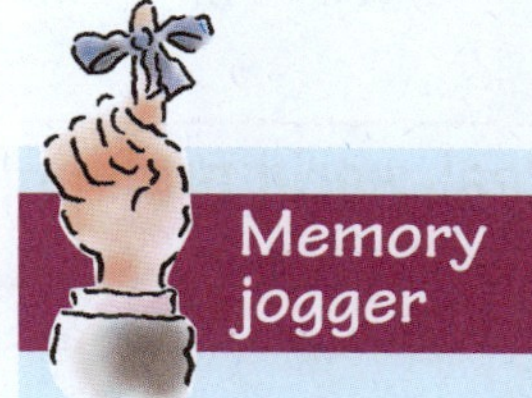

Having trouble remembering which insulin to draw first? Think of the phrase "clear before cloudy." (Who doesn't prefer a clear day to a cloudy day?)

This phrase also helps remind nurses how these medications work: A clear day seems short, but a cloudy day seems to last forever. Clear, regular insulin is short acting and cloudy, and NPH insulin is longer acting (intermediate). Not all long-acting insulin is cloudy though; so be vigilant with insulin!

Calculating continuous insulin infusions

In critical care settings, continuous IV insulin infusion is the most effective method for achieving glycemic targets. Continuous infusion allows close control of insulin administration based on serial measurements of blood glucose levels.

Regular insulin is the only type of insulin that can be administered by the IV route because it has a shorter duration of action than other insulins.

Insulin is usually prescribed in units per hour (units/hr), but it may be ordered in milliliters per hour (mL/hr). In either case, the infusion should be in the lowest concentration of 1 unit/mL to avoid calculation errors that may have serious consequences. An infusion pump must be used to administer IV insulin. The examples here are based on common patient situations.

Real-world problems

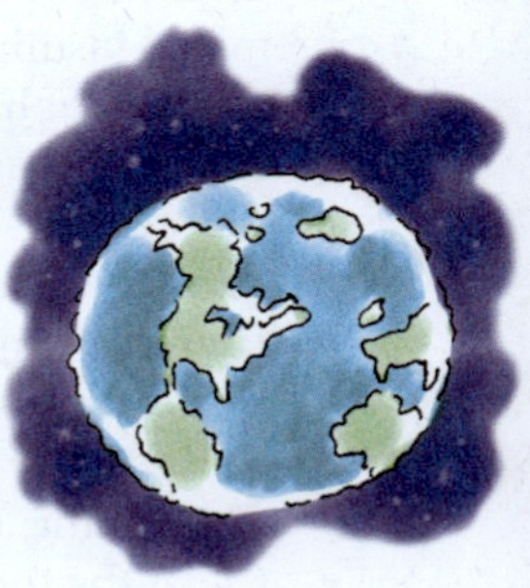

The following examples show how to use the formula, ratio proportion method, and a sliding scale to calculate insulin doses.

Insulin flow #1

A licensed practitioner orders a continuous infusion of 150 units of regular insulin in 150 mL of normal saline at 6 units/hr for a patient. What flow rate will the nurse use to program the IV pump?

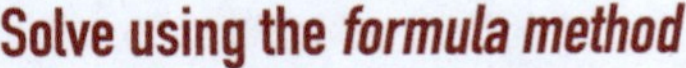

Solve using the *formula method*

Find the flow rate using the *formula method*. Recall the formula:

$$X = \frac{\text{Desired dose (D)}}{\text{Have on hand (H)}} \times \text{Quantity (Q)}$$

Step 1: Set-up the formula with the information provided:

- Desired dose: 6 units/hr
- Have on hand: 150 units
- Quantity: 150 mL

$$X = \frac{6 \text{ units/hr}}{150 \text{ units}} \times 150 \text{ mL}$$

Step 2: Cancel the units that appear in both the numerator and the denominator:

$$X = \frac{6 \cancel{\text{units}} \text{/hr}}{150 \cancel{\text{units}}} \times 150 \text{ mL}$$

Step 3: Multiply the desired dose by quantity (6 × 150):

$$X = \frac{900 \text{ mL/hr}}{150}$$

Step 4: Solve for *X*. Divide the numerator by the denominator (900 ÷ 150):

$$X = 6 \text{ mL/hr}$$

The nurse should set the pump to deliver 6 mL/hr of regular insulin.

Solve using the *ratio proportion method*

Find the flow rate using the *ratio proportion method:*

Step 1: Write a fraction to describe the known solution strength (units/mL of solution):

$$\frac{150 \text{ units}}{150 \text{ mL}}$$

Step 2: Write a second fraction with the infusion rate in the numerator and the unknown flow rate in the denominator:

$$\frac{6 \text{ units/hr}}{X}$$

Step 3: Write the two fractions as a proportion:

$$\frac{150 \text{ units}}{150 \text{ mL}} = \frac{6 \text{ units/hr}}{X}$$

Step 4: Solve for *X* by cross-multiplying:

$$150 \text{ units} \times X = 6 \text{ units/hr} \times 150 \text{ mL}$$

Step 5: Divide each side of the equation by 150 units and cancel units that appear in both the numerator and the denominator:

$$\frac{\cancel{150 \text{ units}} \times X}{\cancel{150 \text{ units}}} = \frac{6 \ \cancel{\text{units}}\text{/hr} \times 150 \text{ mL}}{150 \ \cancel{\text{units}}}$$

$$X = 6 \text{ mL/hr}$$

To administer 6 units/hr of the prescribed insulin, the nurse will set the infusion pump to 6 mL/hr.

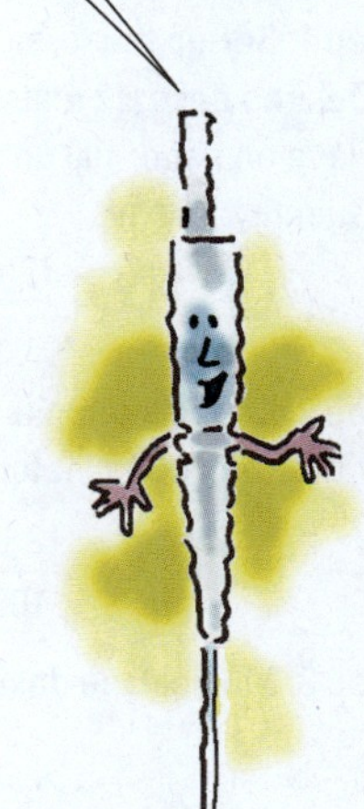
Due to its shorter duration of action, regular insulin is the only insulin administered by the IV route.

Dosage drill

Test your math skills with this drill

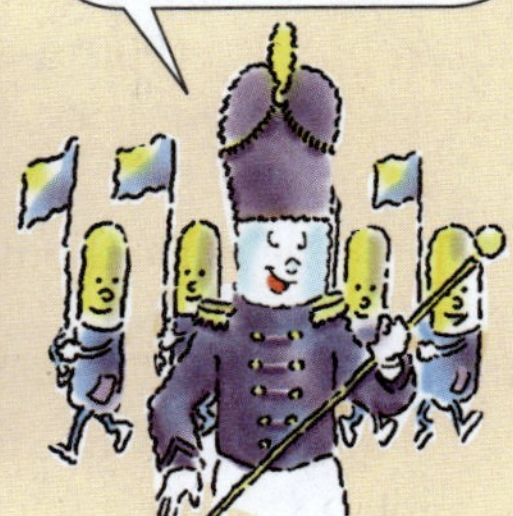
Be sure to show how you arrive at your answer.

A young adult is admitted with complications related to type 1 diabetes. The licensed practitioner orders a continuous infusion of 100 units of regular insulin in 100 mL normal saline at 12 units/hr. What is the hourly flow rate?

Your answer: ________

Find the flow rate using the **formula method:**

Step 1: Set-up the formula with the information provided:

- Desired dose: 12 units/hr
- Have on hand: 100 units
- Quantity: 100 mL

$$X = \frac{12 \text{ units/hr}}{100 \text{ units}} \times 100 \text{ mL}$$

Step 2: Cancel the units that appear in both the numerator and the denominator:

$$X = \frac{12 \cancel{\text{units}}\text{/hr}}{100 \cancel{\text{units}}} \times 100 \text{ mL}$$

Step 3: Multiply the desired dose by quantity (12 × 100):

$$X = \frac{1{,}200 \text{ mL/hr}}{100}$$

Step 4: Solve for X. Divide the numerator by the denominator (1,200 ÷ 100):

$$X = 12 \text{ mL/hr}$$

The hourly flow rate is 12 mL/hr.

Find the flow rate using the **ratio proportion** method:

Step 1: Write a fraction to describe the solution strength:

$$\frac{100 \text{ units}}{100 \text{ mL}}$$

Step 2: Write a second fraction with the infusion rate and the unknown flow rate:

$$\frac{12 \text{ units/hr}}{X}$$

Step 3: Write the two fractions as a proportion:

$$\frac{100 \text{ units}}{100 \text{ mL}} = \frac{12 \text{ units/hr}}{X}$$

Step 4: Solve for X by cross-multiplying:

$$100 \text{ units} \times X = 12 \text{ units/hr} \times 100 \text{ mL}$$

$$\frac{\cancel{100 \text{ units}} \times X}{\cancel{100 \text{ units}}} = \frac{12 \cancel{\text{units}}\text{/hr} \times 100 \text{ mL}}{100 \cancel{\text{units}}}$$

$$X = 12 \text{ mL/hr}$$

The hourly flow rate is 12 mL/hr.

Insulin flow #2

A patient is admitted with diabetes ketone acidosis (DKA) and elevated blood sugars greater than 500. The nurse receives an order to initiate an insulin drip at 0.01 unit/kg/hr. The patient weighs 69 kg. Available is 100 units of insulin added to 100 mL of D_5W solution. What flow rate will the nurse program the IV pump?

Solve using the *formula method*

Find the flow rate using the *formula method*.
Step 1: Determine the dose per hour:

$$X = 0.01 \text{ units/kg/hr}$$
$$X = 0.01 \text{ units} \times 69 \text{ kg/hr}$$
$$X = 0.69 \text{ units/hr}$$

Step 2: Determine the lowest concentration of insulin:

$$X = \frac{100 \text{ units}}{100 \text{ mL}} = 1 \text{ unit/mL}$$

Step 3: Set-up the formula with the information provided:

- Desired dose: 0.69 units/hr
- Have on hand: 1 unit
- Quantity: 1 mL

$$X = \frac{0.69 \text{ units/hr}}{1 \text{ unit}} \times 1 \text{ mL}$$

Step 4: Cancel the units that appear in both the numerator and the denominator:

$$X = \frac{0.69 \cancel{\text{units}} \text{/hr}}{1 \cancel{\text{unit}}} \times 1 \text{ mL}$$

Step 5: Multiply the desired dose by quantity (0.69 × 1):

$$X = \frac{0.69 \text{ mL/hr}}{1}$$

Step 6: Solve for *X*. Divide the numerator by the denominator (0.69 ÷ 1):

$$X = 0.69 \text{ mL/hr}$$

Rounded to the nearest tenth, the nurse should program the IV pump to deliver 0.7 mL/hr.

Solve using the *ratio proportion method*

Find the flow rate using the *ratio proportion method*.
Step 1: Determine the dose in units/hr:

$$69 \text{ kg}{:}X \text{ units/hr}{::}1 \text{ kg}{:}0.01 \text{ units/hr}$$

$$69 \text{ kg} \times 0.01 \text{ units/hr} = 1 \text{ kg} \times X \text{ units/hr}$$

$$\frac{69 \cancel{\text{kg}} \times 0.01 \text{ units/hr}}{1 \cancel{\text{kg}}} = \frac{1 \cancel{\text{kg}} \times X \text{ units/hr}}{1 \cancel{\text{kg}}}$$

$$X = 0.69 \text{ units/hr}$$

Step 2: Determine the lowest concentration of insulin:

$$X = \frac{100 \text{ units}}{100 \text{ mL}} = 1 \text{ unit/mL}$$

Step 3: Write the two fractions as a proportion:

$$\frac{0.69 \text{ units/hr}}{X} = \frac{1 \text{ unit}}{1 \text{ mL}}$$

Step 4: Solve for X by cross-multiplying:

$$0.69 \text{ units/hr} \times 1 \text{ mL} = 1 \text{ units} \times X$$

Step 5: Divide each side of the equation by 1 unit and cancel units that appear in both the numerator and the denominator:

$$\frac{0.69 \cancel{\text{units}}\text{/hr} \times 1 \text{ mL}}{1 \cancel{\text{units}}} = \frac{1 \cancel{\text{units}} \times X}{1 \cancel{\text{units}}}$$

$$X = 0.69 \text{ mL/hr}$$

Rounded to the nearest tenth, the nurse should program the IV pump to deliver 0.7 mL/hr.

Insulin flow #3

A patient is receiving a continuous infusion of insulin at 10 mL/hr. The concentration is 100 units of regular insulin in 100 mL of normal saline. How many units per hour of insulin is the patient receiving?

Solve using the *formula method*

Find the flow rate using the *formula method*.
Step 1: Set-up the formula with the information provided:

- Desired dose: 10 mL/hr
- Have on hand: 100 mL
- Quantity: 100 units

$$X = \frac{10 \text{ mL/hr}}{100 \text{ mL}} \times 100 \text{ units}$$

Step 2: Cancel the units that appear in both the numerator and the denominator:

$$X = \frac{10 \cancel{\text{mL}}/\text{hr}}{100 \cancel{\text{mL}}} \times 100 \text{ units}$$

Step 3: Multiply the desired dose by quantity (10×100):

$$X = \frac{1{,}000 \text{ units/hr}}{100}$$

Step 4: Solve for *X*. Divide the numerator by the denominator ($1{,}000 \div 100$):

$$X = 10 \text{ units/hr}$$

The patient is receiving 10 units/hr of insulin.

Solve using the *ratio proportion method*

Find the flow rate using the *ratio proportion method.*

Step 1: Write a ratio to describe the known solution strength (units/mL):

$$100 \text{ units:}100 \text{ mL}$$

Step 2: Set-up a second ratio comparing the unknown amount of insulin to the prescribed infusion rate:

$$X\text{:}10 \text{ mL/hr}$$

Step 3: Put these ratios into a proportion:

$$100 \text{ units:}100 \text{ mL::}X\text{:}10 \text{ mL/hr}$$

Step 4: Solve for *X*. Multiply the means and the extremes:

$$X \times 100 \text{ mL} = 100 \text{ units} \times 10 \text{ mL/hr}$$

Step 5: Divide each side of the equation by 100 mL and cancel units that appear in both the numerator and the denominator:

$$\frac{X \times \cancel{100 \text{ mL}}}{\cancel{100 \text{ mL}}} = \frac{100 \text{ units} \times 10 \cancel{\text{mL}}/\text{hr}}{100 \cancel{\text{mL}}}$$

$$X = 10 \text{ units/hr}$$

When the insulin infusion runs at 10 mL/hr, the patient receives 10 units/hr.

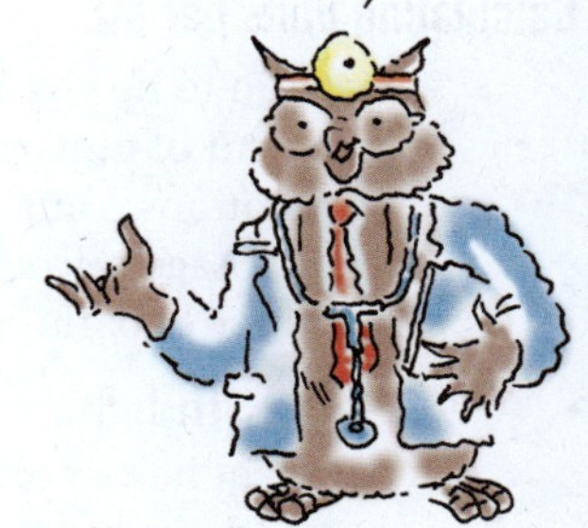

Follow a facility's insulin protocol for how often to check a patient's glucose readings.

Calculating heparin dosages

The anticoagulant heparin can be used to prevent thrombosis and embolism. Like insulin, it requires careful calculation and administration to prevent complications. (See *Heparin hazards*, p. 356.) Depending on the indication, heparin may be ordered to be given subcutaneously or by continuous IV infusion. Either route, nurses must perform calculations to determine the appropriate dose. Like insulin, heparin is a high-alert medication that is prepared in units and may be ordered by the dose or by units per hour.

Heparin monitoring

Heparin may be ordered to prevent the formation of new clots and slows the development of preexisting clots. For DVT (deep vein thrombosis) prophylaxis, heparin is typically ordered to be given subcutaneously several times a day. However, heparin may also be ordered to be administered through a continuous IV infusion and titrated based on a patient's coagulation status through lab values. Monitoring is important to achieve a therapeutic target within the first 24 hours and to maintain therapeutic levels thereafter.

Historically, the most common lab value to monitor unfractionated heparin therapy has been the activated partial thromboplastin time (aPTT). However, more recently, some facilities are now using the anti-Xa assay as the new gold standard for heparin monitoring. This practice change is the result of studies that demonstrated monitoring with the anti-Xa assay rather than the aPTT results in a shorter time to therapeutic anticoagulation, longer maintenance of therapeutic levels, and fewer laboratory tests and heparin dosage changes. No matter which monitoring lab value is utilized, the need for nurses to perform calculations is still necessary.

Calculating units per mL

Heparin to be given subcutaneously or by IV bolus is ordered in measurement of units just like insulin. However, subcutaneous heparin preparations come supplied in mL solutions requiring nurses to perform dosage calculations. Follow these incredibly easy steps to calculate these heparin orders:

Help with heparin

A patient has an order that reads: *Give 4,000 units of heparin subcutaneous q12h.* The heparin vial available contains 5,000 units/mL. How many mL of heparin should the nurse administer?

Solve using the *formula method*

Find the flow rate using the *formula method*. Recall the formula:

$$X = \frac{\text{Desired dose (D)}}{\text{Have on hand (H)}} \times \text{Quantity (Q)}$$

Step 1: Set-up the formula with the information provided:

- Desired dose: 4,000 units
- Have on hand: 5,000 units
- Quantity: 1 mL

$$X = \frac{4{,}000 \text{ units}}{5{,}000 \text{ units}} \times 1 \text{ mL}$$

Step 2: Cancel the units that appear in both the numerator and the denominator:

$$X = \frac{4{,}000 \cancel{\text{units}}}{5{,}000 \cancel{\text{units}}} \times 1 \text{ mL}$$

Step 3: Multiply the desired dose by quantity (4,000 × 1):

$$X = \frac{4{,}000 \text{ mL}}{5{,}000}$$

Step 4: Solve for X. Divide the numerator by the denominator (4,000 ÷ 5,000):

$$X = 0.8 \text{ mL}$$

The nurse should administer 0.8 mL of heparin.

Solve using the *ratio proportion method*

Find the dose using the *ratio proportion method.*
Step 1: Set-up the *first* ratio with the known heparin concentration:

$$5{,}000 \text{ unit}:1 \text{ mL}$$

Step 2: Set-up the *second* ratio with the desired dose and the unknown amount of heparin:

$$4{,}000 \text{ units}:X$$

Step 3: Put these *ratios* into a proportion:

$$5{,}000 \text{ units}:1 \text{ mL}::4{,}000 \text{ units}:X$$

Step 4: Set-up an *equation* by multiplying the means and extremes:

$$1 \text{ mL} \times 4{,}000 \text{ units} = 5{,}000 \text{ units} \times X$$

Step 5: Solve for X. Divide each side of the equation by 5,000 units and cancel units that appear in both the numerator and the denominator:

$$\frac{1 \text{ mL} \times 4{,}000 \cancel{\text{units}}}{5{,}000 \cancel{\text{units}}} = \frac{\cancel{5{,}000 \text{ units}} \times X}{\cancel{5{,}000 \text{ units}}}$$

$$X = 0.8 \text{ mL}$$

The nurse should give the patient 0.8 mL of heparin.

Flow rate

Accurately calculating the flow rate ensures that the heparin dose falls within safe and therapeutic limits.

Follow these incredibly easy steps to calculate the flow rate of heparin.

Go with the flow!

A licensed practitioner orders to start a continuous heparin infusion for a patient. The protocol states to start heparin at 1,000 units/hr. The pharmacy provides heparin 25,000 units added to 500 mL of D_5W. At what flow rate will the nurse start the heparin infusion?

Solve using the *formula method*

Find the flow rate using the *formula method*.

Step 1: Determine the lowest concentration of heparin:

$$X = \frac{25{,}000 \text{ units}}{500 \text{ mL}} = 50 \text{ units/mL}$$

Step 2: Set-up the formula with the information provided:

- Desired dose: 1,000 units/hr
- Have on hand: 50 units
- Quantity: 1 mL

$$X = \frac{1{,}000 \text{ units/hr}}{50 \text{ units}} \times 1 \text{ mL}$$

Step 3: Cancel the units that appear in both the numerator and the denominator:

$$X = \frac{1{,}000 \cancel{\text{ units}} \text{/hr}}{50 \cancel{\text{ units}}} \times 1 \text{ mL}$$

Step 4: Multiply the desired dose by quantity (1,000 × 1):

$$X = \frac{1{,}000 \text{ mL/hr}}{50 \text{ units}}$$

Step 5: Solve for *X*. Divide the numerator by the denominator (1,000 ÷ 50):

$$X = 20 \text{ mL/hr}$$

The hourly flow rate is 20 mL/hr.

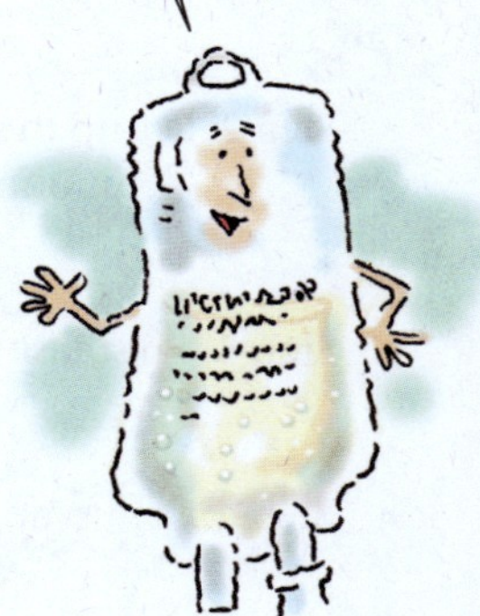
It's important to calculate a heparin infusion rate accurately to ensure the dose falls within safe and therapeutic limits.

Solve using the *ratio proportion method*

Find the dose using the *ratio proportion method*.

Step 1: Write a fraction to express the known solution strength (units of medication divided by milliliters of solution):

$$\frac{25{,}000 \text{ units}}{500 \text{ mL}}$$

Step 2: Write a second fraction with the desired dose of heparin in the numerator and the unknown flow rate in the denominator:

$$\frac{1{,}000 \text{ units/hr}}{X}$$

Step 3: Put these fractions into a proportion:

$$\frac{25{,}000 \text{ units}}{500 \text{ mL}} = \frac{1{,}000 \text{ units/hr}}{X}$$

Step 4: Solve for X by cross-multiplying:

$$25{,}000 \text{ units} \times X = 1{,}000 \text{ units/hr} \times 500 \text{ mL}$$

Step 5: Divide each side of the equation by 25,000 units and cancel units that appear in both the numerator and the denominator:

$$\frac{25{,}000 \cancel{\text{units}} \times X}{25{,}000 \cancel{\text{units}}} = \frac{1{,}000 \cancel{\text{units}}/\text{hr} \times 500 \text{ mL}}{25{,}000 \cancel{\text{units}}}$$

$$X = \frac{500{,}000 \text{ mL/hr}}{25{,}000}$$

$$X = 20 \text{ mL/hr}$$

The nurse should set the flow rate at 20 mL/hr.

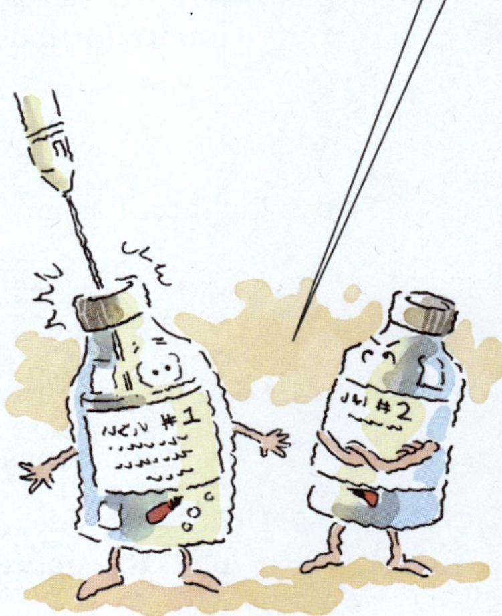
Problems can be simplified by finding the lowest concentration of heparin or insulin before solving the equation.

Know this flow?

A nurse is about to administer a continuous infusion of 25,000 units of heparin in 250 mL of D_5W. If the patient is ordered to receive 600 units/hr, how will the nurse program the IV pump?

Solve using the *formula method*

Find the flow rate using the *formula method*.

Step 1: Determine the lowest concentration of heparin:

$$X = \frac{25{,}000 \text{ units}}{250 \text{ mL}} = 100 \text{ units/mL}$$

Step 2: Set-up the formula with the information provided:

- Desired dose: 600 units/hr
- Have on hand: 100 units
- Quantity: 1 mL

$$X = \frac{600 \text{ units/hr}}{100 \text{ units}} \times 1 \text{ mL}$$

Step 3: Cancel the units that appear in both the numerator and the denominator:

$$X = \frac{600 \cancel{\text{units}}/\text{hr}}{100 \cancel{\text{units}}} \times 1 \text{ mL}$$

Step 4: Multiply the desired dose by quantity (600×1):

$$X = \frac{600 \text{ mL/hr}}{100 \text{ units}}$$

Step 5: Solve for X. Divide the numerator by the denominator ($600 \div 100$):

$$X = 6 \text{ mL/hr}$$

The nurse would program the IV pump to deliver 6 mL/hr of heparin.

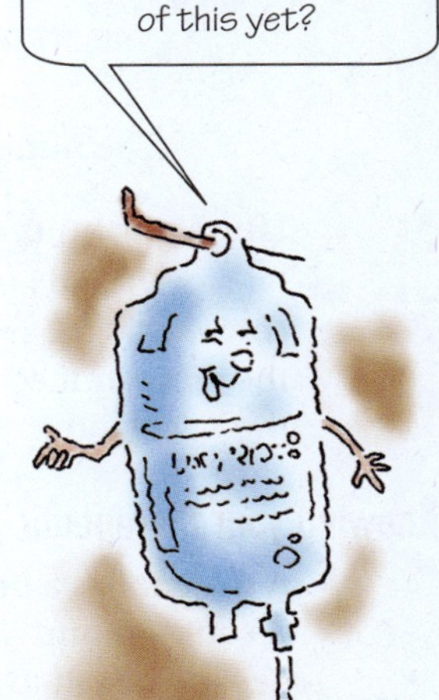

Getting the hang of this yet?

Solve using the *ratio proportion method*

Find the dose using the *ratio proportion method*.

Step 1: Write a fraction to express the known solution strength (units of medication divided by milliliters of solution):

$$\frac{25{,}000 \text{ units}}{250 \text{ mL}}$$

Step 2: Write a second fraction with the desired dose of heparin in the numerator and the unknown flow rate in the denominator:

$$\frac{600 \text{ units/hr}}{X}$$

Step 3: Put these fractions into a proportion:

$$\frac{25{,}000 \text{ units}}{250 \text{ mL}} = \frac{600 \text{ units/hr}}{X}$$

Step 4: Solve for *X* by cross-multiplying:

$$25{,}000 \text{ units} \times X = 600 \text{ units/hr} \times 250 \text{ mL}$$

Step 5: Divide each side of the equation by 40,000 units and cancel units that appear in both the numerator and the denominator:

$$\frac{\cancel{25{,}000 \text{ units}} \times X}{\cancel{25{,}000 \text{ units}}} = \frac{600 \cancel{\text{units}}/\text{hr} \times 250 \text{ mL}}{25{,}000 \cancel{\text{units}}}$$

$$X = \frac{150{,}000 \text{ mL/hr}}{25{,}000}$$

$$X = 6 \text{ mL/hr}$$

The nurse should program the IV pump at 6 mL/hr.

Units per hour

Nurses should also confirm that the programmed flow rate is infusing correctly at the ordered dose. Most IV pumps allow nurses to check the programmed units infusing, but nurses may also want to confirm the calculation.

Knowing your therapeutic range

A patient has a heparin continuous infusion programmed at 30 mL/hr on an IV pump. The heparin concentration hanging is 25,000 units of heparin added to 500 mL of D_5W. How many units/hr of heparin is the patient receiving?

Solve using the *formula method*

Find the flow rate using the *formula method*.

Step 1: Determine the lowest concentration of heparin:

$$X = \frac{25{,}000 \text{ units}}{500 \text{ mL}} = 50 \text{ units/mL}$$

Step 2: Set-up the formula with the information provided:

- Desired dose: 30 mL/hr
- Have on hand: 1 mL
- Quantity: 50 units

$$X = \frac{30 \text{ mL/hr}}{1 \text{ mL}} \times 50 \text{ units}$$

Step 3: Cancel the units that appear in both the numerator and the denominator:

$$X = \frac{30 \cancel{\text{mL}}\text{/hr}}{1 \cancel{\text{mL}}} \times 50 \text{ units}$$

Step 4: Multiply the desired dose by quantity (30 × 50):

$$X = \frac{1{,}500 \text{ units/hr}}{1}$$

Step 5: Solve for *X*. Divide the numerator by the denominator (1,500 ÷ 1):

$$X = 1{,}500 \text{ units/hr}$$

The patient is receiving 1,500 units of heparin an hour.

Solve using the *ratio proportion method*

Find the dose using the *ratio proportion method*.

Step 1: Write a fraction to express the known solution strength (units of medication divided by mL of solution):

$$\frac{25{,}000 \text{ units}}{500 \text{ mL}}$$

Step 2: Set-up the second fraction with the flow rate in the denominator and the unknown dose of heparin in the numerator:

$$\frac{X}{30 \text{ mL/hr}}$$

Step 3: Write these fractions into a proportion:

$$\frac{25{,}000 \text{ units}}{500 \text{ mL}} = \frac{X}{30 \text{ mL/hr}}$$

Step 4: Solve for *X* by cross-multiplying:

$$500 \text{ mL} \times X = 30 \text{ mL/hr} \times 25{,}000 \text{ units}$$

Step 5: Divide each side of the equation by 500 mL and cancel units that appear in both the numerator and the denominator:

$$\frac{\cancel{500\text{ mL}} \times X}{\cancel{500\text{ mL}}} = \frac{30\ \cancel{\text{mL}}/\text{hr} \times 25{,}000\text{ units}}{500\ \cancel{\text{mL}}}$$

$$X = \frac{750{,}000\text{ units/hr}}{500}$$

$$X = 1{,}500\text{ units/hr}$$

With the flow rate set at 30 mL/hr, the patient is receiving 1,500 units/hr of heparin.

Weight-based heparin

Heparin may also be prescribed according to a patient's weight. In this case, nurses will have to obtain a patient's weight in kilograms (kg) to determine the dose and the flow rate.

Weigh in!

A patient diagnosed with a pulmonary embolism (PE) has an order to start a heparin drip using the PE protocol. Per the protocol, the order states to start an infusion at 18 units/kg/hr. The patient weighs 86 kg, and the available heparin solution contains 25,000 units added to 500 mL of D_5W. What flow rate will the nurse program an IV pump for the heparin infusion?

Solve using the *formula method*

Find the flow rate using the *formula method.*

Step 1: Determine the dose per hour:

$$X = 18\text{ units/kg/hr}$$

$$X = 18\text{ units} \times 86\text{ kg/hr}$$

$$X = 1{,}548\text{ units/hr}$$

Step 2: Determine the lowest concentration of heparin:

$$X = \frac{25{,}000\text{ units}}{500\text{ mL}} = 50\text{ units/mL}$$

Step 3: Set up the formula with the information provided:

- Desired dose: 1,548 units/hr
- Have on hand: 50 units
- Quantity: 1 mL

$$X = \frac{1{,}548\text{ units/hr}}{50\text{ units}} \times 1\text{ mL}$$

Step 4: Cancel the units that appear in both the numerator and the denominator:

$$X = \frac{1{,}548\ \cancel{\text{units}}/\text{hr}}{50\ \cancel{\text{units}}} \times 1\text{ mL}$$

Before you give that medication

Heparin hazards

Heparin comes in different concentrations and is considered a high-alert medication. Just like insulin, most facilities require another nurse to witness the calculations and programming of the IV pump for safety and accuracy. Errors in dosage calculations with heparin can cause nontherapeutic anticoagulation levels that can lead to excessive bleeding or increased risk of developing blood clots.

Dosage drill

Test your math skills with this drill

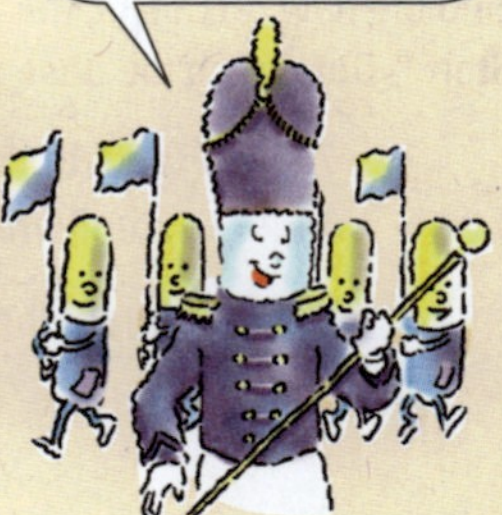
Be sure to show how you arrive at your answer:

An order for a patient who weighs 74 kg states to start a heparin IV infusion at 12 units/kg/hr. The pharmacy sends a bag of 500 mL D_5W containing 25,000 units of heparin. What flow rate should the nurse program the IV pump?

Your answer: ________________

Find the flow rate using the ***formula method:***

Step 1: Determine the dose per hour:

$$X = 12 \text{ units/kg/hr}$$
$$X = 12 \text{ units} \times 74 \text{ kg/hr}$$
$$X = 888 \text{ units/hr}$$

Step 2: Determine the lowest concentration of heparin:

$$X = \frac{25{,}000 \text{ units}}{500 \text{ mL}} = 50 \text{ units/mL}$$

Step 3: Set up the formula with the information provided:

- Desired dose: 888 units/hr
- Have on hand: 50 units
- Quantity: 1 mL

$$X = \frac{888 \text{ units/hr}}{50 \text{ units}} \times 1 \text{ mL}$$

Step 4: Cancel the units that appear in both the numerator and the denominator:

$$X = \frac{888 \cancel{\text{units}}\text{/hr}}{50 \cancel{\text{units}}} \times 1 \text{ mL}$$

Step 5: Multiply the desired dose by quantity (888 × 1):

$$X = \frac{888 \text{ mL/hr}}{50}$$

Step 6: Solve for *X*. Divide the numerator by the denominator (888 ÷ 50):

$$X = 17.76 \text{ mL/hr}$$

Rounding to the nearest tenth space, the flow rate for the IV pump would be 17.8 mL/hr.

(*continued*)

Test your math skills with this drill (*continued*)

Let's try yet another method to verify the correct rate is infusing:

Find the flow rate using the ***ratio proportion method:***

Step 1: Determine the dose in units/hr:

$$74 \text{ kg}:X \text{ units/hr}::1 \text{ kg}:12 \text{ units/hr}$$

$$74 \text{ kg} \times 12 \text{ units/hr} = 1 \text{ kg} \times X \text{ units/hr}$$

$$\frac{74 \cancel{\text{kg}} \times 12 \text{ units/hr}}{1 \cancel{\text{kg}}} = \frac{1 \cancel{\text{kg}} \times X \text{ units/hr}}{1 \cancel{\text{kg}}}$$

$$X = 888 \text{ units/hr}$$

Step 2: Determine the lowest concentration of heparin:

$$X = \frac{25{,}000 \text{ units}}{500 \text{ mL}} = 50 \text{ units/mL}$$

Step 3: Write the two fractions as a proportion:

$$\frac{888 \text{ units/hr}}{X} = \frac{50 \text{ units}}{1 \text{ mL}}$$

Step 4: Solve for X by cross-multiplying:

$$888 \text{ units/hr} \times 1 \text{ mL} = 50 \text{ units} \times X$$

Step 5: Divide each side of the equation by 50 units and cancel units that appear in both the numerator and the denominator:

$$\frac{888 \cancel{\text{units}}/\text{hr} \times 1 \text{ mL}}{50 \cancel{\text{units}}} = \frac{\cancel{50 \text{ units}} \times X}{\cancel{50 \text{ units}}}$$

$$X = \frac{888 \text{ mL/hr}}{50}$$

$$X = 17.76 \text{ mL/hr}$$

Rounding to the nearest tenth space, the flow rate for the IV pump would be 17.8 mL/hr.

Step 5: Multiply the desired dose by quantity $(1{,}548 \times 1)$:

$$X = \frac{1{,}548 \text{ mL/hr}}{50}$$

Step 6: Solve for X. Divide the numerator by the denominator $(1{,}548 \div 50)$:

$$X = 30.96 \text{ mL/hr}$$

Based on the protocol, the nurse should program the IV pump to deliver 31 mL/hr of heparin.

Solve using the *ratio proportion method*

Find the flow rate using the *ratio proportion method.*

Step 1: Determine the dose in units/hr:

$$86 \text{ kg}:X \text{ units/hr}::1 \text{ kg}:18 \text{ units/hr}$$

$$86 \text{ kg} \times 18 \text{ units/hr} = 1 \text{ kg} \times X \text{ units/hr}$$

$$\frac{86 \cancel{\text{kg}} \times 18 \text{ units/hr}}{1 \cancel{\text{kg}}} = \frac{\cancel{1 \text{ kg}} \times X \text{ units/hr}}{\cancel{1 \text{ kg}}}$$

$$X = 1{,}548 \text{ units/hr}$$

Step 2: Determine the lowest concentration of heparin:

$$X = \frac{25{,}000 \text{ units}}{500 \text{ mL}} = 50 \text{ units/mL}$$

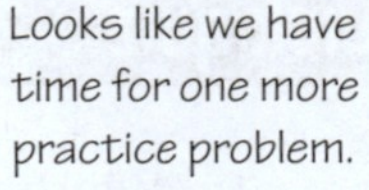

Looks like we have time for one more practice problem.

Step 3: Write the two fractions as a proportion:

$$\frac{1{,}548 \text{ units/hr}}{X} = \frac{50 \text{ units}}{1 \text{ mL}}$$

Step 4: Solve for X by cross-multiplying:

$$1{,}548 \text{ units/hr} \times 1 \text{ mL} = 50 \text{ units} \times X$$

Step 5: Divide each side of the equation by 50 units and cancel units that appear in both the numerator and the denominator:

$$\frac{1{,}548 \cancel{\text{ units}}\text{/hr} \times 1 \text{ mL}}{50 \cancel{\text{ units}}} = \frac{\cancel{50 \text{ units}} \times X}{\cancel{50 \text{ units}}}$$

$$X = \frac{1{,}548 \text{ mL/hr}}{50}$$

$$X = 30.96 \text{ mL/hr}$$

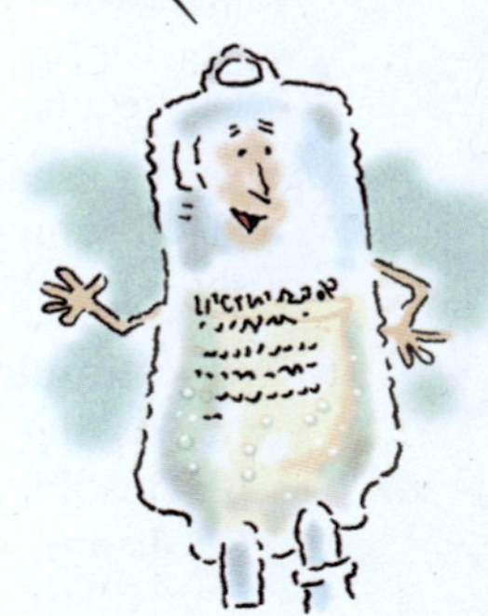

The nurse should program the IV pump to deliver 31 mL/hr of heparin.

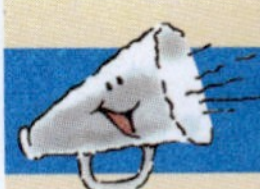

That's a wrap!

Calculating heparin and insulin dosages review

Insulin dosages

- Insulin is a high-alert medication.
- Insulin is measured in units.
- Dosage is based on medication potency (not weight).
- Insulin may be given subcutaneously or by continuous IV infusion.
- Insulin is classified by action time: onset, peak, and duration and by concentration.
- The most common concentration is U-100 insulin.
- Insulin may be ordered by a sliding scale or continuous infusion protocols.
- When combining compatible insulins, draw up clear first then cloudy.

Insulin types

- Rapid acting
- Short acting
- Intermediate acting
- Long acting
- Ultra long acting

Insulin infusions

- Regular insulin is the only type administered by IV route.
- Use an infusion pump.
- For safety, provided in use concentrations of 1 unit/mL.

Heparin dosages

- Heparin may be given subcutaneously or by continuous IV infusion.
- Continuous infusions require close monitoring with coagulation levels.
- Heparin is measured in units and supplied in units/mL solutions.
- Doses may be ordered by units or units/kg.
- Heparin protocols require nurses to be vigilant in their calculations.

Quick quiz

1. Which insulin is the only insulin that can be administered by IV?
   A. NPH
   B. insulin glargine
   C. lispro
   D. regular

Answer: D. Regular insulin is the only insulin that can be given by IV. NPH, insulin glargine, and lispro insulin must be given subcutaneously.

2. Which insulin is classified as a long-acting insulin?
   A. regular
   B. insulin glargine
   C. lispro
   D. NPH

Answer: B. Insulin glargine has a duration of 24 hours. Regular insulin lasts 6 to 8 hours, lispro lasts 3 to 4 hours, and NPH insulin lasts 18 to 24 hours.

3. The nurse starts a continuous infusion of 150 units of regular insulin in 150 mL of normal saline solution. The prescribed dose is 8 units/hr. What's the hourly flow rate?
   A. 8 mL/hr
   B. 10 mL/hr
   C. 18 mL/hr
   D. 80 mL/hr

Answer: A. Solve this problem by setting up the first fraction with the known solution strength and the second fraction with the desired dose and the unknown volume, putting these fractions into a proportion, cross-multiplying, and then dividing and canceling the units of measure that appear in both the numerator and the denominator.

4. Which lab test determines the therapeutic range for heparin?
   A. Activated partial thrombin test
   B. Activated partial thromboplastin time (aPTT)
   C. Partial thrombin activation test
   D. Clotting test

Answer: B. Heparin doses are individualized based on the patient's coagulation status, which is measured by aPTT or antiXa assay.

Scoring

☆☆☆ If you answered all four items correctly, fantastic! You can calculate confidently in critical cases.

☆☆ If you answered two or three items correctly, that isn't bad! You're a cool, calm, and collected calculator.

☆ If you answered fewer than two items correctly, keep at it! You have the best dosage calc. book ever. Keep it with you always and refer to it frequently.

Suggested References

American Diabetes Association. (n.d.). *Statistics about diabetes*. Statistics About Diabetes | ADA. https://diabetes.org/about-diabetes/statistics/about-diabetes

American Diabetes Association. Standards of care in diabetes—2023 abridged for primary care providers. (2022). *Clinical Diabetes*, 41(1), 4–31. https://doi.org/10.2337/cd23-as01

Centeno, E. H., Militello, M., & Gomes, M. P. (2019, June 1). Anti-Xa assays: What is their role today in antithrombotic therapy? *Cleveland Clinic Journal of Medicine*. https://www.ccjm.org/content/86/6/417

Centers for Disease Control and Prevention. (2023, November 14). *National Diabetes Statistics Report*. Centers for Disease Control and Prevention. https://www.cdc.gov/diabetes/data/statistics-report/index.html

ISMP.org. (2017). *2017 ISMP guidelines for optimizing safe subcutaneous insulin use in adults*. Institute for Safe Medical Practices. https://www.ismp.org/sites/default/files/attachments/2018-09/ISMP138D-Insulin%20Guideline-090718.pdf

Neumiller, J. J., Odegard, P. S., & Wysham, C. H. (2009b). Update on insulin management in type 2 diabetes. *Diabetes Spectrum*, 22(2), 85–91. https://doi.org/10.2337/diaspect.22.2.85

Williams-Norwood, T., Caswell, M., Milner, B., Vescera, J. C., Prymicz, K., Ciszak, A. G., Ingle, C., Lacey, C., & Stavrou, E. X. (2020). Design and implementation of an anti–factor XA heparin monitoring protocol. *AACN Advanced Critical Care*, 31(2), 129–137. https://doi.org/10.4037/aacnacc2020132

Appendices and index

Practice makes perfect

1. Which is the correct answer for converting the improper fraction $^{11}/_{2}$ into a mixed number?
   A. $^{2}/_{11}$
   B. $5\,^{1}/_{11}$
   C. $5\,^{1}/_{2}$
   D. $^{22}/_{11}$

2. What is the sum of $^{1}/_{2}$ + $^{3}/_{4}$ + $^{6}/_{10}$?
   A. $1\,^{8}/_{10}$
   B. $1\,^{17}/_{20}$
   C. $2\,^{1}/_{4}$
   D. $^{10}/_{16}$

3. The complex fraction $^{1}/_{75}$ divided by the complex fraction $^{1}/_{25}$ equals which correct answer?
   A. $^{1}/_{3}$
   B. 3
   C. $^{1}/_{100}$
   D. $^{2}/_{3}$

4. What number does dividing the decimal fraction 4.3 by 8.6 yield?
   A. 0.5
   B. 2
   C. 20
   D. 50

5. What is 21.3478 rounded to the nearest hundredth place?
   A. 21.34
   B. 21.3
   C. 21.348
   D. 21.35

6. What is 31% of 105?
   A. 3.15
   B. 31.5
   C. 32.55
   D. 33.3

7. Converting 20% to a decimal fraction becomes which correct answer?
   A. 0.02
   B. 2.0
   C. 0.2
   D. 2.2

8. What is the fraction form for the proportion 1:4::4:16?
   A. $\frac{4}{1} = \frac{4}{16}$
   B. $\frac{1}{4} = \frac{4}{16}$
   C. $\frac{4}{4} = \frac{1}{16}$
   D. $\frac{4}{1} = \frac{16}{4}$

9. A vial contains 20 mg of a medication in 50 mL of solution. How much of the medication is contained in 10 mL of the solution?
   A. 15 mg
   B. 10 mg
   C. 5 mg
   D. 4 mg

10. Solve for X in the proportion 3:9::9:X.
   A. 81
   B. 3
   C. 27
   D. 18

11. How much chlorine bleach should be added to 500 mL of water to make a solution that contains 10 mL of chlorine bleach for every 100 mL of water?
   A. 5 mL
   B. 50 mL
   C. 10 mL
   D. 100 mL

12. How many lb is equal to 70 kg?
   A. 140 lb
   B. 154 lb
   C. 70 lb
   D. 32 lb

13. A patient has been ordered ampicillin 250 mg. The medication is supplied as an oral suspension containing 125 mg per 5 mL. How many mL should the patient receive?
   A. 10 mL
   B. 5 mL
   C. 25 mL
   D. 1 mL

14. How many liters is equal to 0.025 kL?
   A. 250 L
   B. 2.5 L
   C. 0.25 L
   D. 25 L

15. During a 24-hour period, a patient received 600 mL, 1.25 L, and 2.5 L of IV fluid. How many mL of fluid did the patient receive in total?

A. 43,500 mL
B. 43.5 mL
C. 4,350 mL
D. 435 mL

16. An infant weighs 8,300 g. How many kilograms (kg) does this equal?

A. 8,300 kg
B. 8.3 kg
C. 0.83 kg
D. 830 kg

17. A patient received 0.25 mg of digoxin (Lanoxin). How many grams (g) does this equal?

A. 25 g
B. 2.5 g
C. 0.25 g
D. 0.00025 g

18. A patient has an order to receive 2 g of a medication. The medication bottle is labeled 250 mg/mL. How many mL should be given to the patient?

A. 4 mL
B. 6 mL
C. 8 mL
D. 10 mL

19. A patient has an order for 20 mEq of potassium chloride oral solution. The solution contains 60 mEq in every 15 mL. How many mL of the solution should the patient receive?

A. 5 mL
B. 2.5 mL
C. 7.5 mL
D. 3 mL

20. A patient has been prescribed metoprolol tartrate 25 mg PO BID. How should the nurse interpret the order?

A. Give 25 mg of metoprolol tartrate orally every other day.
B. Give 25 mg of metoprolol tartrate orally every day.
C. Give 25 mg of metoprolol tartrate orally three times a day.
D. Give 25 mg of metoprolol tartrate orally twice a day.

21. Which medication order is written incorrectly?

A. *Tylenol elixir 1 tsp PO STAT*
B. *Aspirin 325 PO q A.M.*
C. *Seconal 100 mg PO at bedtime. p.r.n.*
D. *Rocephin 1 g IV daily*

22. The licensed practitioner prescribes metoprolol 5 mg IV q 6 hours for a patient with an acute myocardial infarction. How should this medication be given?

A. Three times per day
B. In a suspension
C. As needed
D. Intravenously

23. A nurse is preparing to administer a stool softener scheduled to be given at 0800. The nurse understands that this type of noncritical medication can be given during what time frame?

A. The medication can be given one-half hour before or after the ordered time.
B. Give the medication 1 hour before or after the ordered time.
C. The medication can be given 15 minutes before or after the ordered time.
D. Give the medication exactly at the ordered time.

24. A nurse is preparing to administer a patient's scheduled 0900 medications. When should the nurse document the administration time of the medication?

A. Document before giving the medication to the patient.
B. Document after giving the medication to the patient.
C. Document at the beginning of the shift.
D. Document at the end of the shift.

25. A patient tells the nurse that they take two ibuprofen tablets at a time for menstrual cramps. If one tablet of the ibuprofen tablets contains 200 mg, how many mg does the patient take at a time?

A. 500 mg
B. 600 mg
C. 400 mg
D. 300 mg

26. What name listed on a medication's label is referred to as the medication's nonproprietary name?

A. Trade name
B. Generic name
C. Manufacturer name
D. Chemical name

27. The licensed practitioner orders *minoxidil 5 mg PO daily* for treatment of hypertension in a 52-year-old patient. The medication comes supplied in 2.5 mg tablets. How many tablets should be administered?

A. ½ tablet
B. 1 tablet
C. 1½ tablets
D. 2 tablets

28. The licensed practitioner orders *Milk of Magnesia 1½ tbs PO at bedtime* for a patient experiencing constipation. How many mL of medication will the nurse tell the patient to take at bedtime?

A. 17.5 mL
B. 15.5 mL
C. 22.5 mL
D. 7.5 mL

29. A patient is ordered *Tylenol 240 mg supp per rectum* to treat a fever. The medication comes available as 120 mg suppositories. How many suppositories should the nurse administer?

A. 1½ supp
B. 1 supp
C. 2 supp
D. ½ supp

30. A patient has an order to apply a lidocaine 5% patch at 0900 and to remove the patch at 2100. Which reason does the rationale of the 12-hours-on and 12-hours-off application directions include?

A. To prevent it from falling off while the patient sleeps
B. To prevent it from irritating the patient's skin
C. To prevent the patient from developing a tolerance to the drug
D. To prevent toxicity

31. A patient has an order to receive hydromorphone 0.5 mg IV every 4 hours prn for postoperative pain. The medication is available in a prefilled syringe containing 1 mg of hydromorphone per 1 mL. How many mL should the nurse administer?

A. 1 mL
B. 0.75 mL
C. 0.5 mL
D. 0.25 mL

32. A licensed practitioner orders fentanyl 25 mcg IV to be given now to a patient undergoing a procedure. The medication comes available in a vial containing fentanyl 100 mcg in 2 mL. How many mL of fentanyl will the nurse need to ***waste***?

A. 0.5 mL
B. 0.75 mL
C. 1 mL
D. 1.5 mL

33. A nurse has an order to administer heparin 5,000 units subcut *q8h* for a patient. The heparin available is 5,000 units in 1 mL. How many mL of heparin should be administered?

A. 1 mL
B. 0.75 mL
C. 0.5 mL
D. 0.25 mL

34. A nurse has an order to start an infusion on a patient of D5W at 100 mL/hr. The available gravity tubing is calibrated at 15 gtt/mL. What should be the calculated drip rate?

A. 31 gtt/min
B. 33 gtt/min
C. 25 gtt/min
D. 30 gtt/min

35. A nurse has an order to administer 2,000 mL of normal saline IV fluids over 24 hours. Using an IV pump, what flow rate will the nurse set the pump?

A. 150 mL/hr
B. 125 mL/hr
C. 110 mL/hr
D. 83 mL/hr

36. A patient has an infusion of 25,000 units of heparin in 500 mL of 0.45% NS solution infusing at 750 units/hr. What flow rate should be programmed in the IV pump?

A. 25 mL/hr
B. 15 mL/hr
C. 10 mL/hr
D. 5 mL/hr

37. A 4-year-old patient weighs 46 lb. How many kg does this child weigh?

A. 21 kg
B. 20 kg
C. 23 kg
D. 12 kg

38. The licensed practitioner orders a single dose of acetaminophen 10 mg/kg/dose oral suspension for a child with a fever who weighs 6 kg. How many mg will the nurse administer?

A. 1.6 mg
B. 16 mg
C. 60 mg
D. 80 mg

39. A child weighing 66 lb is admitted with appendicitis. How much maintenance IV fluid should the child receive in 24 hours?

A. 1,500 mL/day
B. 1,700 mL/day
C. 1,800 mL/day
D. 1,900 mL/day

40. A 25-year-old primigravida has been in labor for 20 hours with little progress. The licensed practitioner prescribes oxytocin. The order reads *10 units oxytocin in 1,000 mL NS to infuse via pump at 1 mU/min for 15 minutes; then increase flow rate to 2 mU/min.* How will the nurse program the IV pump to deliver 1 mU/min for 15 minutes?

A. 4 mL/hr
B. 6 mL/hr
C. 8 mL/hr
D. 12 mL/hr

41. Using the information in the previous problem, what will be the new flow rate to deliver 2 mU/min?

A. 10 mL/hr
B. 20 mL/hr
C. 12 mL/hr
D. 15 mL/hr

42. A patient with preeclampsia has an order to deliver *4 g magnesium sulfate in 250 mL D_5W to infuse at 1 g/hr.* What flow rate will the nurse use to program an IV pump?

A. 125 mL/hr
B. 250 mL/hr
C. 25 mL/hr
D. 63 mL/hr

43. A 170-lb patient with minimal urine output has an order to receive dopamine at 5 mcg/kg/min. The premixed bag of dopamine contains 800 mg in 500 mL D_5W. How many mL of solution containing dopamine will the patient receive each hour?

A. 17 mL
B. 16 mL
C. 15 mL
D. 14 mL

44. A patient experiencing an acute myocardial infarction is to receive nitroglycerin 10 mcg/min IV. The IV solution contains 250 mL D_5W with 25 mg nitroglycerin. How many mL should the patient receive each hour?

A. 16 mL
B. 10 mL
C. 6 mL
D. 4 mL

45. A patient has an order for a continuous infusion of 3 mg/min of lidocaine. Lidocaine comes available in a solution containing *1 g lidocaine in 250 mL D_5W*. What flow rate will the nurse use to program an infusion pump?

   A. 30 mL/hr
   B. 45 mL/hr
   C. 60 mL/hr
   D. 70 mL/hr

46. A licensed practitioner prescribes an order for 2 L of Lactated Ringer solution to be infused over 16 hours. The drop factor of the gravity administration set is 20 gtt/mL. What drip rate will the nurse use to deliver the fluids?

   A. 25 gtt/min
   B. 33 gtt/min
   C. 20 gtt/min
   D. 42 gtt/min

47. The nurse is to administer vancomycin 1.25 g in 250 mL to infuse over 90 minutes. What hourly flow rate should the nurse set the infusion pump to deliver the medication?

   A. 167 mL/hr
   B. 65 mL/hr
   C. 35 mL/hr
   D. 15 mL/hr

48. The nurse receives an order to administer 4,000 mL of normal saline solution IV over 12 hours. What should the drip rate be if the drop factor of the tubing is 15 gtt/mL?

   A. 46 gtt/min
   B. 91 gtt/min
   C. 166 gtt/min
   D. 83 gtt/min

49. A patient has a single-dose order for ketorolac tromethamine 15 mg IV for pain. Ketorolac tromethamine is available in a vial containing 60 mg/2 mL. How many mL should the nurse administer?

   A. 0.5 mL
   B. 5 mL
   C. 0.2 mL
   D. 2 mL

50. A 150-lb patient is to receive gentamicin 3 mg/kg/daily in three equally divided doses. Gentamicin is available in 80 mg/2 mL. How many mL should the nurse administer every 8 hours?

   A. 1.7 mL
   B. 4 mL
   C. 2.7 mL
   D. 1.3 mL

51. A patient has an order for digoxin 250 mcg PO every day. The pharmacy stocks digoxin 0.5-mg scored tablets. How many tablets should the nurse administer?

A. ¼ tab
B. 1 tab
C. ½ tab
D. 2 tabs

52. The licensed practitioner orders phenytoin sodium suspension 300 mg PO every day. Phenytoin is available in a suspension of 125 mg/5 mL. How many mL should the nurse administer per dose?

A. 18 mL
B. 12 mL
C. 6 mL
D. 2.1 mL

53. A patient has an order for azathioprine (Imuran) 75 mg PO every day. Imuran is available in 50-mg unscored tablets. How should the nurse administer the dose?

A. Administer 2 tablets.
B. Administer 1½ tablets.
C. Administer 1 tablet.
D. Withhold the dose until the pharmacy sends a 75-mg tablet.

54. An infant weighing 2.3 kg has an order to receive gentamicin 2.5 mg/kg/dose IV q12h. The pharmacy stocks gentamicin in a solution of 2 mg/mL. How many mL of the solution should the nurse administer for each dose?

A. 3.2 mL
B. 2.6 mL
C. 1.9 mL
D. 2.9 mL

55. An infant weighing 8 lb is about to receive a blood transfusion of 15 mL/kg of packed red blood cells (PRBCs) over 4 hours. What hourly flow rate should the nurse set the infusion pump to deliver the PRBCs?

A. 8 mL/hr
B. 10.6 mL/hr
C. 13.5 mL/hr
D. 15.2 mL/hr

Answers

1. C. Divide the numerator (11) by the denominator (2). The calculation looks like this:

$$\frac{11}{2} = 11 \div 2 = 5\tfrac{1}{2}$$

This results in 5 with 1 left over. The 1 becomes the new numerator and the denominator remains the same.

2. B. Step 1: Determine the lowest common denominator (20) then convert each to the lowest common denominator: $\frac{1}{2} = \frac{10}{20}$, $\frac{3}{4} = \frac{15}{20}$, $\frac{6}{10} = \frac{12}{20}$.
Step 2: Add all the numerators and place over the denominators:

$$\frac{10}{20} + \frac{15}{20} + \frac{12}{20} = \frac{37}{20}.$$

Step 3: Reduce to lowest terms: $1\frac{17}{20}$.

3. A. Step 1: Divide the dividend $\frac{1}{75}$ by the divisor $\frac{1}{25}$.
Step 2: Invert the divisor ($\frac{1}{25}$) and multiply. $\frac{1}{75} \times \frac{25}{1} = \frac{25}{75}$.
Step 3: Reduce to lowest terms: $\frac{1}{3}$.

4. A. Step 1: Move the decimal points of both the divisor and the dividend one place to the right before dividing.
Step 2: Place the quotient's decimal point over the new decimal point in the dividend.

5. D. The number 4 is in the hundredth place. Since the number to the right of it is 7, which is greater than 5; add 1 to 4 to round off the number.

6. C. Step 1: Restate the question as a decimal fraction by removing the percent sign and moving the decimal point two places to the left (The decimal fraction is 0.31).
Step 2: Multiply 0.31 by 105.

7. C. Step 1: Remove the percent sign.
Step 2: Move the decimal point two places to the left.

8. B. Step 1: Make the ratio on both sides into fractions by substituting slashes for colons.
Step 2: Replace the double colon in the center with an equal sign.

9. D. Solving using the Ratio Proportion Method
Step 1: Substitute X for the amount of medication in 10 mL of solution.
Step 2: Set up a proportion with ratios or fractions.
Step 3: Solve for X:

$$X\text{:10 mL::20 mg:50 mL} \quad \text{or} \quad \frac{X}{10 \text{ mL}} = \frac{20 \text{ mg}}{50 \text{ mL}}$$

Solving using the Formula Method (desired over have method)

Step 1: Set up the formula using the components of the formula:
D = 10 mL; H = 50 mL; Q = 20 mg

$$X = \frac{10 \cancel{mL}}{50 \cancel{mL}} \times 20 \text{ mg}$$

Step 2: Solve for X. Divide 10 by 50 = 0.2.
Step 3: Multiply 0.2 × 20 = 4 mg.

10. C. Step 1: Multiply the means and the extremes.
Step 2: Put the products of the means and extremes into an equation.
Step 3: Solve for X by dividing both sides by 3. The calculation looks like this:

$$9 \times 9 = 3 \times X$$
$$81 = 3X$$
$$X = 27$$

11. B. Solving using the Ratio Proportion Method
Step 1: Substitute X for the amount of chlorine bleach in 500 mL of water.
Step 2: Set up a proportion with ratios or fractions.
Step 3: Solve for X. The setup looks like this:

X mL bleach:500 mL water::10 mL bleach:100 mL water

Solving using the Formula Method
Step 1: Set up the formula using the components of the formula:
D = 500 mL; H = 100 mL; Q = 10 mL

$$X = \frac{500 \cancel{mL}}{100 \cancel{mL}} \times 10 \text{ mL}$$

Step 2: Solve for X. Divide 500 by 100 = 5.
Step 3: Multiply 5 × 10 = 50 mL.

12. B. Using the conversion factor 1 kg = 2.2 lb, multiply 70 kg by 2.2.

13. A. Solving using the Ratio Proportion Method
Step 1: Substitute X for the amount of medication in 5 mL of solution.
Step 2: Set up a proportion with ratios or fractions.
Step 3: Divide both sides by 125.
Step 4: Solve for X:

250 mg:X mL::125 mg:5 mL
125 X = 1,250 mL

Solving using the Formula Method
Step 1: Set up the formula using the components of the formula:
D = 250 mg; H = 125 mg; Q = 5 mL

$$X = \frac{250 \cancel{mg}}{125 \cancel{mg}} \times 5 \text{ mL}$$

Step 2: Solve for *X*. Divide 250 by 125 = 2.
Step 3: Multiply 2 × 5 = 10 mL.

14. D. Using the *Amazing metric decimal place finder*, p. 86, count the number of places to the right or left of kiloliters (kL) to reach liters (L). In this case, it's three places to the right, therefore, move the decimal three places to the right. Another way is to multiply the kL by 1,000 since 1 kL = 1,000 L.

15. C. Knowing that there are 1,000 mL in 1 L, convert all the measurements to mL and add the numbers together.

16. B. Using the *Amazing metric decimal place finder*, p. 86, count the number of places to the right or left of kilograms (kg) to reach grams (g). In this case, it's three places to the left, therefore, move the decimal three places to the left. Another way is to divide the g by 1,000 since 1 kg = 1,000 g.

17. D. Using the *Amazing metric decimal place finder*, p. 86, count the number of places to the right or left of milligrams (mg) to reach grams (g). In this case, it's three places to the left, therefore, move the decimal three places to the left. Another way is to divide the mg by 1,000 since 1 g = 1,000 mg.

18. C. Solving using the Ratio Proportion Method
Step 1: Convert g to mg. Recall that 1 g = 1,000 mg.
Step 2: Set up a proportion with ratios or fractions.
Step 3: Multiply the means and the extremes.
Step 4: Divide both sides by 250.
Step 5: Solve for *X*.

$$2{,}000 \text{ mg}:X \text{ mL}::250 \text{ mg}:1 \text{ mL}$$

$$2{,}000 \text{ mL} = 250\,X$$

Solving using the Formula Method
Step 1: Set up the formula using the components of the formula and cancel the units that appear in both the numerator and the denominator.
D = 2,000 mg; H = 250 mg; Q = 1 mL

$$X = \frac{2{,}000 \cancel{\text{mg}}}{250 \cancel{\text{mg}}} \times 1 \text{ mL}$$

Step 2: Solve for *X*. Divide 2,000 by 250 = 8.
Step 3: Multiply 8 × 1 = 8 mL.

19. A. Solving using the Ratio Proportion Method
Step 1: Set up the equation using *X* as the unknown quantity:

$$\frac{X}{20 \text{ mEq}} = \frac{15 \text{ mL}}{60 \text{ mEq}}$$

Step 2: Cross-multiply the fractions.
Step 3: Solve for X. Divide both sides by 60 mEq to isolate X and cancel like units.
Step 4: Finish the math.
Solving using the Formula Method
Step 1: Set up the formula using the components of the formula and cancel the units that appear in both the numerator and the denominator.

a. D = 20 mEq; H = 60 mEq; Q = 15 mL

$$X = \frac{20\ \cancel{\text{mEq}}}{60\ \cancel{\text{mEq}}} \times 15\ \text{mL}$$

Step 2: Solve for X. Divide 20 by 60 = 0.3333.
Step 3: Multiply 0.3333 × 10 = 4.9995 = 5 mL.

20. **D.** In the correct answer, BID stands for "twice a day."

21. **B.** In this order, the unit of measure for the dose is missing.

22. **D.** IV is the abbreviation for intravenous, which means the medication should be injected through an intravenous catheter.

23. **B.** Noncritical scheduled medications are considered on time if they're given one hour before or after the ordered time.

24. **B.** Document the time of the medication administration immediately after giving the medication to the patient to keep from mistakenly giving it again.

25. **C.** Solve using the Ratio Proportion Method
Step 1: Set up the equation with 200 mg/1 tablet as the known amount and X as the unknown factor:

$$\frac{200\ \text{mg}}{1\ \text{tablet}} = \frac{X}{2\ \text{tablet}}$$

Step 2: Solve for X. Cross-multiply the fractions.
Step 3: Divide both sides by 1 tablet to isolate X and cancel like units.
Step 4: Finish the math.
Solve using the Formula Method
Step 1: Set up the formula using the components of the formula and cancel the units that appear in both the numerator and the denominator.

a. D = 2 tablets; H = 1 tablet; Q = 200 mg

$$X = \frac{2\ \cancel{\text{tabs}}}{1\ \cancel{\text{tabs}}} \times 200\ \text{mg}$$

Step 2: Solve for X. Divide 2 by 1 = 2.
Step 3: Multiply 2 × 200 = 400 mg.

26. **B.** The generic name is the accepted nonproprietary name, which is a simplified form of the medication's chemical name.

27. **D.** Solve using the Ratio Proportion Method

Step 1: Set up the equation with 2.5 mg equals 1 tablet as the known factor and *X* as the unknown factor:

$$\frac{2.5 \text{ mg}}{1 \text{ tablet}} = \frac{5 \text{ mg}}{X}$$

Step 2: Solve for *X*. Cross-multiply the fractions.

Step 3: Divide both sides by 2.5 mg to isolate *X* and cancel like units.

Step 4: Finish the math.

Solve using the Formula Method

Step 1: Set up the formula using the components of the formula and cancel the units that appear in both the numerator and the denominator.

a. D = 5 mg; H = 2.5 mg; Q = 1 tablet

$$X = \frac{5 \cancel{\text{mg}}}{2.5 \cancel{\text{mg}}} \times 1 \text{ tablet}$$

Step 2: Solve for *X*. Divide 5 by 2.5 = 2.

Step 3: Multiply 2 × 1 = 2 tablets.

28. **C.** Solve using the Ratio Proportion Method

Step 1: Set up the equation with 1 tbs equals 15 mL as the known factor and *X* as the unknown factor:

$$\frac{1 \text{ tbs}}{15 \text{ mL}} = \frac{1.5 \text{ tbs}}{X}$$

Step 2: Solve for *X*. Cross-multiply the fractions.

Step 3: Divide both sides by 1 tbs to isolate *X* and cancel like units.

Step 4: Finish the math.

Solve using the Formula Method

Step 1: Recall that 1 tbs = 30 mL. Set up the formula using the components of the formula:

a. D = 1.5 tbs; H = 1 tbs; Q = 15 mL

$$X = \frac{1.5 \cancel{\text{tbs}}}{1 \cancel{\text{tbs}}} \times 15 \text{ mL}$$

Step 2: Solve for *X*. Divide 1.5 by 1 = 1.5.

Step 3: Multiply 1.5 × 15 = 22.5 mL.

29. **C.** Solve using the Ratio Proportion Method

Step 1: Set up the equation with 120 mg/1 supp as the known factor and *X* as the unknown factor:

$$\frac{120 \text{ mg}}{1 \text{ supp}} = \frac{240 \text{ mg}}{X}$$

Step 2: Solve for *X*. Cross-multiply the fractions.
Step 3: Divide both sides by 100 units to isolate *X* and cancel like units.
Step 4: Finish the math.
Solve using the Formula Method
Step 1: Set up the formula using the components of the formula and cancel the units that appear in both the numerator and the denominator.
a. D = 240 mg; H = 120 mg; Q = 1 suppository

$$X = \frac{240 \cancel{\text{mg}}}{120 \cancel{\text{mg}}} \times 1 \text{ supp}$$

Step 2: Solve for *X*. Divide 240 by 120 = 2.
Step 3: Multiply 2 × 1 = 2 supp.

30. C. Drug tolerance is a reduced reaction or diminished response to a medication following its repeated use. A new patch is applied daily and removed after 12 to 14 hours to prevent the patient from developing a tolerance to the medication.

31. C. Solve using the Ratio Proportion Method
Step 1: Set up the equation with 1 mg/1 mL as the known factor and *X* as the unknown factor:

$$\frac{1 \text{ mg}}{1 \text{ mL}} = \frac{0.5 \text{ mg}}{X}$$

Step 2: Solve for *X*. Cross-multiply the fractions.
Step 3: Divide both sides by 1 mg to isolate *X* and cancel like units.
Step 4: Finish the math.
Solve using the Formula Method
Step 1: Set up the formula using the components of the formula and cancel the units that appear in both the numerator and the denominator.
a. D = 0.5 mg; H = 1 mg; Q = 1 mL

$$X = \frac{0.5 \cancel{\text{mg}}}{1 \cancel{\text{mg}}} \times 1 \text{ mL}$$

Step 2: Solve for *X*. Divide 0.5 by 1 = 0.5.
Step 3: Multiply 0.5 × 1 = 0.5 mL.

32. D. Solve using the Ratio Proportion Method
Step 1: Set up the equation with 100 mcg/2 mL as the known factor and *X* as the unknown factor:

$$\frac{100 \text{ mcg}}{2 \text{ mL}} = \frac{25 \text{ mcg}}{X}$$

Step 2: Solve for X. Cross-multiply the fractions.
Step 3: Divide both sides by 100 mcg to isolate X and cancel like units.
Step 4: Finish the math.
Step 5: Subtract 2 mL – X. The nurse will waste 1.5 mL of fentanyl.
Solve using the Formula Method
Step 1: Set up the formula using the components of the formula and cancel the units that appear in both the numerator and the denominator.
a. D = 25 mcg; H = 100 mcg; Q = 2 mL

$$X = \frac{25\ \cancel{\text{mcg}}}{100\ \cancel{\text{mcg}}} \times 2\ \text{mL}$$

Step 2: Solve for X. Divide 25 by 100 = 0.25.
Step 3: Multiply 0.25 × 2 = 0.5 mL.
Step 4: Subtract 2 mL – 0.5 mL = 1.5 mL.

33. **A.** Solve using the Ratio Proportion Method
Step 1: Set up the equation with 5,000 units/1 mL as the known factor and X as the unknown factor:

$$\frac{5{,}000\ \text{units}}{1\ \text{mL}} = \frac{5{,}000\ \text{units}}{X}$$

Step 2: Solve for X. Cross-multiply the fractions.
Step 3: Divide both sides by 5,000 units to isolate X and cancel like units.
Step 4: Finish the math.
Solve using the Formula Method
Step 1: Set up the formula using the components of the formula and cancel the units that appear in both the numerator and the denominator.
a. D = 5,000 units; H = 5,000 units; Q = 1 mL

$$X = \frac{5{,}000\ \text{units}}{5{,}000\ \text{units}} \times 1\ \text{mL}$$

Step 2: Solve for X. Divide 5,000 by 5,000 = 1.
Step 3: Multiply 1 × 1 = 1 mL.

34. **C.** Recall the drip rate formula:

$$\text{Drip rate (gtts/min)} = \frac{\text{Volume to be infused (in mL)}}{\text{Time (in minutes)}} \times \text{Drop factor (gtts/mL)}$$

Step 1: Convert 1 hour to 60 minutes to fit the formula.
Step 2: Set up the formula with the information provided and cancel the units that appear in both the numerator and the denominator.

$$X = \frac{100\ \cancel{\text{mL}}}{60\ \text{min}} \times \frac{15\ \text{gtt}}{1\ \cancel{\text{mL}}}$$

Step 3: Multiply the volume by the drop factor (100 by 15).

$$X = \frac{1{,}500 \text{ gtt}}{60 \text{ min}}$$

Step 4: Solve for X. Divide the numerator by the denominator (1,500 ÷ 60).

$$X = 25 \text{ gtt/min}$$

35. D. Recall the flow rate formula:

$$\text{Flow rate (mL/hr)} = \frac{\text{Total volume ordered (in mL)}}{\text{Total time (in hours)}}$$

Step 1: Set up the formula using the components of the formula.

$$X = \frac{2{,}000 \text{ mL}}{24 \text{ hours}} = 83.33 \text{ mL/hr}$$

Step 2: Solve for X. Round to the nearest whole number.

36. B. Solve using the Ratio Proportion Method

Step 1: Set up the equation with 25,000 units/500 mL as the known factor and X mL as the unknown factor:

$$\frac{25{,}000 \text{ units}}{500 \text{ mL}} = \frac{750 \text{ units/hr}}{X}$$

Step 2: Solve for X. Cross-multiply the fractions.

Step 3: Divide both sides by 25,000 units to isolate X and cancel like units.

Step 4: Finish the math.

Find the flow rate using the formula method.

Step 1: Determine the lowest concentration of heparin:

$$X = \frac{25{,}000 \text{ units}}{500 \text{ mL}} = 50 \text{ units/mL}$$

Step 2: Set up the formula with the information provided and cancel the units that appear in both the numerator and the denominator.

a. D = 750 units/hr; H = 50 units; Q = 1 mL

$$X = \frac{750 \cancel{\text{units}}\text{/hr}}{50 \cancel{\text{units}}} \times 1 \text{ mL}$$

Step 3: Multiply the desired dose by quantity (750 × 1):

$$X = \frac{750 \text{ mL/hr}}{50}$$

Step 4: Solve for X. Divide the numerator by the denominator (750 ÷ 50)

$$X = 15 \text{ mL/hr}$$

37. **A.** Step 1: Divide the weight in pounds by 2.2 kg (1 kg = 2.2 lb).
Step 2: Round off the answer (20.9) to 21.

38. **C.** Determine the number of mg per dose to give by multiplying the child's weight by the ordered dose (6 kg × 10 mg = 60 mg/dose).

39. **B.** Step 1: Convert the child's weight to kg by dividing 66 lb by 2.2 = 30 kg.
Step 2: Calculate the dosage:
a. The first 20 kg of a child's weight requires 1,500 mL.
b. Each additional kg of weight requires 20 mL/kg.
c. Since this child weighs 30 kg, they will need 1,500 mL for the first 20 kg and 200 mL for the additional 10 kg of weight.

40. **B.** Solve using the Ratio Proportion Method
Step 1: Determine the concentration of the solution by setting up the equation with 10 units/1,000 mL as the known factor and X as the unknown factor:

$$\frac{10 \text{ units}}{1{,}000 \text{ mL}} = \frac{X}{1 \text{ mL}}$$

Step 2: Cross-multiply and solve for X.
Step 3: Convert to milliunits (mU) by multiplying by 1,000.
Step 4: Determine the flow rate by setting up the equation with 10 mU/1 mL as the known factor and 15 mU/X as the unknown factor:

$$\frac{10 \text{ milliunits}}{1 \text{ mL}} = \frac{15 \text{ milliunits}}{X}$$

Step 5: Cross-multiply and solve for X.
Step 6: Convert to an hourly rate by multiplying by 4 (60 minutes/15 minutes = 4).
Another option to solve: Recall the formula:

$$X = \frac{\text{Ordered amount in units/min}}{\text{Medication concentration (units/mL)}} \times 60 \text{ min/hr}$$

Step 1: Convert mU to units (1 mU = 1,000 units)
Step 2: Set up the formula using the components of the formula and cancel the units that appear in both the numerator and the denominator:

$$X = \frac{1{,}000 \cancel{\text{units}}/\cancel{\text{min}}}{10 \cancel{\text{units}}/1{,}000 \text{ mL}} \times 60 \cancel{\text{min}}/\text{hr}$$

Step 3: Multiply 10 × 1,000 mL = 10,000 mL.
Step 4: Divide 1,000 by 10,000 = 0.1 mL.
Step 5: Solve for *X*. Multiply 0.1 × 60 = 6 mL/hr.

41. C. Solve using the Ratio Proportion Method
Step 1: Using the calculation for the solution above, 10 mU/1 mL, determine that the patient needs 120 mU in 1 hr (2 mU/min × 60 min). Set up the equation with 10 mU/1 mL as the known factor and 120 mU/*X* as the unknown factor:

$$\frac{10 \text{ milliunits}}{1 \text{ mL}} = \frac{120 \text{ milliunits}}{X}$$

Step 2: Cross-multiply and solve for *X*.
Use the provided formula:
Step 1: Convert mU to units (2 mU = 2,000 units)
Step 2: Set up the formula using the components of the formula and cancel the units that appear in both the numerator and the denominator:

$$X = \frac{2{,}000 \cancel{\text{units}}/\cancel{\text{min}}}{10 \cancel{\text{units}}/1{,}000 \text{ mL}} \times 60 \cancel{\text{min}}/\text{hr}$$

Step 3: Multiply 10 × 1,000 = 10,000.
Step 4: Divide 2,000 by 10,000.
Step 5: Solve for *X*. Multiply 0.2 × 60 = 12 mL/hr.

42. D. Find the flow rate using the Ratio Proportion Method
Step 1: Set up the equation with 4 g/250 mL as the known factor and 1 g/*X* as the unknown factor:

$$\frac{4 \text{ g}}{250 \text{ mL}} = \frac{1 \text{ g}}{X}$$

Step 2: Cross-multiply and solve for *X*.
Step 3: Round off the answer.
Find the flow rate using the Formula Method.
Step 1: Set up the formula using the components of the formula and cancel the units that appear in both the numerator and the denominator:
a. D = 1 g/hr; H = 4 g; Q = 250 mL

$$X = \frac{1 \cancel{\text{g}}/\text{hr}}{4 \cancel{\text{g}}} \times 250 \text{ mL}$$

Step 2: Solve for *X*. Divide 1 by 4 = 0.25.

$$X = \frac{250 \text{mL/hr}}{4}$$

Step 3: Multiply 0.25 × 250 = 62.5. Rounded to the whole number = 63 mL.

43. D. Step 1: Convert the patient's weight to kg by dividing the weight in lb by 2.2 kg (170 ÷ 2.2 = 77 kg).

Step 2: Determine the concentration of medication in mcg by multiplying mg by 1,000.

Step 3: Divide by 500 mL to determine the concentration in 1 mL.

$$\frac{800 \text{ mg}}{500 \text{ mL}} \times \frac{1{,}000 \text{ mcg}}{1 \text{ mg}} = \frac{800{,}000 \text{ mcg}}{500 \text{ mL}} = \frac{1{,}600 \text{ mcg}}{1 \text{ mL}}$$

Step 4: To find out how many mL/hr should be given, use the formula: weight in kg × dose in mcg/kg/min × 60 (minutes in 1 hour) ÷ concentration in 1 mL of solution:

$$\frac{77 \text{ kg}}{1} \times \frac{5 \text{ mcg}}{\text{kg/min}} = \frac{385 \text{ mcg}}{1 \text{ min}}$$

$$\frac{385 \text{ mcg}}{\text{min}} \times \frac{60 \text{ min}}{1 \text{ hr}} = \frac{23{,}100 \text{ mcg}}{1 \text{ hr}}$$

$$\frac{23{,}100 \text{ mcg/hr}}{1{,}600 \text{ mcg/mL}} = 14.43 \text{ mL/hr}$$

Step 5: Round off the answer.

Another option to solve: Recall the formula:

$$X = \frac{\text{Ordered amount in mg or mcg/min}}{\text{Medication concentration (mg or mcg/mL)}} \times 60 \text{ min/hr}$$

Step 1: Convert the patient's weight into kg:

$$X = \frac{170 \text{ lb}}{2.2 \text{ kg}} = 77 \text{ kg}$$

Step 2: Determine the dose per minute:

$$X = 5 \text{ mcg/kg/min}$$
$$X = 5 \times 77 \text{ kg/min}$$
$$X = 385 \text{ kg/min}$$

Step 3: Determine the lowest concentration of dopamine:

$$X = \frac{800 \text{ mg}}{500 \text{ mL}} = 1.6 \text{ mg/mL}$$

Step 4: Since dopamine is ordered in mcg, convert 1.6 mg to mcg (1.6 × 1,000) = 1,600 mcg/mL

Step 5: Set up the formula with the information provided and cancel the units that appear in both the numerator and the denominator:

$$X = \frac{385 \text{ mcg/min}}{1{,}600 \text{ mcg/mL}} \times 60 \text{ min/hr}$$

Step 6: Solve for X. Divide 385 by 1,600 = 0.2406.
Step 7: Multiply 0.2406 by 60 = 14.436.

$$X = 14.4375 = 14 \text{ mL/hr}$$

44. C. Step 1: Determine the concentration. Convert the 25 mg of nitroglycerin to mcg by multiplying by 1,000 and divide by the amount of solution.

$$\frac{25{,}000 \text{ mcg}}{250 \text{ mL}} = 100 \text{ mcg/mL}$$

Step 2: Set up the equation and cross multiply:

$$\frac{100 \text{ mcg}}{1 \text{ mL}} = \frac{10 \text{ mcg}}{X}$$

$$10 \text{ mcg} \times 1 \text{ mL} = 100 \text{ mcg} \times X \text{ (mL)}$$

$$\frac{10 \cancel{\text{mcg}} \times 1 \text{ mL}}{100 \cancel{\text{mcg}}} = \frac{\cancel{100} \cancel{\text{mcg}} \times X \text{ mL}}{\cancel{100} \cancel{\text{mcg}}}$$

Step 3: Solve for X. Determine mL/hour by multiplying the ordered dose by 60 minutes and dividing by the concentration.

$$X = 0.1 \text{ mL} \times 60 \text{ min}$$

Another option to solve: Recall the formula:

$$X = \frac{\text{Ordered amount in mg or mcg/min}}{\text{Medication concentration (mg or mcg/mL)}} \times 60 \text{ min/hr}$$

Step 1: Convert 25 mg of nitroglycerin to mcg (25 mg = 25,000 mcg).
Step 2: Determine the lowest concentration of nitroglycerin:

$$\frac{25{,}000 \text{ mcg}}{250 \text{ mL}} = 100 \text{ mcg/mL}$$

Step 3: Set up the formula using the components of the formula and cancel the units that appear in both the numerator and the denominator:

$$X = \frac{10 \cancel{\text{mcg}}/\cancel{\text{min}}}{100 \cancel{\text{mcg}}/\text{mL}} \times 60 \cancel{\text{min}}/\text{hr}$$

Step 4: Solve for X. Divide 10 by 100 = 0.1.
Step 5: Multiply 0.1 by 60 = 6 mL.

45. B. Step 1: Convert 1 g to mg (1 g × 1,000).

Step 2: Set up the equation with 1,000 mg/250 mL as the known factor and *X* as the unknown factor to determine the concentration in 1 mL:

$$\frac{1{,}000 \text{ mg}}{250 \text{ mL}} = \frac{X}{1 \text{ mL}}$$

Step 3: Cross-multiply and solve for *X*.

Step 4: Using this information, set up an equation with the concentration per mL as the known factor and 3 mg/*X* as the unknown factor:

$$\frac{4 \text{ mg}}{1 \text{ mL}} = \frac{3 \text{ mg}}{X}$$

Step 5: Cross-multiply and solve for *X*.

Step 6: Using 0.75 mL for 3 mg of lidocaine, set up the final equation to determine hourly flow rate with 0.75 mL/1 minute and *X*/60 minutes.

Step 7: Cross-multiply and solve for *X*.

Another option to solve: Recall the formula:

$$X = \frac{\text{Ordered amount in mg or mcg/min}}{\text{Medication concentration (mg or mcg/mL)}} \times 60 \text{ min/hr}$$

Step 1: Convert 1 g of lidocaine to mg (1 g × 1,000 = 1,000 mg).

Step 2: Determine the lowest concentration of lidocaine:

$$\frac{1{,}000 \text{ mg}}{250 \text{ mL}} = 4 \text{ mg/mL}$$

Step 3: Set up the formula using the components of the formula and cancel the units that appear in both the numerator and the denominator:

$$X = \frac{3 \cancel{\text{mg}}/\cancel{\text{min}}}{4 \cancel{\text{mg}}/\text{mL}} \times 60 \cancel{\text{min}}/\text{hr}$$

Step 4: Solve for *X*. Divide 3 by 4 = 0.75.

Step 5: Multiply 0.75 by 60 = 45 mL/hr

46. D. Step 1: Convert 2 L to mL by setting up an equation with the conversion of 1,000 mL/1 L:

$$\frac{1 \text{ L}}{1{,}000 \text{ mL}} = \frac{2 \text{ L}}{X}$$

The total to be infused is 2,000 mL.

Step 2: Convert 16 hours to minutes to determine how many minutes the solution needs to be infused over (16 × 60 = 960 minutes).

Recall the formula:

$$\text{Drip rate (gtts/ min)} = \frac{\text{Volume to be infused (in mL)}}{\text{Time (in minutes)}} \times \text{Drop factor (gtts/mL)}$$

Step 3: Set up the formula using the components of the formula and cancel the units that appear in both the numerator and the denominator.

$$X = \frac{2{,}000\ \cancel{\text{mL}}}{960\ \text{min}} \times 20\ \text{gtt}/\cancel{\text{mL}}$$

Step 4: Solve for *X*. Divide 2,000 by 960 = 2.083.
Step 5: Multiply 2.083 × 20 = 41.66. Rounded to the nearest whole number: 42 gtt/min.

47. A. Recall the formula:

$$\text{Flow rate (mL/hr)} = \frac{\text{Total volume ordered (in mL)}}{\text{Total time (in hours)}}$$

Step 1: Covert 90 minutes to hours (90 ÷ 60 = 1.5)
Step 2: Set up the formula with the information provided:

$$X = \frac{250\ \text{mL}}{1.5\ \text{hr}} = 166.67\ \text{mL/hr}$$

Step 3: Round off the answer.

48. D. Step 1: Convert 12 hours to minutes to determine how many minutes the solution needs to be infused over (12 × 60 = 720 minutes).

Recall the formula:

$$\text{Drip rate (gtts/min)} = \frac{\text{Volume to be infused (in mL)}}{\text{Time (in minutes)}} \times \text{Drop factor (gtts/mL)}$$

Step 2: Set up the formula using the components of the formula and cancel the units that appear in both the numerator and the denominator.

$$X = \frac{4{,}000\ \cancel{\text{mL}}}{720\ \text{min}} \times 15\ \text{gtt}/\cancel{\text{mL}}$$

Step 3: Solve for *X*. Divide 4,000 by 720 = 5.5555.
Step 4: Multiply 5.5555 by 15 = 83.33. Rounded to the nearest whole number = 83 gtt/min.

49. **A.** Solve using the Ratio Proportion Method

Step 1: Set up an equation using 60 mg/2 mL as the known factor and 15 mg/*X* as the unknown factor:

$$\frac{60\text{ mg}}{2\text{ mL}} = \frac{15\text{ mg}}{X}$$

Step 2: Cross-multiply and solve for *X*.

Step 3: Divide both sides of the equation by 60 mg and cancel units that appear in both the numerator and denominator.

Solve using the Formula Method

Step 1: Set up the formula using the components of the formula and cancel the units that appear in both the numerator and the denominator.

a. D = 15 mg; H = 60 mg; Q = 2 mL

$$X = \frac{15\cancel{\text{ mg}}}{60\cancel{\text{ mg}}} \times 2\text{ mL}$$

Step 2: Solve for *X*. Divide 15 by 60 = 0.25.

Step 3: Multiply 0.25 × 2 = 0.5 mL.

50. **A.** Step 1: Convert the patient's weight to kg by dividing the weight in lb by 2.2 kg (150 ÷ 2.2 = 68 kg).

Step 2: Determine the number of mg the patient is to receive per day by multiplying the desired dose per day by the weight in kg (68 kg × 3 mg = 204 mg).

Step 3: Determine the number of mg to administer every 8 hours by dividing the total amount of mg/day by 3 (204 ÷ 3 = 68).

Step 4: Determine the number of mL to administer every 8 hours by cross-multiplying the available concentration (80 mg/2 mL) and the unknown factor (68 mg/*X*) and solving for *X*.

Solve using the Formula Method

Complete Steps 1–3 as outlined above.

Step 5: Set up the formula using the components of the formula and cancel the units that appear in both the numerator and the denominator.

a. D = 68 mg; H = 80 mg; Q = 2 mL

$$X = \frac{68\cancel{\text{ mg}}}{80\cancel{\text{ mg}}} \times 2\text{ mL}$$

Step 6: Solve for *X*. Divide 68 by 80 = 0.85.

Step 7: Multiply 0.85 × 2 = 1.7 mL.

51. **C.** Solve using the Ratio Proportion Method

Step 1: Convert the dose in mcg to mg by dividing by 1,000 (1 mg = 1,000 mcg).

Step 2: Set up an equation using 0.5 mg/tablet as the known factor, and 0.25 mg/X as the unknown factor:

$$\frac{0.5 \text{ mg}}{1 \text{ tab}} = \frac{0.25 \text{ mg}}{X}$$

Step 3: Solve for X by cross-multiplying.

Step 4: Divide both sides by 0.5 mg and cancel units that appear in both the numerator and denominator.

Since the tablet is scored, the nurse can safely administer the dose.

Solve using the Formula Method

Step 1: Convert the dose in mcg to mg by dividing by 1,000 (1 mg = 1,000 mcg).

Step 2: Set up the formula using the components of the formula and cancel the units that appear in both the numerator and the denominator.

a. D = 0.25 mg; H = 0.5 mg; Q = 1 tablet

$$X = \frac{0.25 \cancel{\text{mg}}}{0.5 \cancel{\text{mg}}} \times 1 \text{ tablet}$$

Step 3: Solve for X. Divide 0.25 by 0.5 = 0.5.

Step 4: Multiply 0.5 × 1 = 0.5 tablet.

52. **B.** Solve using the Ratio Proportion Method

Step 1: Set up an equation using 125 mg/5 mL as the known factor and 300 mg/X as the unknown factor:

$$\frac{125 \text{ mg}}{5 \text{ mL}} = \frac{300 \text{ mg}}{X}$$

Step 2: Cross-multiply and solve for X.

Step 3: Divide both sides of the equation by 125 mg and cancel units that appear in both the numerator and denominator.

Solve using the Formula Method

Step 1: Set up the formula using the components of the formula and cancel the units that appear in both the numerator and the denominator.

a. D = 300 mg; H = 125 mg; Q = 5 mL

$$X = \frac{300 \cancel{\text{mg}}}{125 \cancel{\text{mg}}} \times 5 \text{ mL}$$

Step 2: Solve for X. Divide 300 by 125 = 2.4.

Step 3: Multiply 2.4 × 5 = 12 mL.

53. **D.** Determine the number of tablets to administer by setting up an equation using 50 mg/tablet as the known factor and 75 mg/X as the unknown factor, and solve for X.

Since the tablet is unscored, the nurse shouldn't break it in half to administer the prescribed dose. The nurse must call the pharmacy to have the dose sent as a single tablet. If this is not available, the nurse needs to contact the licensed practitioner for an alternative form of the medication. In some cases, the patient may have to bring their own medication into the hospital to be administered, but only after it has been sent to the pharmacy first!

54. D. Step 1: Determine the number of mg per dose to give by multiplying the infant's weight by the ordered dose (2.3 kg × 2.5 mg = 5.75 mg/dose).

Step 2: Determine the number of mL to administer by cross-multiply the known drug concentration (2 mg/1 mL) by the unknown factor (5.75 mg/X) and solve for X.

Solve using the Formula Method

Complete Steps 1–2 as outlined above.

Step 3: Set up the formula using the components of the formula and cancel the units that appear in both the numerator and the denominator.

a. D = 5.75 mg; H = 2 mg; Q = 2 mL

$$X = \frac{5.75 \cancel{mg}}{2 \cancel{mg}} \times 1 \text{ mL}$$

Step 4: Solve for X. Divide 5.75 by 2 = 2.875.

Step 5: Multiply 2.875 × 1 = 2.875 = 2.9 mL.

55. C. Step 1: Convert the infant's weight to kg by dividing the weight in lb by 2.2 kg (8 ÷ 2.2 = 3.6 kg).

Step 2: Determine the total volume of PRBC that needs to be infused (3.6 kg × 15 mL = 54 mL).

Step 3: Calculate the hourly flow rate by dividing the total volume of the transfusion (54 mL) by the number of hours (54 ÷ 4 = 13.5 mL/hr).

Medication therapy conversions

Common metric measures

Metric measure of weight

1 kilogram (kg) = 1,000 grams (g)
1 g = 1,000 milligrams (mg)
1 mg = 1,000 micrograms (mcg)
1,000,000 mcg = 1 g

Metric measure of volume

1 liter (L) = 1,000 milliliters (mL)
1 cubic centimeter (cc) = 1,000 milliliters (mL)
1 kilogram (kg) = 1,000 grams (g)
1 g = 1,000 milligrams (mg)
1 mg = 1,000 micrograms (mcg)
1,000,000 mcg = 1 g

Metric household equivalents

Metric measure		Household measure
1 teaspoon (tsp)	=	5 mL
1 tablespoon (T or tbs)	=	15 mL
2 tbs	=	30 mL
1 ounce (oz)	=	30 mL
8 ounces (1 cup)	=	240 mL
1 pint (pt)	=	473 mL
1 quart (qt)	=	946 mL
1 gallon (gal)	=	3,785 mL
1 kilogram (kg)	=	2.2 lb
2.5 centimeters (cm)	=	1 inch
1 foot	=	12 inches

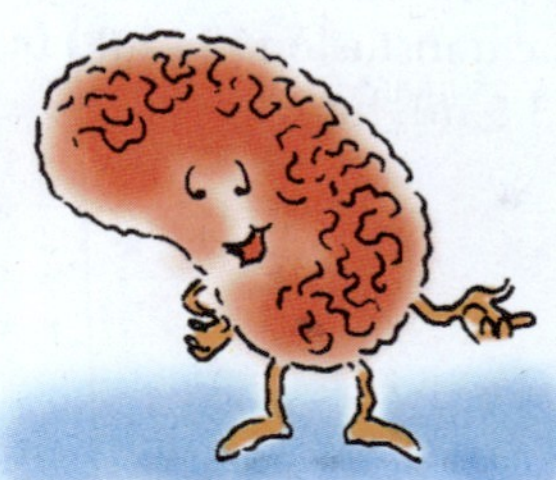

Dosage calculations are a snap with these conversion charts!

Weight conversion

To convert a patient's weight in pounds (lb) to kilograms (kg):

- Divide the number of lb by 2.2 kg

To convert a patient's weight in kilograms (kg) to pounds (lb)

- Multiply the number of kg by 2.2 lb.

Pounds	Kilograms
10	4.5
20	9.1
30	13.6
40	18.2
50	22.7
60	27.3
70	31.8
80	36.4
90	40.9
100	45.5
110	50
120	54.5
130	59.1
140	63.6
150	68.2
160	72.7
170	77.3
180	81.8
190	86.4
200	90.9

Temperature conversion

To convert Fahrenheit to Celsius:

- Subtract 32 from the temperature in Fahrenheit and then divide by 1.8

To convert Celsius to Fahrenheit:

- Multiply the temperature in Celsius by 1.8 and then add 32.

$$(F - 32) \div 1.8 = \text{degrees Celsius}$$
$$(C \times 1.8) + 32 = \text{degrees Fahrenheit}$$

Degrees Fahrenheit (°F)	Degrees Celsius (°C)
89.6	32
91.4	33
93.2	34
94.3	34.6
95	35
95.4	35.2
96.2	35.7
96.8	36
97.2	36.2
97.6	36.4
98	36.7
98.6	37
99	37.2
99.3	37.4
99.7	37.6
100	37.8
100.4	38
100.8	38.2

Degrees Fahrenheit (°F)	Degrees Celsius (°C)
101	38.3
101.2	38.4
101.4	38.6
101.8	38.8
102	38.9
102.2	39
102.6	39.2
102.8	39.3
103	39.4
103.2	39.6
103.4	39.7
103.6	39.8
104	40
104.4	40.2
104.6	40.3
104.8	40.4
105	40.6

Dosage calculation formulas

Common calculation formulas

Calculation methods

Ratio proportion method

$$H : V = D : V$$

Means

Extremes

H = Have on Hand
D = Desired Dose
H = Have on Hand
V = Vehicle (form of medication)

The rule is that the product of the Means is equal to the product of the Extremes

Formula method (Desired over have)

$$X = \frac{\text{Desired dose (D)}}{\text{Have on hand (H)}} \times \text{Quantity (Q)}$$

Dimensional analysis

$$\cancel{\text{Unit 1}} \times \frac{\text{Unit 2}}{\cancel{\text{Unit 1}}} = \text{Unit 2}$$

Given Unit × Conversion Factor = Needed Unit

Intravenous calculation formulas

Drip Rate

$$\underset{\text{(gtts/min)}}{\text{Drip rate}} = \frac{\text{Volume to be infused (in mL)}}{\text{Time (in minutes)}} \times \underset{\text{(gtts/mL)}}{\text{Drop factor}}$$

Flow Rate

$$\text{Flow rate (mL/hr)} = \frac{\text{Total volume ordered (in mL)}}{\text{Total time (in hours)}}$$

Infusion Time

$$\text{Infusion Time} = \frac{\text{Total volume ordered (in mL)}}{\text{Flow rate (mL/hr)}}$$

Total Volume

$$\text{Total volume (mL)} = \text{Flow rate (mL/hr)} \times 1 \text{ mL}$$

Lowest Concentration

$$X = \frac{\text{Amount of medication (mg or mcg)}}{\text{Amount of fluid (mL)}}$$

Critical Care Flow Rates

Orders for Mg or Mcg/Minute

$$X = \frac{\text{Ordered amount in mg or mcg/min}}{\text{Medication concentration (mg or mcg/mL)}} \times 60 \text{ min/hr}$$

Orders for Units/Minute

$$X = \frac{\text{Ordered amount in units/min}}{\text{Medication concentration (units/mL)}} \times 60 \text{ min/hr}$$

Glossary

antineoplastic drugs: medications that stop or block the growth of tumor cells

apothecaries' system: system used to measure liquid volumes and solid weights based on the units *dro*, *minim*, and *grain*, with amounts expressed in Roman numerals; used before the metric system was established

atrial fibrillation: a type of irregular heartbeat that can cause blood clots, stroke, and heart failure

automated medication dispensing system: state-of-the-art automated medication management system designed to improve medication management, enhance patient safety, and streamline workflow for health care professionals

avoirdupois system: measurement system used to order certain pharmaceutical products and to weigh patients; based on the units: *grain*, *ounce*, and *pound*

barcoding: a technology that uses a series of parallel lines, numbers, and symbols to encode information on products or items such a patient identification bands and medications.

body surface area (BSA): the area covered by a person's external skin calculated in square meters (m^2) according to height and weight; used to calculate safe pediatric dosages for all medications and safe dosages for adult patients receiving extremely potent medications or medications requiring great precision, such as antineoplastic and chemotherapeutic agents

common factor: a number that's a factor of two different numbers (e.g., 2 is a common factor of 4 and 6.)

common fraction: fraction with a whole number in both the numerator and denominator (such as $\frac{2}{3}$)

complex fraction: fraction in which the numerator and the denominator are fractions such as:

$$\frac{\frac{2}{7}}{\frac{5}{16}}$$

concentration: ratio that expresses the amount of a medication in a solution; sometimes called *drug strength*

computer physician order entry (CPOE): the process of providers entering and sending treatment instructions including medication, laboratory, and radiology orders via a computer application rather than paper, fax, or telephone

denominator: the bottom number in a fraction, which represents the total number of equal parts of a whole (e.g., in the fraction $\frac{7}{10}$, the denominator is 10.)

dividend: in division, the number to be divided (e.g., in the problem $33 \div 7$, 33 is the dividend.)

divisor: in division, the number by which the dividend is divided (e.g., in the problem $33 \div 7$, 7 is the divisor.)

dosage: the amount, frequency, and number of doses of a medication

dose: the amount of a medication to be given at one time

drip rate: the number of drops of IV solution to be infused per minute (gtt/min); based on the drop factor (number of drops delivered per mL) and calibrated for the selected IV tubing

drop factor: the number of drops to be delivered per milliliters of solution in an IV administration set; measured in gtt/mL (drops per milliliter); listed on the package containing the IV tubing administration set

drug: any natural or artificially made chemical that is used as a medicine

Drug Enforcement Agency (DEA): a federal law enforcement agency that enforces the United States' controlled substance laws and regulations and aims to reduce the supply of and demand for such substances

enteral route: within or by way of the digestive system, usually nutrition

equianalgesic dose: amount of an opioid analgesic that provides the same pain relief as 10 mg of IM morphine; used to recalculate the necessary dose when substituting one analgesic for another

flow rate: the number of milliliters of IV fluid to administer over 1 hour (mL/hr); based on the total volume to be infused in milliliters and the amount of time for the infusion

fraction: representation of the division of one number by another number; mathematical expression for parts of a whole, with the bottom number (denominator) describing the total number of parts and the top number (numerator) describing the parts of the whole being considered (e.g., $\frac{1}{2}$, $\frac{1}{3}$, $\frac{7}{18}$)

generic name: accepted nonproprietary name, which is a simplified form of the medication's chemical name

glucometer: device used to calculate blood glucose levels—and, thereby, insulin levels—from one drop of blood

grain (gr): the basic unit for measuring solid weight in the Apothecaries' system

gram (g): basic unit of weight in the metric system; represents the weight of one cubic centimeter of water at 4°C

high-alert medications: medications that have a heightened risk of causing significant patient harm when they are used in error.

household system: system that uses familiar household items, such as teaspoons, to measure medications

improper fraction: fraction in which the numerator is larger than or equal to the denominator, such as $\frac{3}{2}$, $\frac{10}{7}$, and $\frac{5}{5}$

independent double-check: process that requires two people to separately check the targeted components of the work process, without knowing the results of their college—this process is typically used to prevent medication errors on high-alert medications

International System of Units: system adopted in 1960 by the International Bureau of Weights and Measures to promote the use of standard metric abbreviations to prevent medication transcription errors

intradermal route: medication administration into the dermis of the skin

intramuscular (IM) route: medication administration into a muscle

intravenous (IV) route: medication administration into a vein

largest common divisor: in a fraction, the largest whole number that can be divided into both the numerator and denominator of a fraction (e.g., in the fraction $\frac{8}{10}$, the largest common divisor is 2.)

licensed practitioner: An individual who is licensed and qualified to direct or provide care, treatment, and services in accordance with state law and regulation, applicable federal law and regulation, and organizational policy

liter (L): basic unit of fluid volume in the metric system; equivalent to $\frac{1}{10}$ of a cubic meter

lowest common denominator: smallest number that's a multiple of all denominators in a set of fractions; also called *least common multiple* (e.g., for the fractions, $\frac{1}{100}$ and $\frac{3}{150}$, the lowest common denominator is 300.)

lowest terms: in a fraction, the smallest numbers possible in the numerator and denominator (Reduce a fraction to its lowest terms by dividing the numerator and denominator by the largest common divisor. e.g., in the fraction $\frac{3}{15}$, divide both the numerator and denominator by 3, the largest common divisor, to find $\frac{1}{5}$, the lowest terms of this fraction.)

medication: the use or application of medicine; a medicinal substance

medication administration record (MAR): a report that serves as a legal record of the medications administered to a patient at a facility by a health care professional

medication reconciliation: a process that compares the medication a patient is taking before and after a transition in care such as on admission, transfer, or discharge

meter (m): basic unit of length in the metric system; equivalent to 39.37 inches

metric system: decimal-based measurement system that uses the units: *meter* (for length), *liter* (for volume), and *gram* (for weight); most widely used system for measuring amounts of medications

military time: a format for expressing time, based on the 24-hour clock

milliequivalent (mEq): number of grams of a solute in 1 mL of normal solution; used to measure electrolytes

minim: basic unit for measuring liquid volume in the Apothecaries' system

mixed number: number that consists of a whole number and a fraction (such as $1\frac{1}{2}$)

multiplied common denominator: for a set of fractions, the product of all the denominators, which is found by multiplying all the denominators together (e.g., for the fractions, $\frac{1}{2}$, $\frac{2}{3}$, and $\frac{3}{5}$, multiply the denominators together to find the multiplied common denominator, which is 30 [$2 \times 3 \times 5 = 30$].)

nonparenteral medications: medications administered by the oral, topical, or rectal route, as opposed to medications administered by the parenteral route

nomogram: chart used to determine body surface area in square meters, based on the patient's height and weight

numerator: the top number in a fraction, which represents the number of parts being considered (e.g., in the fraction $\frac{7}{10}$, the numerator is 7.)

oral route (P.O.): medication administration through the mouth

parenteral route: medication administration through a route other than the digestive tract, such as IV, IM, and subcut

percentage: a quantity stated as a part per hundred; written with a percent sign (%), which means "for every hundred" (e.g., 50% represents 50 parts out of 100 total parts.)

prime factor: prime numbers that can be divided into some part of a mathematical expression such as the denominators in a set of fractions; used to find the lowest common denominator for a set of fractions (e.g., the prime factors for the denominators in the fractions $\frac{1}{10}$ and $\frac{2}{3}$ are 5, 2, and 3.)

prime number: whole number that's evenly divisible only by 1 and itself, such as 2, 3, 5, and 7

product: the answer of a multiplication problem (e.g., in the equation, $4 \times 5 = 20$, the product is 20.)

proper fraction: fraction with a numerator that's smaller than the denominator (such as $\frac{1}{2}$)

proportion: set of equivalent ratios or fractions (An example of a proportion expressed by ratios is 2:3::8:12, which is read as "2 is to 3 as 8 is to 12." The same proportion expressed with fractions is $\frac{2}{3} = \frac{8}{12}$.)

quotient: the answer of a division problem (e.g., in the equation $20 \div 5 = 4$, the quotient is 4.)

ratio: numerical way to compare items or show a relationship between numbers, with numbers separated by a colon, which represents the words, "is to" (e.g., **the ratio 4:** 5 is read as "4 is to 5." Ratios are commonly used to describe the relative proportions of ingredients such as the amount of medication relative to its solution.)

reciprocal: inverted fraction; used when dividing fractions (e.g., to divide $\frac{1}{2}$ by $\frac{2}{3}$, multiply $\frac{1}{2}$ by the reciprocal of $\frac{2}{3}$, which is $\frac{3}{2}$; in other words, $\frac{1}{2} \div \frac{2}{3} = \frac{1}{2} \times \frac{3}{2} = \frac{3}{4}$. When a fraction is multiplied by its reciprocal, the product is 1; e.g., the reciprocal of the fraction $\frac{2}{3}$ is $\frac{3}{2}$, and $\frac{2}{3} \times \frac{3}{2} = \frac{6}{6}$ or 1.)

rectal route (PR): medication administration (usually by suppository) through the rectum

reconstitute: to restore a dried substance to a fluid form that can be used for injection; the process of adding a diluent to a powdered medication to prepare a solution or suspension

reduce: to simplify a numerical expression by using the lowest possible numbers—or lowest terms—to describe it (e.g., the fraction $\frac{15}{45}$ may be reduced to $\frac{1}{3}$.)

rounding off: reducing the number of decimal places used to express a number (e.g., a decimal fraction that's expressed in thousandths may be rounded off to the nearest hundredths or tenths; the number 12.827 rounded off to the nearest hundredths is 12.83. The same number rounded off to the nearest tenths is 12.8.)

subcutaneous (subcut) route: medication administration into the subcutaneous tissue

The Joint Commission: a nonprofit organization that accredits health care organizations and programs in the United States and internationally

topical route: medication administration through the skin (after absorption through the skin layers, the medication enters circulation), usually in cream, ointment, or transdermal patch form

trade name: the medication's name given by the manufacturer; also called the *brand* or *proprietary name*

transcribe: to write or type a copy of something; to record information by hand, tape-recorder, or computer

transdermal route: medication administration in which the medication is absorbed continuously through the skin and enters the systemic system

unit system: measurement system that expresses the amount of a medication in units, United States Pharmacopeia (USP) units, or International Units. Examples of medications measured in units include insulin, heparin, the topical antibiotic bacitracin, and penicillins G and V. Some forms of vitamins A and D are measured in USP units. The hormone calcitonin and the fat-soluble vitamins A, D, and E are measured in International Units.

ventricular fibrillation: a life-threatening arrhythmia that causes the heart to quiver instead of beating normally

Index

Note: t refers to a table; i refers to an illustration.

E

F

Note: t refers to a table; i refers to an illustration.

Note: t refers to a table; i refers to an illustration.

Note: t refers to a table; i refers to an illustration.

Q

R

S

T

Note: t refers to a table; i refers to an illustration.

Note: t refers to a table; i refers to an illustration.